Oral Manifestations of Systemic Diseases

Editor

JOEL J. NAPEÑAS

ATLAS OF THE ORAL AND MAXILLOFACIAL SURGERY CLINICS OF NORTH AMERICA

www.oralmaxsurgeryatlas.theclinics.com

Consulting Editor
RICHARD H. HAUG

September 2017 • Volume 25 • Number 2

ELSEVIER

1600 John F. Kennedy Boulevard • Suite 1800 • Philadelphia, Pennsylvania, 19103-2899
http://www.oralmaxsurgeryatlas.theclinics.com

ATLAS OF THE ORAL AND MAXILLOFACIAL SURGERY CLINICS OF NORTH AMERICA Volume 25, Number 2 September 2017 ISSN 1061-3315 ISBN-13: 978-0-323-54542-6

Editor: John Vassallo; j.vassallo@elsevier.com
Developmental Editor: Colleen Dietzler

Reprints. For copies of 100 or more of articles in this publication, please contact the Commercial Reprints Department, Elsevier Inc., 360 Park Avenue South, New York, NY 10010-1710. Tel.: 212-633-3874; Fax: 212-633-3820; E-mail: reprints@elsevier.com.

Atlas of the Oral and Maxillofacial Surgery Clinics of North America (ISSN 1061-3315) is published biannually by Elsevier, 360 Park Avenue South, New York, NY 10010-1710. Months of issue are March and September. Periodicals postage paid at New York, NY and additional mailing offices. Subscription prices are $455.00 for international individual, $370.00 for US individual and Canadian individual; $220.00 for international student and Canadian student, $100.00 for US student; $504.00 for international institution, $530.00 for Canadian institution, $410.00 for US institution. Foreign air speed delivery is included in all *Clinics* subscription prices. All prices are subject to change without notice. POSTMASTER: Send address changes to *Atlas of the Oral and Maxillofacial Surgery Clinics of North America*, Health Sciences Division, Subscription Customer Service, 3251 Riverport Lane, Maryland Heights, MO 63043. Tel: 1-800-654-2452 (U.S. and Canada); 314-447-8871 (outside U.S. and Canada). Fax: 314-417-8029. E-mail: journalscustomerservice-usa@elsevier.com (for print support); journalsonline support-usa@elsevier.com (for online support).

Atlas of the Oral and Maxillofacial Surgery Clinics of North America is covered in *MEDLINE/PubMed (Index Medicus)*.

Printed in the United States of America.

Contributors

CONSULTING EDITOR

RICHARD H. HAUG, DDS
Professor and Chief, Oral Maxillofacial Surgery, Carolinas Medical Center, Charlotte, North Carolina, USA

EDITOR

JOEL J. NAPEÑAS, DDS, FDS RCSEd
Associate Professor of Oral Medicine, Director, Oral Medicine Residency Program, Department of Oral Medicine, Carolinas HealthCare System, Carolinas Medical Center, Charlotte, North Carolina, USA

AUTHORS

PAOLO G. ARDUINO, DDS, MSc, PhDs
Department of Surgical Sciences, CIR-Dental School, University of Turin, Turin, Italy

LEAH BOWERS, BSc, DMD
Clinical Assistant Professor, Oral and Maxillofacial Surgery, University of California, San Francisco School of Dentistry, San Francisco, California, USA

GRACE BRADLEY, DDS, MSc, FRCD(C)
Professor, Oral Pathology and Oral Medicine, Faculty of Dentistry, University of Toronto, Toronto, Ontario, Canada

MICHAEL BRENNAN, DDS, MHS
Professor and Chair, Department of Oral Medicine, Carolinas Medical Center, Carolinas HealthCare System, Charlotte, North Carolina, USA

AMR BUGSHAN, BDS, PhD
Senior Resident, Division of Oral Medicine, Department of Diagnostic Sciences, Tufts University School of Dental Medicine, Boston, Massachusetts, USA; Teaching Assistant, College of Dentistry, Imam Abdulrahman Bin Faisal University, Damman, Kingdom of Saudi Arabia

BHAVIK DESAI, DMD, PhD
Assistant Professor, Division of Oral Medicine, Department of Diagnostic Sciences, Tufts University School of Dental Medicine, Boston, Massachusetts, USA

MARY HIL EDENS, DDS
Resident, Oral Medicine Residency Program, Department of Oral Medicine, Carolinas HealthCare System, Charlotte, North Carolina, USA

SHARON ELAD, DMD, MSc
Professor and Chair, Department of Oral Medicine, Eastman Institute for Oral Health, University of Rochester Medical Center, Rochester, New York, USA

ARWA M. FARAG, BDS, DMSc, FDS RCSEd
Assistant Professor, Division of Oral Medicine, Department of Diagnostic Sciences, Tufts University School of Dental Medicine, Boston, Massachusetts, USA; Assistant Professor, Department of Oral Medicine, Faculty of Dentistry, King AbdulAziz University, Jeddah, Kingdom of Saudi Arabia

MAHNAZ FATAHZADEH, DMD, MSD
Professor of Oral Medicine, Department of Diagnostic Sciences, Rutgers School of Dental Medicine, Newark, New Jersey, USA

KENTARO IKEDA, DDS, MPH, FDS RCSEd
Assistant Professor, Department of Diagnostics and Biological Sciences, University of Colorado School of Dental Medicine, Assistant Professor, Department of Family Medicine, University of Colorado School of Medicine, Aurora, Colorado, USA

LISA JOHNSON, DDS, MSc, FRCD(C)
Assistant Professor, Department of Oral and Maxillofacial Sciences, Faculty of Dentistry, Dalhousie University, Halifax, Nova Scotia, Canada

YASSER KHALED, BDS, MDSc, MMSc
Resident, Oral Medicine Residency Program, Department of Oral Medicine, Carolinas HealthCare System, Charlotte, North Carolina, USA

IONA LEONG, BDS, MSc, FRCD(C)
Assistant Professor, Oral Pathology and Oral Medicine, Faculty of Dentistry, University of Toronto, Toronto, Ontario, Canada

CHRISTINA McCORD, DDS, MSc, FRCD(C)
Assistant Professor, Division of Oral Pathology, Department of Pathology and Laboratory Medicine, Schulich School of Medicine and Dentistry, Western University, London, Ontario, Canada

LINA MARIA MEJIA, DDS, MPH
Assistant Professor, Department of Oral Medicine and Diagnostic Sciences, College of Dental Medicine, Nova Southeastern University, Fort Lauderdale, Florida, USA

JOEL J. NAPEÑAS, DDS, FDS RCSEd
Associate Professor of Oral Medicine, Director, Oral Medicine Residency Program, Department of Oral Medicine, Carolinas HealthCare System, Carolinas Medical Center, Charlotte, North Carolina, USA

MARCEL NOUJEIM, DDS, MS
Professor and Program Director, Oral and Maxillofacial Radiology, Department of Comprehensive Dentistry, UT Health San Antonio, San Antonio, Texas, USA

KRISTINA PERSCHBACHER, DDS, MSc, FRCD(C)
Assistant Professor, Oral Pathology and Oral Medicine, Faculty of Dentistry, University of Toronto, Toronto, Ontario, Canada

VIDYA SANKAR, DMD, MHS
Member of the Faculty, Department of Oral Medicine, Infection and Immunity, Harvard School of Dental Medicine, Associate Surgeon, Division of Oral Medicine and Dentistry, Department of Surgery, Brigham and Women's Hospital, Boston, Massachusetts, USA

ALESSANDRO VILLA, DDS, MPH, PhD
Division of Oral Medicine and Dentistry, Brigham and Women's Hospital, Boston, Massachusetts, USA

ELIZABETH WARING, DMD
Division of Oral Medicine and Dentistry, Brigham and Women's Hospital, Boston, Massachusetts, USA

NOAM YAROM, DMD
Head, Oral Medicine Unit, Sheba Medical Center, Tel Hashomer, Israel; Senior Lecturer, Department of Oral Pathology and Oral Medicine, School of Dental Medicine, Tel Aviv University, Tel Aviv, Israel

YEHUDA ZADIK, DMD, MHA
Head, Oral Medicine Clinic for Hematologic and Oncologic Patients, Department of Oral Medicine, Sedation and Maxillofacial Imaging, Hebrew University-Hadassah School of Dental Medicine, Jerusalem, Israel; Head, Department of Oral Medicine, Oral and Maxillofacial Center, Medical Corps, Israel Defense Forces, Tel Hashomer, Israel

Contents

ATLAS OF THE ORAL AND MAXILLOFACIAL SURGERY CLINICS OF NORTH AMERICA

FORTHCOMING ISSUES

March 2018

Fat Grafting for Aesthetic Facial Surgery
Shahrokh C. Bagheri, Husain Ali Khan, and Behnam Bohluli, *Editors*

September 2018

Sialendoscopy
Michael D. Turner and Maria J. Troulis, *Editors*

PREVIOUS ISSUES

March 2017

Advances in the Management of Mandibular Condylar Fractures
Martin B. Steed, *Editor*

September 2016

Upper Facial Rejuvenation
Faisal A. Quereshy, *Editor*

RELATED INTEREST

Dental Clinics, January 2016, Volume 60, Issue 1
Oral Radiology: Interpretation and Diagnostic Strategies
Mel Mupparapu, *Editor*
Available at: http://www.dental.theclinics.com

Preface

Oral Manifestations of Systemic Diseases

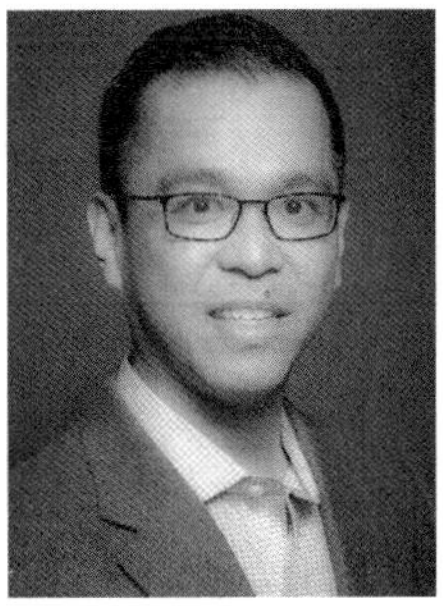

Joel J. Napeñas, DDS, FDS RCSEd
Editor

The orofacial region comprises an intricate combination of components seen in other organ systems in the body, to include mucous membranes, skin, nerves, muscles, ligaments, bone, and exocrine glands. This is in addition to the unique features of the oral cavity to include the dentition, periodontium, and salivary milieu. Consequently, the orofacial region reflects an individual's overall systemic health, and issues that arise here may be the initial presentation or a complication of a systemic condition. For instance, enlarged gingiva may be an early manifestation of a hematologic malignancy through leukemic infiltration of the gingiva. When a unique orofacial abnormality and condition presents that necessitates a thorough history taking and workup, the process may uncover a systemic condition that would impact any subsequent dental or surgical management of the patient, by affecting either their ability to tolerate or recover from treatment or the prognosis or outcome of the proposed treatment.

The goal of this issue of the *Atlas of the Oral and Maxillofacial Surgery Clinics of North America* is to provide a brief comprehensive overview to aid providers in the approach to and identification of systemic conditions that appear in the orofacial region, as presented by international oral medicine experts. This begins with an overview of the fundamentals in approaching a patient, which would necessitate a thorough medical history, comprehensive medical evaluation, and appropriate subsequent tests (eg, laboratory and imaging studies, biopsies, cultures).

The individual articles in this issue are delineated by organ systems and disease states. The oral cavity, at the one end of the gastrointestinal tract, would naturally be prone to lesions from a gastrointestinal disorder, such as oral ulcers and cobblestone lesions seen in patients with inflammatory bowel disease. Immunodeficient patients may be more prone to orofacial infections or unique lesions of infectious causes. Patients with high caries rate and salivary hypofunction may provide an initial opportunity to diagnose an underlying autoimmune condition such as Sjögren's syndrome. Therapies and drugs targeted toward systemic disorders may cause oral complications in the form of hyposalivation, immunosuppression, allergic reactions, osteonecrosis, and/or other oral lesions. Hematologic disorders may result in increased oral bleeding that would impact dental and surgical care, or may have initial oral manifestations such as enlarged gingiva, as previously mentioned. Naturally, the mouth, with its complex oral ecosystem, is commonly subject to viral, bacterial, and fungal infections. Multiorgan disorders, or disorders of the endocrine system, have various manifestations in the oral cavity and orofacial region. Dermatologic disorders have unique presentation in the oral cavity, as evidenced by various mucosal conditions such as lichen planus.

The information and images of more common and/or significant conditions in this issue are intended to serve as a quick reference for providers as they encounter them in their clinical practice. This array of conditions further emphasizes the orofacial region and oral cavity as a reflection of a patient's overall health.

Joel J. Napeñas, DDS, FDS RCSEd
Department of Oral Medicine
Carolinas HealthCare System
Carolinas Medical Center
PO Box 32861
Charlotte, NC 28232, USA

E-mail address:
joel.napenas@carolinashealthcare.org

Atlas Oral Maxillofacial Surg Clin N Am 25 (2017) xiii
1061-3315/17/© 2017 Published by Elsevier Inc.
http://dx.doi.org/10.1016/j.cxom.2017.06.001

Introduction to Oral Manifestations of Systemic Diseases

Evaluation of the Patient

Mary Hil Edens, DDS , Yasser Khaled, BDS, MDSc, MMSc ,
Joel J. Napeñas, DDS, FDS RCSEd*

KEYWORDS

• Medical history • Review of systems • Imaging studies • Radiographs • Oral diagnosis • Laboratory tests

KEY POINTS

- For all complaints related to the orofacial region, a detailed evaluation is to be performed.
- The diagnosis is often delivered solely after obtaining a thorough medical history.
- The physical clinical examination should be conducted in a systematic and repeatable fashion, and in a manner to disprove the original provisional diagnosis obtained from the medical history, and to obtain a provisional differential diagnosis.
- Investigations may be required to confirm a diagnosis and prognosis, exclude some diagnoses, or aid in guiding treatment course.

Orofacial manifestations of systemic diseases of various types and causes have similar symptoms and clinical appearances that may make them difficult to diagnose solely on signs and symptoms. Thus, for all complaints related to the orofacial region, a detailed medical evaluation is to be performed, which would entail a detailed medical and dental history, comprehensive examination, performing appropriate tests (eg, imaging studies, laboratory studies, biopsy), or trial therapeutic regimens to obtain a differential diagnosis and a final diagnosis. This article provides a brief overview and review of the general approach to such patients.

History of present condition and medical history

The major sections of patient interviewing include the following:[1]

Source and reliability

- The patient should be the source of information.
- If an interpreter is required, then an official accredited translator should be used rather than a family member. The name of the interpreter and license number should be included in the notes.

The authors have nothing to disclose.
Oral Medicine Residency Program, Department of Oral Medicine, Carolinas HealthCare System, PO Box 32861, Charlotte, NC 28232, USA
* Corresponding author.
E-mail address: joel.napenas@carolinashealthcare.org

Atlas Oral Maxillofacial Surg Clin N Am 25 (2017) 85-92

http://dx.doi.org/10.1016/j.cxom.2017.04.001

Chief complaint

- This is the patient's brief statement, in their own words, explaining why he or she sought medical attention

History of present illness

History of present illness refers to recent changes in health that led the patient to seek care. It should describe the information relevant to the chief complaint:

- Time of onset
- Initiating factors or incidences that proceeded onset (eg, illnesses, injury, activities, new medications)
- The interviewer must determine if there are any debilitating symptoms that might impact the patient:[1]
  - Pain
  - Constipation
  - Weakness
  - Nausea
  - Shortness of breath
  - Depression
- Anatomic location (as noted by patient)
- Degree of pain (for example, using a 0 [none] to 10 [worst] scale) currently, average, and at worst
- Temporality of symptoms: continuous versus intermittent, times of day
- Exacerbating and alleviating factors
- Previous providers whom they sought care for this condition
- Previous treatments performed, and their response to therapy

Past medical, family, and social history

An overall assessment of the patient's health before the present illness should be performed and should include the following:

- Medical
  - General current state of health
  - Past: Illnesses, injuries or accidents, hospitalizations, surgeries, immunizations
    - The record of the past illnesses should include childhood and adult problems
  - Allergies (medications, food, environmental)
- Current medications
- Complementary/alternative therapies to include supplements
- Immunizations
- Social
  - Tobacco use (past and current)
  - Alcohol use (past and current)
  - Substance abuse
  - Diet
  - Sleep patterns
  - Current occupation
- Family
  - Information about the entire family, living and deceased, history of significant illnesses (eg, diabetes, cardiac, cancer, autoimmune conditions)
  - Attention to possible genetic and environmental aspects of disease should be considered
  - Considerations also include country of origin of family members, whether the patient grew up in a rural or urban setting, in what country did he or she grow up, at what age did the patient emigrate, the patient's native language, and the ethnicity of the spouse
- Psychological history
  - Information about the education, life experiences, and personal relationships of the patient
  - Information about the patient's lifestyle, schooling, military service, religious beliefs, and marital relationships[2]

Occupational and environmental history

- Inquire about all occupations and the duration of each and temporal relationship between the onset of illness and exposure. Exposure to potential disease-producing substances should be considered.
- Occupational exposures account for an estimated 50,000 to 70,000 deaths annually in the United States.
- More than 350,000 new cases of occupational disease are recognized each year.
- Inquire whether the patient resides or ever resided near mines, farms, factories, or shipyards.[2]

Review of systems

- The review of symptoms should summarize all symptoms the patient is currently experiencing and is best organized from the head to the extremities. The review of systems should include the following: general, skin, head, eyes, ears, nose, mouth, throat, neck, chest, cardiac, vascular, breasts, gastrointestinal, urinary, genitalia, musculoskeletal, and neurologic.[3]
- Examples of systemic conditions elicited from the medical history or review of systems that manifest in the orofacial area or impact dental treatment are outlined in Table 1.

Examination

A systematic and thorough approach should be used to examine the patient, executing the examination in the same sequence each time to avoid skipping steps. The purpose of the examination is to disprove or test any bias or conclusions that the provider elicits from their interview.

Vital signs

A thorough examination often begins by taking vital signs, which often include pulse, blood pressure, temperature, conscious state, and respiration rate. Normal values are listed below.[3]

- Normal average temperature for an adult: 36.6°C, 97.8°F
- Normal average blood pressure for an adult: 120/80 mmHg
- Normal pulse for an adult: 60 to 80 bpm

- Elevated temperature may indicate an infectious process
- If the pulse rate is significantly high, a provider should explore causes such as fear/anxiety, physical exertion, cardiac problems, or hyperthyroidism

General evaluation

- Provider should make an assessment of the patient's orientation to person, place, and time.
- Start with the most general aspect and include assessing the patient's overall appearance.
- Overall affect: Do they look well? Distressed? Anxious? Alert?
  - Because there can be strong correlations between psychological stressors and some conditions such as orofacial pain, a provider should make an attempt to gauge any psychological stressors that might be contributing and might affect treatment.[4]
- The skin should also be examined for rashes, pallor, erythema, lesions, and discolorations. The patient's hands should be visualized for evidence of arthritis and Raynaud syndrome, and the patient's nails evaluated for changes in shape/color[3]
- If significant weight loss is noted, this could be a sign of an eating disorder, nutritional problem, or systemic disease, and the patient should be questioned further.

Cranial nerve examination

- Damage to one of the cranial nerves may result in a motor or sensory deficiency (Table 2).

American Society of Anesthesiologists classification of physical status

This classification is summarized by the following:

- Class I: Healthy
- Class II: Controlled, mild systemic disease

Table 1 Select systemic conditions and potential orofacial manifestations

Condition	Potential orofacial manifestations
Anemia	Sore mouth; burning mouth; glossitis; oral ulcerations; angular stomatitis
Autoimmune disorders	Systemic lupus erythematosus: Oral lesions, hyposalivation, secondary Sjögren's syndrome Rheumatoid arthritis: Secondary Sjögren's syndrome, temporomandibular disorder
Bleeding disorders	Oral bleeding; petechiae; caution or contraindication for invasive procedures or nonsteroidal anti-inflammatory drugs
Blood-borne infections	HIV: Increased susceptibility for fungal, viral processes (eg,: candidiasis, herpetic); periodontal disease; Kaposi sarcoma; oral ulcerations; petechiae secondary to thrombocytopenia; salivary gland disorders Hepatitis B and C: Association with lichen planus, sialadenitis, salivary gland disorders, oral bleeding
Cardiovascular disease	Medications causing hyposalivation; gingival hyperplasia; lichenoid drug reaction from various medications for hypertension (angiotensin-converting-enzyme inhibitors, beta-blockers, nifedipine, hydrochlorothiazide, furosemide, spironolactone)
Diabetes	Sialosis; dry mouth; periodontal disease; impaired healing; susceptibility to infection
Gastrointestinal disorders	Inflammatory bowel disease: Oral ulcerations; "cobblestone" lesions; orofacial granulomatosis; gingival enlargement; fissured tongue; pyostomatitis vegetans
History of cancer with previous radiotherapy and chemotherapy	Pain and sensory changes; salivary gland hypofunction; increased caries rate, osteoradionecrosis; medication-related osteonecrosis of the jaw
History of solid organ transplant	Increased risk of infection, neoplasm; graft-versus-host disease; gingival hyperplasia
Hyperparathyroidism	Bony changes as seen in radiographs: Radiolucencies/rarefaction; loss of lamina dura, central giant cell granulomas, hypercalcemia
Kidney disease	Oral bleeding
Liver disease	Oral bleeding; jaundice
Neurologic disorders	Gingival hyperplasia secondary to medication; trigeminal neuralgia
Pregnancy	Oral aphthae; Behçet syndrome; gingivitis; epulides

- Class III: Severe systemic disease
- Class IV: Life-threatening systemic disease
- Class V: Severe disease such that patient not expected to live more than 24 hours
- Class VI: Organ donor

Head and neck examination

Lymph nodes

- The neck and lymph nodes should be carefully examined for any swellings, areas of induration or asymmetry (unilateral or bilateral), or swollen/fixed lymph nodes.
- The following lymph nodes should be assessed in a head/neck examination: preauricular, postauricular, sub-occipital, middle cervical, posterior cervical, supraclavicular, juguloomohyoid, submental, submandibular, and facial.
- The jugulodigastric lymph node is particularly important to palpate and assess because it is the most common one connected with oral cancers and infections of the tonsils.
- Tenderness to palpation should be assessed, because this may indicate inflammation or infection[3]

Muscles of mastication

- The following muscles of mastication, neck and shoulder, should be palpated and assessed: temporalis, masseter,

Table 2 Cranial nerve testing

Cranial nerve	Test
I Olfactory	Ask patient to identify a classic smell
II Optic	Compare patient's vision to provider's
III Oculomotor	Check that pupils are equal, round, and reactive to light and accommodation
IV (Trochlear) & VI (Abducens)	Ask the patient to move their eyes up, down, and to each side
V (Trigeminal)	Sensory: Light touch to forehead, malar and mandibular areas, and corneal reflex Motor: Symmetry and tension of masseters when clenching teeth
VII (Facial)	Ask patient to wrinkle forehead, tightly close eyes, and smile
VIII (Vestibular)	Light brushing of fingers by each ear to see if the patient can hear from each ear
IX (Glossopharyngeal) &X (Vagus)	Gag reflex, ask patient to say "ahhh" to check for soft palate mobility
XI (Accessory)	Ask patient to shrug shoulders to determine if sternocleidomastoid muscle and trapezius have normal function
XII (Hypoglossal)	Tongue: Check deviation with protrusion

medial pterygoid, suprahyoid, temporal tendon, sternocleidomastoid, and trapezius.

- A provider should note any tenderness to palpation using a 0 to 3 scale:
  - 0: No tenderness
  - 1: Patient says it feels slightly tender to palpation
  - 2: Patient says it is painful to palpation, usually indicated with facial reaction
  - 3: Patient withdraws in pain as a result of palpation
- Palpate for the presence of myofascial "trigger points," which are tight bands of muscle tissue that are typically a source of pain at site of palpation or referred elsewhere.
- If there is pain with palpation of the temporal arteries, this could suggest giant cell arteritis and further evaluation should be done[4]

Temporomandibular joints

- When evaluating the temporomandibular joints, the provider should palpate the joint at rest and while the patient opens and closes their mouth several times.
- This will allow for the detection of pops, clicks, or crepitus.
- The ranges of movement are most easily measured with a millimeter ruler and should be recorded in order to assess the patient's range over multiple visits.
  - Normal opening range is 40 to 50 mm with normal lateral movement at 12 mm, although it is variable based on patient's size.
  - The active range measures how much the patient can open without assistance, whereas the passive range is the maximum opening with assistance.
  - The active range can decrease with age and is less in women, which should be taken into consideration[4]
  - It should also be noted if the patient experiences pain with any of these movements.
  - The provider should also note if there is deviation or deflection with opening and to which side.

Salivary glands

- The parotid and submandibular salivary glands should also be palpated, and the exudate examined out of the 4 major ducts (Wharton and Stenson ducts) intraorally (Fig. 1).
- If there is no salivary flow noted, this might indicate hyposalivation or a blockage in the duct.

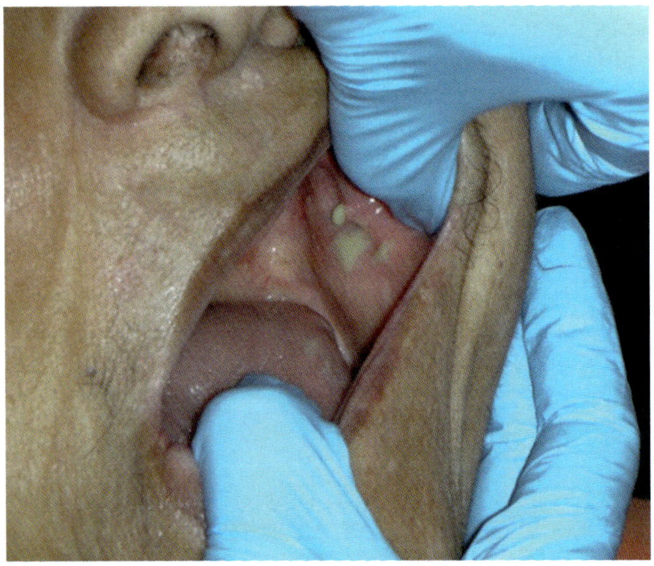

Fig. 1 Purulent exudate from an infection of the left parotid salivary gland.

- If the flow from the salivary glands is not clear, then a bacterial culture of this fluid might be recommended to determine if there is an infection of the salivary gland.

Intraoral examination

- The lips, buccal mucosa, labial mucosa, dorsal and ventral tongue, floor of mouth, soft and hard palate, tonsillar pillars, gingivae, and teeth should all be carefully evaluated.
- It is also crucial to examine the patient's oropharynx with good illumination noting any abnormalities of the soft palate, uvula, tonsils, and pharynx.
- A clinical photograph can also be invaluable with the patient's chart to monitor changes.
- Photography can be an invaluable imaging tool for the clinician. Having good-quality photographs of a lesion as a baseline reference can allow the provider to objectively monitor for any changes in size, shape, and color (Fig. 2). Having a good camera and adequate light will produce the best photographs that should become part of the patient's file[3]
- Checking the patient's occlusion for any abnormalities is also important[4]

Imaging studies

Although the amount of radiation exposure from oral imaging has improved over time and the risks are relatively low, risks still exist, and it is important for a provider to order imaging only when necessary for diagnosis.

Intraoral radiographs

- A periapical radiograph is appropriate when the root or apical area is suspected of a pathologic process (eg, abscess, granuloma, cyst, trabecular changes) (Fig. 3).
- A bitewing radiograph is appropriate for evaluating proximal caries and bone loss via the alveolar crest.
- Occlusal films can be used to evaluate for buccal or lingual expansion from cystic processes.
- Panoramic radiographs are appropriate when anatomy, such as the temporomandibular joints, sinuses, inferior alveolar nerve canal, and angle of the mandible, needs to be visualized (Fig. 4).
  - Panoramic radiographs are not typically helpful in the diagnosis of features directly in the midline because this area is typically blurred in the image.

Three-dimensional imaging

- Three-dimensional imaging is helpful in the diagnosis of oral manifestations of systemic disease by using volumetric data to differentiate bone and soft tissue based on their different densities.
- Computed tomography (CT) scans (Fig. 5)
  - CT allows a provider to focus in on certain areas of concern in "cut-away views" and manipulate the image from different angulations, and separate different structures to view individually
  - If soft tissue abnormalities are suspected, the patient should have intravenous iodinated contrast dye injected for better visualization.
  - CT perfusion is often used to detect growth of new vasculature and to determine how well a patient has responded to radiation or chemotherapy. This technique

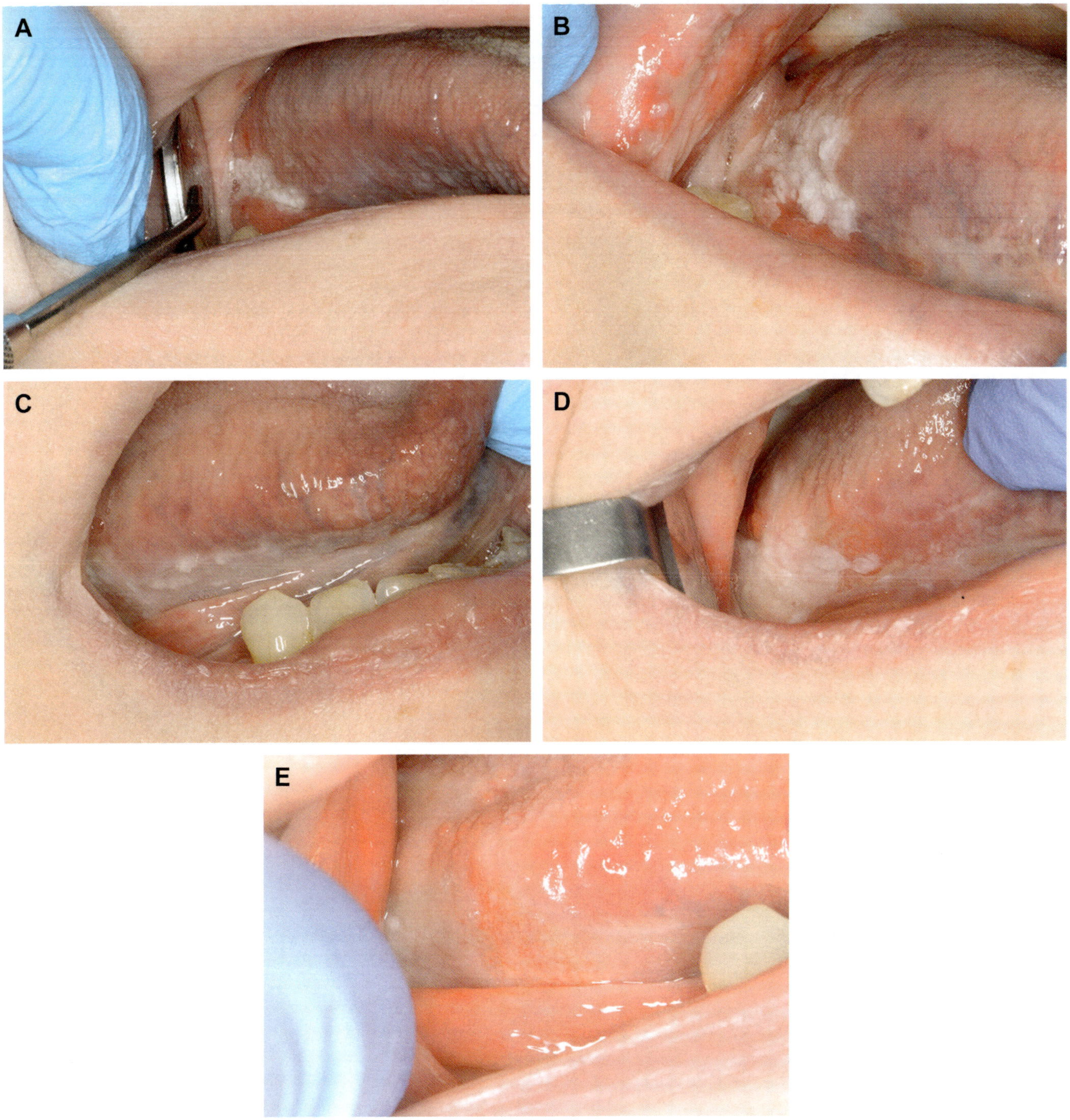

Fig. 2 Serial clinical photographs of same patient seen over a period of 6 years, showing the progression from lichen planus to squamous cell carcinoma of the right lateral posterior tongue. (*A*) 2010, (*B*) 2011, (*C*) 2013, (*D*) 2015, (*E*) 2016.

uses a fast injection rate followed by a quick succession of scans to calculate blood flow and blood volume[5]

- Magnetic resonance imaging (MRI) (Fig. 6)
    - It uses the proton distribution in tissues within a magnetic field.
    - It is most ideal for diagnosis of soft tissue abnormality as well as the spaces surrounding the temporomandibular joint.[3]
    - The provider should also ensure that the patient does not have a pacemaker in place, nerve stimulators, cochlear implants, or prosthetic cardiac valves containing metal, because they are contraindicated for an MRI[5]
    - Diffusion-weighted imaging (DWI) is a type of MRI that uses the diffusion of water molecules to analyze suspected abnormality. This type of imaging is ideal when monitoring a patient with a history of head/neck cancer due to the fact that DWI can help the provider differentiate between postsurgical or postradiation scarring and a potential new lesion[5]
- Positive emission tomography (PET) scan (Fig. 7)
    - PET is a form of imaging that typically uses a radiotracer called fluorodeoxyglucose, which is absorbed by metabolically active cells based on either blood flow or glucose utilization. Malignant lesions can demonstrate

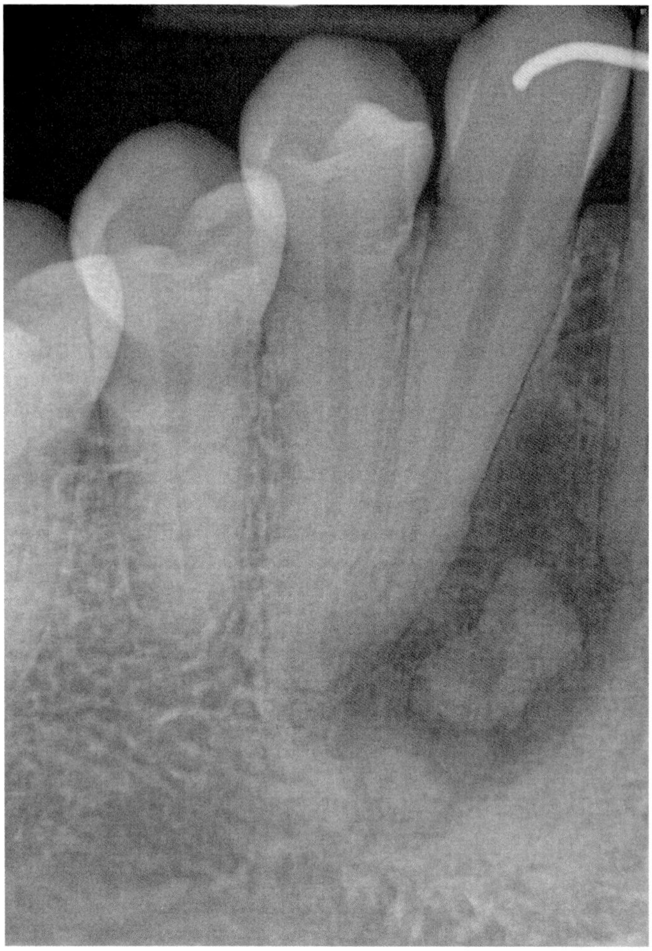

Fig. 3 Periapical radiograph showing a compound odontoma.

high concentrations of the radiotracer material and therefore be identified on an image.
  - It is used in conjunction with a CT scan so that anatomy can be identified, and analysis is used to determine staging of a cancer or possible metastases.
  - Unfortunately, false positives and false negatives are somewhat common within PET imaging in areas of inflammation or necrosis[5]
- Ultrasonography
  - Ultrasonographycan be helpful for the diagnosis of superficial neck structures and can guide clinicians performing fine needle aspiration/biopsy or cytology.
  - This technique depends on measurements based on the reflection of high-frequency (2–15 MHz) sound wavelengths (0.6–0.01 mm)[3]
  - It may be limited in giving a definitive diagnosis, but it can be helpful in suggesting whether the neck or salivary mass being examined has a benign or malignant nature[5]
- Sonoelastography
  - Sonoelastographyis a technique that measures tissue elasticity and helps differentiate lesions based on the fact that malignant lesions are typically more dense and less elastic than benign lesions[5]
- Sialography
  - Sialography is another type of imaging that can be helpful in diagnosis, particularly if a salivary gland obstruction is suspected.
  - This type of imaging involves a radiopaque dye being injected in the salivary duct, and radiographs are taken from different angulations[5]

Diagnostic tests and studies

The following diagnostic tests and studies may be needed to reach an accurate diagnosis if certain conditions are suspected.

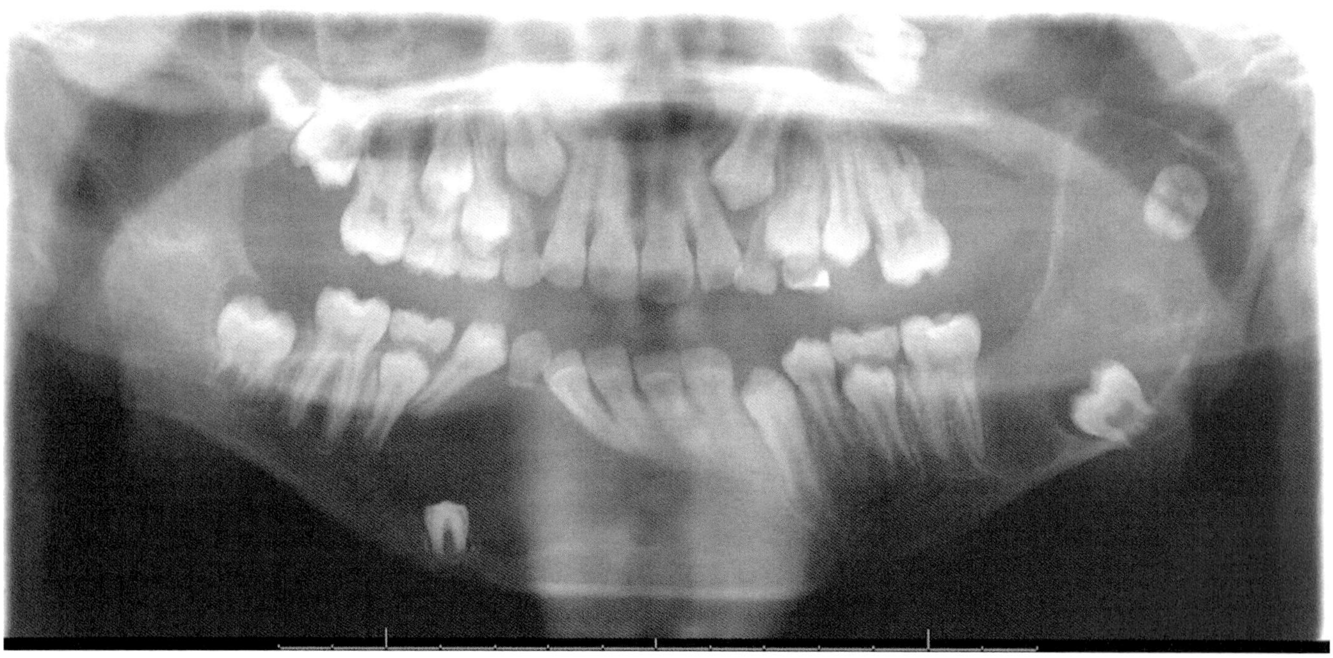

Fig. 4 Panoramic radiograph of a 12-year-old patient with Gorlin syndrome. Odontogenic keratocysts are on the left maxilla and the left ramus that has displaced multiple teeth.

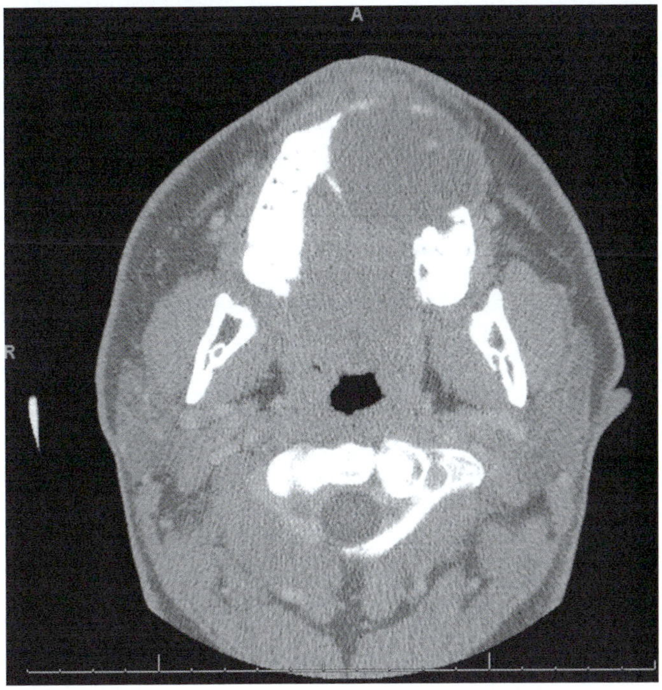

Fig. 5 Axial view CT scan showing a nasopalatine duct cyst of the maxilla.

Urinalysis

A urinalysis, routinely used with "dipsticks," may show glycosuria (diabetes), ketonuria (diabetes), bilirubin/urobilinogen (hepatobiliary disorders), proteinuria (menstruation or renal, urinary tract, or cardiac disease), or hematuria (menstruation or renal, urinary tract disease).

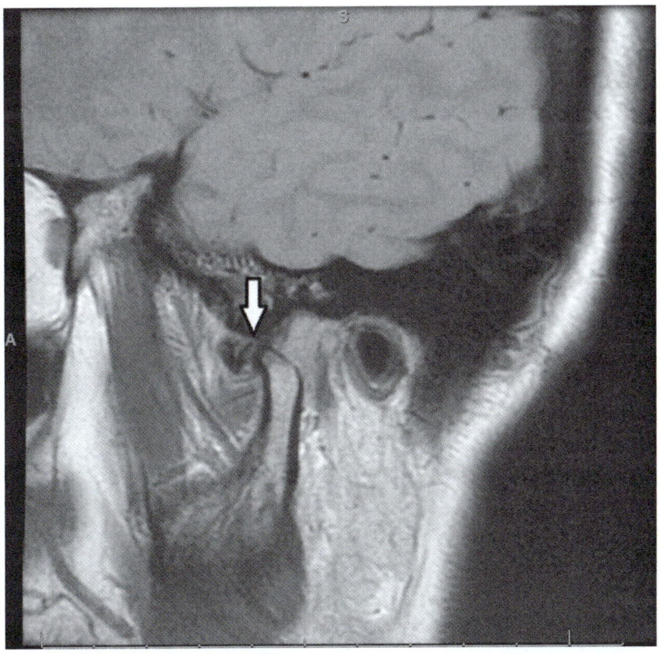

Fig. 6 MRI of the temporomandibular joint without contrast, open-mouth image. Image shows mild degenerative change of the condyle articular surface and anterior displacement of the articular disc (*arrow*) that is not recaptured on opening.

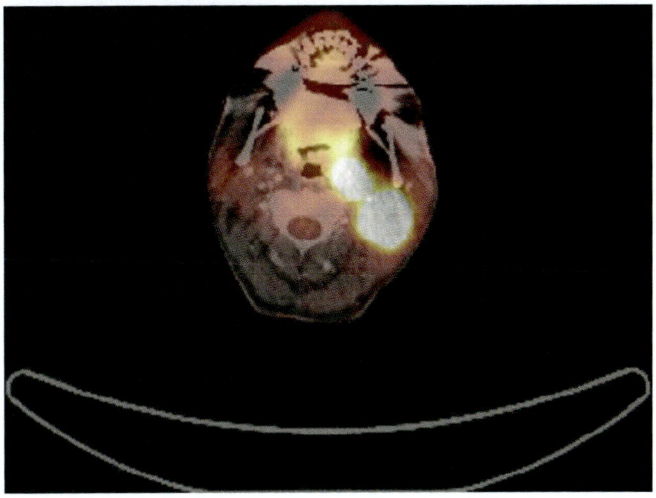

Fig. 7 PET/CT scan in axial view at the level of the mandible showing a large left tonsillar mass. Bright yellow areas indicate areas of hypermetabolism, indicating a malignant process.

Blood testing

The most common blood tests are the following[6]:

- Complete blood count: For example, anemias, infection, hematologic malignancies, thrombocytopenia, pancytopenia
- Erythrocyte sedimentation rate: Inflammatory processes, anemia
- Coagulation panel (prothrombin time, international normalization ratio, partial thromboplastin time): Bleeding disorders
- Ferritin, iron, transferrin, foliate, vitamin B12: Hematinic deficiencies
- Blood glucose: Diabetes
- Serum urea, creatinine, electrolyte levels
- Serum liver function tests (eg, aspartate aminotransferase, alanine aminotransferase): Liver disease
- Serum calcium, phosphate, alkaline phosphatase, and serology
- Autoantibodies: If autoimmune condition (eg, systemic lupus erythematosus, Sjogren syndrome) is suspected (the presence of autoantibodies does not always indicate disease):
  - Antinuclear antibodies (ANA)
  - DNA antibodies (double-stranded DNA)
  - Sjögren's antibodies (soluble substance A [SSA] and soluble substance B [SSB])
  - Scleroderma: Nucleolus-specific RNA, Sc1-70 (antitopisomerase)
  - Pemphigus: antibodies to Desmogleins 1 (DG1) and 3 (DG3)

Smear and culture

- Bacteriologic smear and culture: Positive culture does not necessarily confer causal relation with disease
- Fungal smear: *Candida hyphae* suggest that Candida species are pathogenic
- Viral culture: Indicates in some acute ulcerative or vesicular lesions; high degree of false negative results

Biopsy

Indications for biopsy include lesions with neoplastic or premalignant features, persistent lesions of unknown cause, lesions that do not respond to treatment, focal lesions involving the gingiva and periodontium, confirmation of a clinical diagnosis, or lesions causing the patient extreme concern.

Biopsy techniques

- Usually a single biopsy is taken, but sometimes multiple biopsies may be indicated for additional investigations, certain malignant diseases, or widespread leukoplakic or erythroplakic field changes.
- There are biopsy techniques that can be done without anesthesia (eg, exfoliative cytology and brush biopsy)
- The techniques requiring anesthesia include the following:
  - Incisional and excisional scalpel or tissue punch
  - Curettage
  - Needle biopsy with 14-G Tru-Cut needle, 16-G Vim Silverman needle, 18G TSK SURECUT needle, or 22/25-G standard disposable needle

Mucosal biopsies

- Excisional biopsies in which removal of complete lesion is performed are preferred for small, isolated, benign lesions.
- Incisional biopsies, which take a sample of part of the lesion, should include normal and lesional tissue. The punch is better used for incisional biopsies; however, if a larger piece of tissue is needed, a scalpel is preferred[3]

Immunostaining and immunofluorescence

- This is indicated if differential diagnosis includes immune-mediated conditions, such as pemphigus, pemphigoid, or linear immunoglobulin A (IgA) disease.
- Specimens for immunostaining should not be fixed in formalin but must be either handed immediately to laboratory staff for freezing, immediately snap-frozen, or placed in Michel's solution if to be transported to a distant site laboratory.
- Direct immunofluorescence is a qualitative technique used to detect immune deposits on excised tissue, using antibodies to label a specific antigen with a fluorescent dye.
- Indirect immunofluorescence is a qualitative and quantitative technique used to detect the presence of autoantibodies in a patient's bloodstream. In this case, a blood draw of the patient is performed.

Oral smears for cytology

- Smears can last for up to 3 weeks and can be done on wooden, metal, or dental plastic instruments.

Oral brush biopsy

- A brush biopsy is designed to obtain a transepithelial specimen containing cells from all 3 layers of the epithelium, including the base, intermediate, and superficial layers. This distinguishes it from cytology, which only samples cells from the surface of the lesion.

Labial salivary gland

- Labial minor salivary gland biopsy is performed for evaluation and workup for Sjögren's syndrome.
- At least 4 lobules of salivary gland should be excised, and the patient must be warned of possible postoperative mild hypoesthesia.

References

1. Swartz M. Textbook of physical diagnosis: history and examination. 7th edition. Philadelphia: WB Saunders; 2010. p. 129–36.
2. Lockhart P. Dental care of the medically complex patient. 5th edition. Philadelphia: Elsevier Health Sciences; 2004.
3. Scully C. Oral and maxillofacial medicine: the basis of diagnosis and treatment. Philadelphia: Elsevier Health Sciences; 2004.
4. de Leeuw R, Klasser GD. Orofacial pain: guidelines for assessment, diagnosis and management. 5th edition. Hanover Park: Quintessence Publishing; 2008.
5. Webb D. Diagnosis and management of neck masses. Atlas Oral Maxillofac Surg Clin North Am 2015;23:2–5.
6. Alexander RE, Wright JM, Thiebaud S. Evaluating, documenting and following up oral pathological conditions. A suggested protocol. J Am Dent Assoc 2001;132(3):329–35.

Oral Manifestations of Gastrointestinal Disorders

Lina Maria Mejia, DDS, MPH

KEYWORDS

• Gastrointestinal • Gastroesophageal • Ulcerative colitis • Crohn's disease • Extra-abdominal • Pyostomatitis vegetans • Aphthous ulcers • Hepatitis

KEY POINTS

- Dentists are often the first health care professionals to identify a systemic disease. Oral manifestations can be the initial indication of gastrointestinal (GI) disease and allow for an early diagnosis, treatment, and improved prognosis.
- The oral lesions associated with GI disease are multiple.
- Dental erosion is related to patients with gastroesophageal reflux disease, bulimia, or anorexia. Oral ulcerations, diffuse mucosal swelling, cobblestone mucosa, mucogingivitis, pyostomatitis vegetans, and others are lesions associated with IBD (Crohn's disease and ulcerative colitis).
- Crohn's disease is a chronic inflammatory process that can involve any part of the GI tract.
- Liver disease can cause bleeding abnormalities; care must be exercised when prescribing medications that are metabolized in the liver.

Introduction

The oral cavity is a mirror that reflects many of the human body's internal secrets; this concept was highlighted in the US Surgeon General's report Oral Health in America in 2000.[1]

The oral cavity is diagnostically accessible, so alterations can be the first indication of systemic diseases and may possibly allow for an early diagnosis, treatment, and enhanced prognosis.[2–5]

Astute dentists may be the first health care professionals to identify a systemic disease through observation of its oral manifestations. Through the inspection of the oral cavity, signs and symptoms such as persistent pain, halitosis, ulcerations, swelling, bleeding, and/or xerostomia might raise suspicion of systemic disease that includes the gastrointestinal (GI) tract.[6,7]

The oral lesions may be the first sign of GI disease, sometimes before the clinically apparent onset of the abdominal disease. These oral signs maybe present during the disease process or persist even after the abdominal disease has resolved. As an example, in the inflammatory bowel diseases (IBDs) Crohn's disease (CD) and ulcerative colitis (UC), oral manifestations, such as oral ulcerations, diffuse mucosal swelling, cobblestone mucosa, and localized mucogingivitis, may be the first sign of GI disease. Gastroesophageal reflux disease (GERD), bulimia, or anorexia, may cause irreversible dental erosion due to the exposure of tooth enamel to acidic gastric content.[8]

The most common oral changes identified in GI diseases are dental erosion, erythema at various sites of the oral cavity, oral ulcers, gingivitis, periodontitis, and glossitis.[9] Oral health care professionals are responsible for identifying, diagnosing, and treating oral conditions associated with GI diseases, along with providing appropriate dental care. This article reviews the oral changes observed in commonly occurring GI diseases.

Gastroesophageal reflux disease

GERD is caused by the rise of gastric contents, acidic and nonacidic, above the gastroesophageal junction (esophagus). GERD is a common condition in adults, affecting men and women equally, and occurs in all age groups. The prevalence increases in people older than 40 years.[10,11] In the United States, approximately 20% of the population has GERD.[12]

The cause of GERD is multifactorial. The following are conditions that can increase risk of GERD:[13,14]

- Obesity
- Certain foods and beverages, including chocolate, peppermint, fried or fatty foods, coffee, or alcoholic beverages
- Hiatal hernia
- Delayed stomach emptying
- Pregnancy
- Smoking
- Asthma
- Diabetes
- Dry mouth
- Connective tissue disorders, such as progressive systemic sclerosis (scleroderma).

Disclosures: No relationship with a commercial company.

Department of Oral Medicine and Diagnostic Sciences, College of Dental Medicine, Nova Southeastern University, 3200 South University Drive, Fort Lauderdale, FL 33328-2018, USA

E-mail addresses: lm1273@nova.edu, Lina.Mejia@nova.edu

Atlas Oral Maxillofacial Surg Clin N Am 25 (2017) 93-104

http://dx.doi.org/10.1016/j.cxom.2017.04.002

The typical symptoms of GERD include heartburn, regurgitation, dysphagia, and retrosternal pain. Furthermore, abnormal reflux can cause a wide range of atypical symptoms, including sleep disturbance, coughing, laryngitis, hoarseness, asthma, chronic obstructive pulmonary disease, unexplained chest pain, angina, sinusitis, otalgia, halitosis, dental erosion, and other dental manifestations (Box 1).[15–17] The frequency in which patients experience symptoms is varied.[18] Approximately 7% to 10% of Americans experience symptoms of GERD on a daily basis, and it has been reported that 25% to 40% of Americans experience symptomatic GERD at some point during their lives.[19,20] The number of individuals affected is probably higher due to the control of symptoms with over-the-counter (OTC) medications without consulting a medical professional.[21]

GERD complications include premalignant and malignant conditions of the esophagus. One of the main purposes in evaluating patients with chronic symptoms of GERD is to recognize Barrett esophagus (BE). BE is a precursor to esophageal adenocarcinoma (EAC). In EAC, there is squamous metaplasia from the normal squamous epithelial lining to columnar epithelium containing goblet cells.[22–24] Fortunately, approximately half of the patients examined do not manifest macroscopic changes of the esophageal mucosa. Serious endoscopic findings are identified in 10% of patients. BE is a complication with a 30-fold higher risk of development of EAC when compared with patients without this condition.[25,26] On the other hand, most patients with BE die from reasons unrelated to adenocarcinoma of the esophagus.[26,27]

Long-standing GERD is the main risk factor for the development of BE. Other risk factors, such male gender, advanced age, white race, obesity, hiatal hernia, and smoking, have to be considered to assess and counsel the patient effectively. Patient counseling is provided to reduce modifiable risks, such as nutrition and tobacco use, and to determine the need for endoscopy and biopsy.[23,28]

Medical management

The initial management of GERD relies on reviewing and eliminating modifiable factors, and/or providing safe efficacious acid suppressive therapy. For instance, advise weight loss for obese patients with GERD. Study outcomes show that weight loss over a 6-month period led to a significant improvement in GERD symptoms in 81% of the subjects; 65% had complete resolution and 15% had partial resolution of reflux symptoms.[13,29–31] GERD symptoms are improved with tobacco cessation due to the increase of saliva production. Moreover, patients suffering from GERD symptoms during the night should be coached to avoid late-night snacks and meals with high fat content. Fatty meals delay gastric emptying and produce distention and reflux. Sleeping with the head raised on 2 or 3 pillows or tilting the bed frame might dramatically improve symptoms.

Several medications are available to treat GERD, including antacids such Maalox, Mylanta, Rolaids, histamine 2 (H2) receptor antagonists (RAs), and proton pump inhibitors (PPIs).[32] H2RAs have been used since the mid-1970s to treat GERD and peptic ulcer disease. In patients with GERD, H2RAs improve the symptoms of heartburn and regurgitation and heal mild to moderate esophagitis. Types of H2 blockers include cimetidine, famotidine, nizatidine, and ranitidine. PPIs are the most common pharmacologic treatment used for GERD because of their potent acid suppression.[33] PPIs heal erosive esophagitis more efficaciously than do H2RAs and provide resolution of signs and symptoms, including ulcers and/or esophageal damage. PPIs, such as omeprazole (also available OTC), lansoprazole, esomeprazole, pantoprazole, and rabeprazole, are available by prescription.

Surgical treatment is reserved for patients who do not respond to medical therapy. Patients with a good initial response to medical therapy but who have severe functional and anatomic abnormalities of the gastroesophageal junction are those who are most commonly treated with surgery.[29,34]

Box 1. Gastroesophageal reflux disease signs and symptoms

Primary symptoms
- Heartburn
- Regurgitation
- Dysphagia

Abnormal reflux atypical symptoms
- Coughing and/or wheezing
- Hoarseness, sore throat, laryngitis
- Asthma
- Otitis media
- Noncardiac chest pain
- Enamel erosion or other dental manifestations
- Halitosis (bad breath)

Oral manifestations and considerations

Oral findings in patients with GERD include periodic increase in salivation, xerostomia (dry mouth), burning sensation, tongue sensitivity, halitosis, palatal erythema, oral ulcers(gingiva), dysgeusia (foul taste), gingivitis, periodontitis, dental thermal sensitivity and/or pulpitis, and dental erosion.[17] Dental erosion is defined as the loss of tooth substance by chemical processes (acid exposure) not involving bacteria. Repeated or prolonged exposure of teeth to acid leads to selective dissolution of specific components of the tooth surface, with eventual loss of tooth substance, hypersensitivity, functional impairment, and even tooth fracture. The degree of dental erosion due to GERD is associated with the extent of the disease, frequency of reflux, the pH and type of acid, and the quantity and quality of saliva.[7,9,11]

The distribution of erosion in patients with GERD affects the occlusal surfaces of the posterior mandibular teeth and the palatal surfaces of the maxillary anterior teeth. Affected teeth exhibit worn, smooth, silky glazed, or shiny enamel. They may appear yellow and become sensitive to temperature changes as the underlying dentin becomes exposed. More advanced stages of dental erosion disclose changes in the tooth morphology, resulting in a concavity in the enamel, the width of which clearly exceeds its depth. Further progression of occlusal erosion leads to a rounding of the cusps and, in severe cases, the whole occlusal morphology disappears and pulp exposure may occur (Figs. 1–3).[9,17,35]

Dental erosion is irreversible and may require dental restorative treatment. Soft tissue oral findings will usually resolve with medical management of GERD.[8,11,16,35]

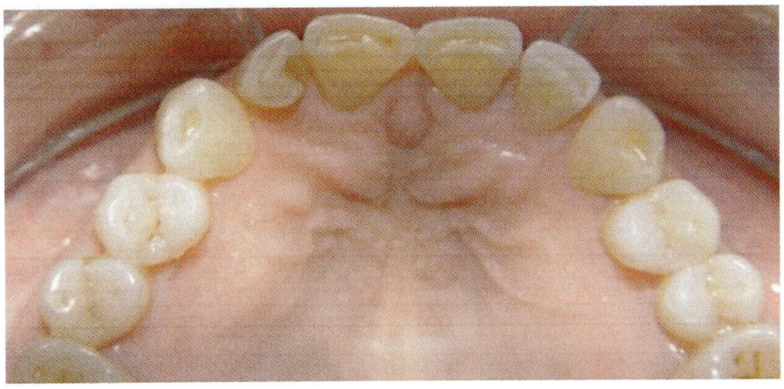

Fig. 1 Dental erosion in a patient with GERD. Lingual surfaces of the anterior superior teeth present areas of erosion, which gives them an opaque appearance.

Inflammatory bowel disease

IBD is a group of chronic inflammatory diseases, including CD and UC, which affect the GI tract.[36,37]

The incidence and prevalence of IBD varies by geographic location. IBD is more common in the United States and Europe than in Asia and Africa. IBD occurs more frequently among Jews and whites than in African Americans.[38] Approximately 1 million Americans are affected.[39] Men and women are equally affected. The onset of IBD is between 20 and 40 years of age.[37,40] The cause of IBD is believed to be multifactorial, including immune system, environmental factors, and genetics.[41] Experimental and clinical evidence suggest that IBD results from an immune reaction in individuals genetically susceptible to dysregulation of the normal gut flora, with sensitization and destruction of the colon mucosa.[37] Besides the expected GI symptoms, 20% of patients present with diverse extra-abdominal manifestations. Some of the most common organs involved are joints, skin, eyes, and biliary tract.[36,42] Oral manifestations in patients with IBD can be present years before the appearance of the intestinal disease.[36,43]

Ulcerative colitis

UC is an inflammatory reaction that may affect all or part of the large intestine characterized by remissions and exacerbations. Macroscopically, in mild disease the mucosa may have a granular appearance. Advanced disease may include stripping of the mucosa, with areas of sloughing, ulceration, and bleeding.[40] The cause of UC remains unknown. The 3 prominent features of UC are

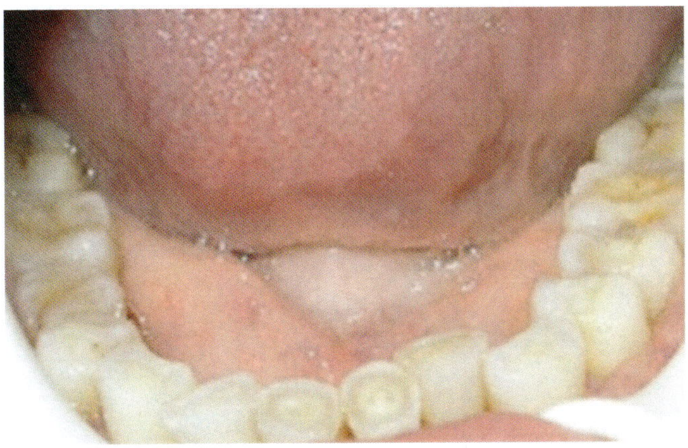

Fig. 2 Dental erosion in a patient with GERD. Different degrees of dental erosion can be seen in the incisal and occlusal surfaces of the lower teeth.

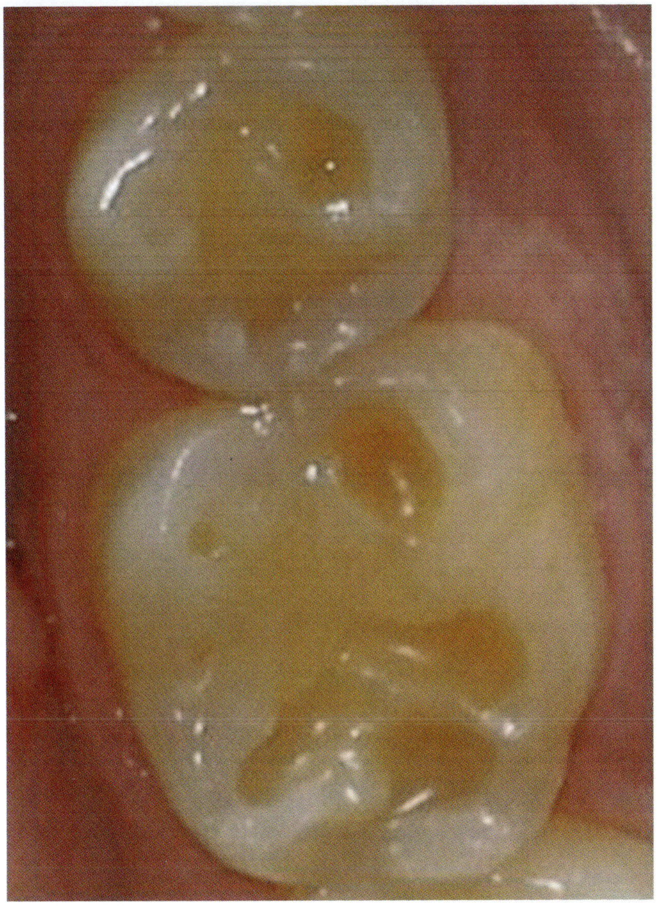

Fig. 3 Dental erosion in a patient with GERD, occlusal changes in the morphology result in a concavity in the enamel.

attacks of diarrhea, rectal bleeding, and abdominal cramps.[20,44] Patients are frequently dehydrated. UC patients may also present with fatigue, weight loss, and fever due to the malabsorption of water and electrolytes. The frequency of bowel movements and the amount of blood present reflect the activity of the disease. Often, the diarrhea is severe with 5 to 8 bowel movements in a 24-hour period. The crampy pain is present in both abdominal quadrants and is usually present before bowel movements. Extra-abdominal manifestations are frequently present. Erythema nodosum is characterized by red swollen nodules that are usually on the thighs and legs. Eye disorders, such as episcleritis, uveitis, corneal ulcers, and retinitis, may cause pain and photophobia. Joint symptoms, frequently affecting the ankles, knees, and wrists, occur in up to 20% of patients with the disease. Liver disease is a serious complication of UC. Anemia is commonly associated with UC. It is most likely caused by blood loss and is typically a microcytic hypochromic anemia of iron deficiency. Leukocytosis occurs in active disease and is usually associated with intra-abdominal abscess. Electrolyte imbalances, hypoalbuminemia, and low serum magnesium and potassium levels may occur because of the severe chronic diarrhea.[20,44–46]

Medical management

The aim of the UC therapy is to reduce inflammation and manage the deleterious effects of the disease. Anti-inflammatory medications are generally the first-line drugs prescribed. Sulfasalazine is used to initiate and maintain a remission in UC. Its active moiety, 5-aminosalicylate, has a direct anti-inflammatory effect on intestinal tissues without altering the colon flora. Corticosteroids and corticotropin are used in patients who have not responded satisfactorily to sulfasalazine. The steroid medications are prescribed in high doses (eg, 40–60 mg of oral prednisone daily initially and then maintenance doses of 10–20 mg of prednisone daily). Immunosuppressive agents, such as azathioprine, cyclosporine, and mercaptopurine, are used in patients who do not respond to traditional medical therapy. Also, Remicade (infliximab) 5 mg/kg is an intravenous medication used in adults with moderate to severe active UC or CD who have had an inadequate response to conventional therapy. This medication helps reduce signs and symptoms, inducing and keeping clinical remission and mucosal healing, and eliminating the steroid medication.[47]

Approximately 15% to 20% of patients receive surgery for intractable disease. Proctocolectomy combined with ileostomy is a curative procedure for UC. Today, new disposable ileostomy equipment is offered, most patients can look forward to an active lifestyle and normal life expectancy.[44,45,48]

Oral manifestations and considerations

The oral changes in UC cases have about 8% of incidence and are nonspecific and uncommon. Oral health care providers can discover them on the clinical examination in a patient with UC. The following are oral findings.

- Pyostomatitis vegetans

  Oral lesions of pyostomatitis vegetans (PV) are not premalignant and consist of multiple small white or yellow pustules on an erythematous and edematous mucosal background. The pustules can break, coalesce, and lead to a scattered, clumped, or typical snail-track appearance.[49] Pustules can involve almost all parts of the oral cavity. The most commonly involved areas are the buccal gingiva, labial, and buccal mucosa, and the least affected are the tongue and floor of the mouth (Fig. 4).[50] Histologic features are intraepithelial and subepithelial microabscesses with large numbers of eosinophils and neutrophils. Hyperkeratosis and acanthosis can be present as well.[49,51] Direct immunofluorescence is useful for the differential diagnosis of PV from pemphigus vulgaris, the result is negative in PV for deposits of immunoglobulin (Ig) A, Ig G, and complement (C) 3.[36,52] PV lesions can be painless or they can cause severe oral discomfort, which is not related to clinical activity of UC. There is a preference for men with a male/female ratio of nearly 3:1. PV can occur at any age, being more prevalent between 20 and 59 years old, with an average age of 34 years.[36,53] PV can involve almost any part of the oral cavity but is most frequently observed on the labial attached gingiva, soft and hard palate, buccal mucosa, and vestibular gingivae. The least affected locations are the floor of the mouth and the tongue. The intestinal symptoms usually precede oral PV by several months or years.[36,50] Clinically, the patient could present with fever, enlarged and tender submandibular lymph nodes, and pain (intensity is variable). Some patients with extensive chronic oral lesions may not have any pain. The main laboratory result seen in up to 90% of patients is peripheral eosinophilia.[36,50,52]
- Pyoderma gangrenosum

  These are deep ulcers, sometimes through the tonsillar pillar.[54]
- Aphthous stomatitis or aphthous ulcerations

  The size, depth, and duration are classified as major, minor, and herpetiform (see later discussion).[55]
- Hairy leukoplakia

  This lesion is commonly associated with human immunodeficiency virus (HIV) disease. This lesion probably serves as a marker of severe immunosuppression and may result from the use of corticosteroids or other immunosuppressive agents (Fig. 5).[56]
- Halitosis

  Prolonged glucocorticosteroids use can cause adrenal suppression and reduce the patient's capacity to respond to stress. For major operative or surgical procedures, the dose must be properly adjusted in consultation with the patient's physician. Routine dental treatments, such as cleanings or simple restorations, are not affected by steroid or immunosuppressive therapy.[44,55] Medical consultation is advised before surgical procedures.

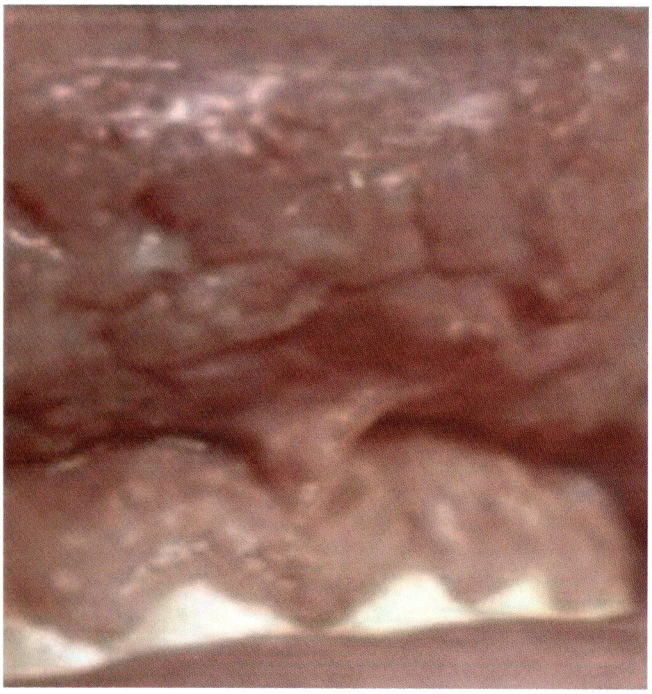

Fig. 4 Lesions on the labial mucosa and gingiva in a patient with PV.

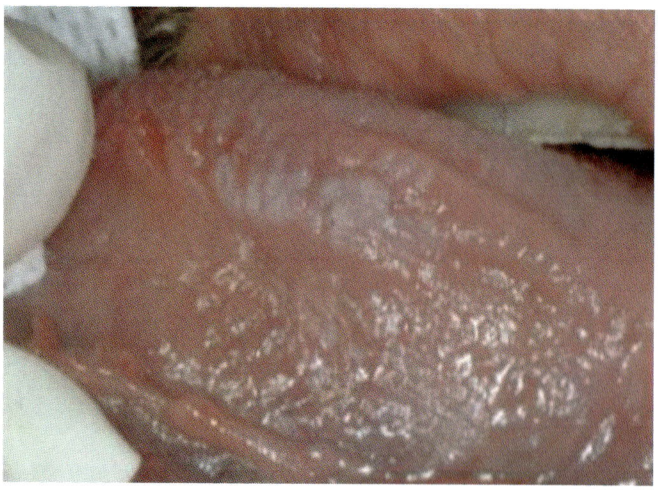

Fig. 5 Hairy leukoplakia.

- Ulcerative colitis

  UC is related to chronic bleeding due to vitamin K–dependent liver factors. Blood work-up that includes hemoglobin, hematocrit, platelet count, and a red blood cell count should be performed before dental procedures to rule out anemia (macrocytic and microcytic) and bleeding propensity.[46] Liver function tests should be done. Abnormal results dictate that management modification is necessary according to the potential for altered drug metabolism and coagulation. Patients who have extensive bowel surgery may suffer from malabsorption of vitamin K, vitamin B_{12}, and folic acid. They should be evaluated for bleeding disorders from insufficient levels of vitamin K (fibrin clot formation). Prothrombin time (PT) or international normalized ratio (INR) and a partial thromboplastin time will provide information about the patient's ability clot formation.

Crohn's disease

CD is a chronic inflammatory disease of the GI tract, involving predominantly the small or large intestine; the distal ileum and proximal colon are affected most frequently. The inflammation involves all the layers of the gut. It is characterized by segmental distribution of intestinal ulcers interrupted by normal appearing mucosa. This distribution has been described as skip lesions. Granulomas are present in about 50% of patients.[49,57,58]

The incidence of CD most studies have found nearly even rates in men and women and it affects all ages. CD occurs most frequently in urban women aged 20 to 39 years.[38–40]

Researchers suggest that a cause of CD might be an autoimmune reaction. The bacteria in the GI tract trigger the immune system, leading to CD symptoms to include chronic inflammation and mucosal ulceration. The following factors may play a role in the cause of CD[40,55]:

- Genetic (having a family member, most often a sibling or parent, with IBD)
- Stress
- Diet (high-fat)
- Smoking.

The clinical presentation of CD depends on the extent of inflammation and on the location of intestinal involvement. Clinical symptoms include intermittent episodes of abdominal distress, fever, vomiting, crampy abdominal pain, diarrhea, fatigue, weight loss, and growth failure in children.[40,49,58]

Intestinal complications from CD include transmural fibrosis, intestinal fissuring, abscess formation. Malabsorption is another complication resulting in weight loss, anemia, growth failure, clubbing fingers, and reduced bone mineral density.[59] Because of the skip lesion distribution, lesions of CD are not as amenable to surgery as those of UC.

Oral manifestations and considerations

Oral lesions prevalence ranges from 0.5% to 20% of CD patients. Most oral manifestations of CD occur in patients with active intestinal disease, and their presence frequently correlates with disease activity. In 60% of patients, oral symptoms precede the intestinal manifestations.[8,37] Recurrent aphthous ulcers are the most common oral manifestation of CD.[59]

Oral manifestations of CD can be classified as specific and nonspecific lesions according to the granulomatous changes noted on the histopathology.[36,40,49,60] Boxes 2 and 3 present a brief description of these lesions.

Granulomatous changes that constitute the hallmark of CD are observed in PV, cobblestone mucosal architecture, and minor salivary gland duct disease. CD patients develop diffuse swelling of the lips and face, inflammatory hyperplasia of the oral mucosa with a cobblestone pattern, indurated polypoid tag-like lesions in the vestibule and retromolar pad area, and persistent deep linear ulcerations with hyperplastic margins. Oral lesions can present pain, impair appropriate oral function, or even cause psychological issues.[49] Other clinical findings in CD are pallor, angular cheilitis, glossitis, candidiasis, perioral dermatitis, lichenoid reactions, and increased risk of dental caries.[3,36,37,74]

Oral lesions can be treated with palliative rinses, ointment, and topical steroids.[55] The patient must be advised that prolonged use of topical steroids will result in mucosal atrophy, and an increased incidence of mucosal candidiasis.

Dental management

Dental management of CD includes

- Frequent preventive and routine dental care to monitor oral health and to prevent the destruction of hard and soft tissue

Box 2. Specific oral lesions in Crohn's disease

Indurated tag-like lesions
- These are white reticular tags, which are referred as mucosal tags, epithelial tags, or folds.[36]
- These lesions are found generally in the labial vestibules, and in the retromolar regions.[61]
- Up to 75% of these lesions may show noncaseating granulomas on histopathology.[62]
- There has been no specific direct association of these lesions with intestinal CD activity reported.

Cobblestone surface appearance (Fig. 6)
- Fissured swollen buccal mucosa with corrugation and hyperplastic appearance of the mucosa.
- Generally, these mucosa-colored firm plaques are found on the buccal mucosa and palate.[36,59,62]
- Lesions can be painful, causing difficulty eating or speaking.[36]
- Lesions are pathognomonic for CD but are not necessarily concurrent with the intestinal activity in CD.[43]
- Treatment involves the use of topical or systemic corticosteroids.[59]

Mucogingivitis[49,63]
- Gingiva may become edematous, granular, and hyperplastic in CD, with or without ulceration. Lesions can involve the entire body of the attached gingiva.
- This lesion has no connotation with intestinal CD activity.

Other specific lesions[60,64,65]
- Lip swelling with vertical fissures
- Deep linear ulcerations (usually in the buccal sulci with hyperplastic folds)
- Midline lip fissuring

Box 3. Nonspecific oral lesions in Crohn's disease

Aphthous ulcers or aphthous stomatitis (Figs. 7 and 8)

- Aphthous ulcers lesions clinically manifest as small, hallow, round or oval, painful, self-healing ulcerations with circumscribed margins, erythematous haloes, and central fibrinous exudate (yellow or gray floors).[66]
- These lesions may occur in 20% to 25% of the general population. Oral ulcers happen in 20% to 30% of patients with CD, and 10% in patients with UC. The presence of aphthous ulcers does not always correlate with disease activity. During active disease lesions can be more severe. However, this correlation is not clear.[36,49,67]
- The cause of aphthous ulcers lesions is unclear but several local (eg, smoking) and microbial factors have been proposed as causative agents.[68] These include Behçet disease, mouth and genital ulcers with inflamed cartilage (MAGIC) syndrome, CD, UC, HIV infection, Marshall syndrome, cyclic neutropenia, stress, psychological imbalance, menstrual cycle, immunologic (cytokines; eg, IL-2, IL-10, and, particularly, tumor necrosis factor-alpha), genetic, allergic, and nutritional factors (eg, gluten-sensitive enteropathy, iron, folic acid, zinc deficiencies, vitamin B1, B2, B6, and B12 deficiencies).
- Aphthous stomatitis has been associated with ankylosing spondylitis, uveitis, peripheral arthritis, and erythema nodosum.[69] Aphthous ulcers are not specific for IBD and may be observed in other disorders, including celiac sprue, HIV and acquired immune deficiency syndrome (AIDS), Behçet disease, and Reiter syndrome, as well as common aphthae seen in the normal population.[36,70]
- Control of the systemic disease CD is generally sufficient to control the aphthous ulcer. Effective treatment includes occlusive barriers, amlexanox, laser, topical or systemic corticosteroids, intralesional steroids, immunosuppressants, or a combination of these modalities, depending on the severity of the ulcerations. Some of the topical steroids preparations (ointment, gel, cream, rinse) are triamcinolone acetonide 0.1%, fluocinonide 0.05%, clobetasol propionate 0.05%, and dexamethasone elixir (0.5 mg/5 mL spit or swish). These are used up to 3 times per day. Continuous use of topical steroids, longer than 2 weeks, can cause mucosal atrophy and candidiasis, and increase the risk of systemic absorption.[71–73]

PV and other nonspecific lesions

PV can occur in both UC and CD but is more common UC.

Other nonspecific oral findings of CD[36,41,49,74,75]

- Angular cheilitis (Fig. 9)
- Persistent submandibular lymphadenopathy
- Sicca syndrome and reduced salivation
- Halitosis
- Dental caries and periodontal involvement
- Candidiasis (Fig.10)
- Odynophagia
- Dysphagia
- Minor salivary gland enlargement
- Perioral erythema with scaling
- Recurrent buccal abscesses
- Glossitis (Fig.11)
- Mucosal discoloration
- Lichen planus (Figs.12 and 13)
- Metallic dysgeusia

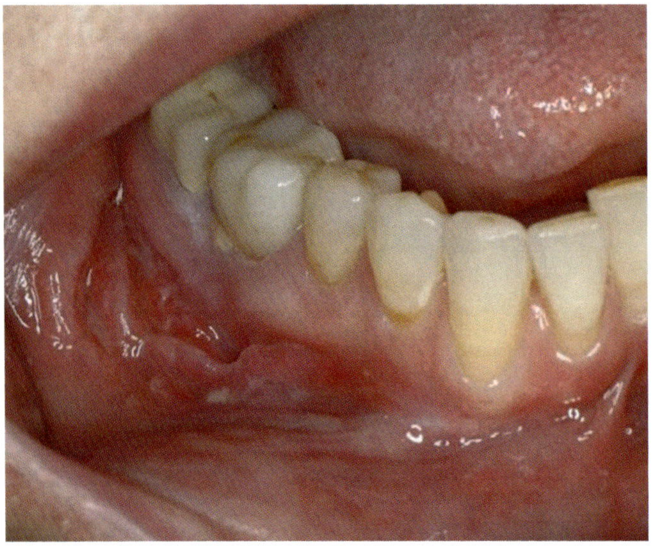

Fig. 6 Cobblestone appearance in CD.

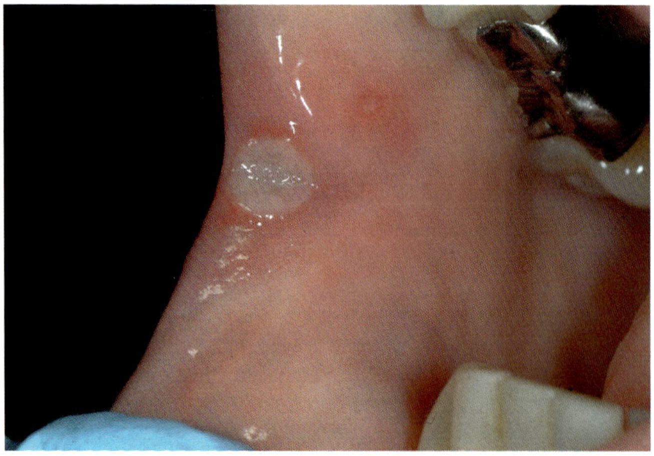

Fig. 7 Aphthous ulcers.

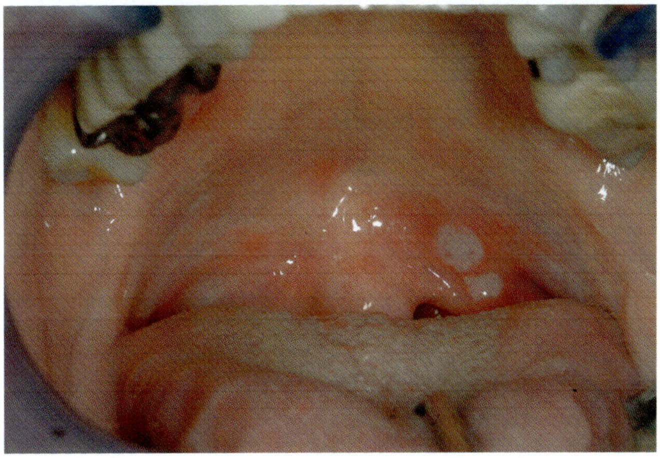

Fig. 8 Aphthous ulcers.

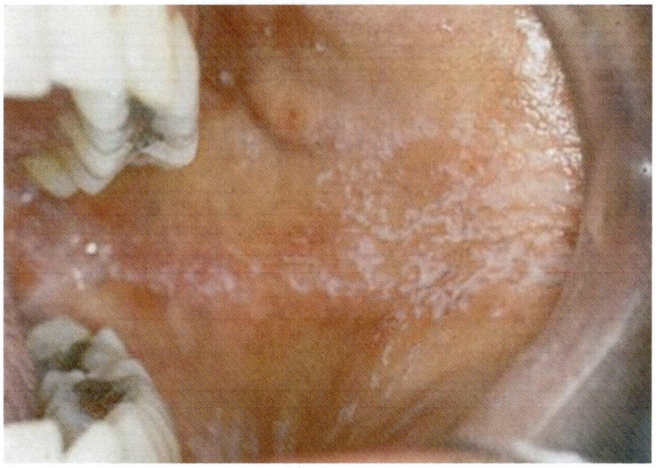

Fig. 10 Candidiasis (pseudomembranous).

- Management of glucocorticosteroid therapy in consultation with the patient's physician
- Screening, diagnosis, and treatment of any oral inflammatory, infectious, or granulomatous lesions as necessary
- Palliative rinses such as sodium bicarbonate mouth rinses (one-half teaspoon of baking soda in 8 ounces of warm water) may be used to swish and expectorate
- Topical steroid therapy[65,71]
  - Moderate-potency topical steroid, such as fluocinonide 0.05%, desoximetasone, and triamcinolone (can be topically applied to the lesions, 4 times a day; not to exceed 2 continuous weeks)
  - Ultrapotent preparations (can be topically applied to the lesions, 4 times a day), such as clobetasol and halobetasol
  - Dexamethasone elixir 0.5 mg/5 mL can be used as a rinse or gargle for 1 minute, 4 times daily, and expectorated
- Knowledge of drug interactions of patient's medications
- Consultation with patient's physician as needed.

Liver disease

The liver serves as the major organ for protein synthesis, catabolic functions, and detoxifying activities in the body. The liver is essential in the excretion of heme pigments and participates in the immune response. All intermediary metabolism of food occurs here. The liver regulates gluconeogenesis. Lipids are metabolized in the liver to form cholesterol and triglycerides. Proteins, albumin, and clotting factors (factors I, II, V, VII, IX, and X) are synthesized and stored in the liver. Because some of the clotting factors also depend on vitamin K (eg, II, VII, IX, and X), coagulopathy can occur from hepatocyte dysfunction and/or vitamin K malabsorption. The metabolism of drugs is principally performed by the cytochrome P-450 microsomal enzyme system in the hepatocyte. Local anesthetics, analgesics, sedatives, antibiotics, and antifungals are all metabolized in the liver. Consequently, cautious use of these drugs in a person with liver dysfunction is essential. The liver inactivates or metabolizes hormones such as insulin, aldosterone, antidiuretic hormone, estrogens, and androgens. Clearly, liver dysfunction can express itself through multiple signs and symptoms. Liver disease commonly manifests itself through jaundice, and the disease progression can lead to liver failure and death. Liver functions are summarized in Box 4.[72,76–78]

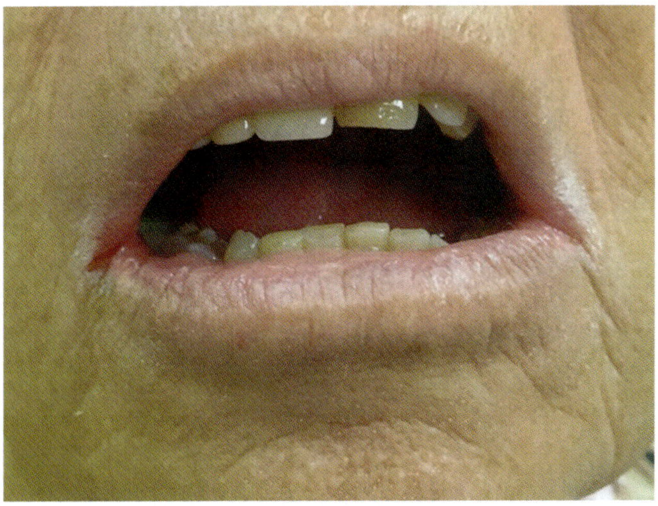

Fig. 9 Angular cheilitis.

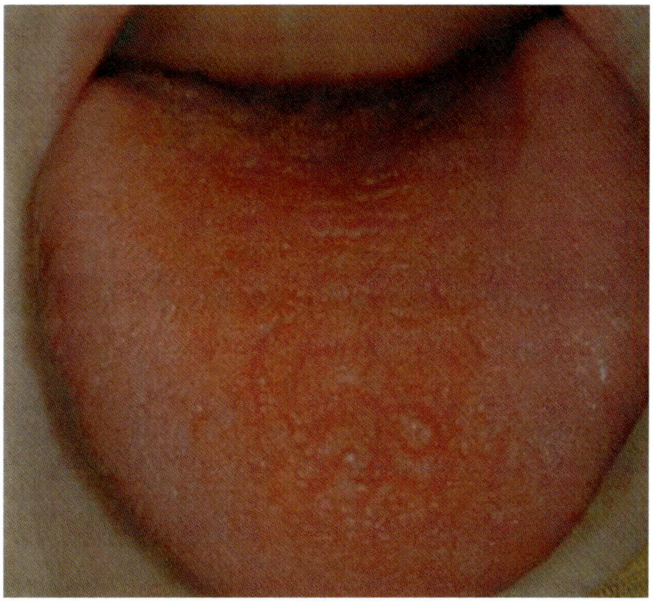

Fig. 11 Glossitis.

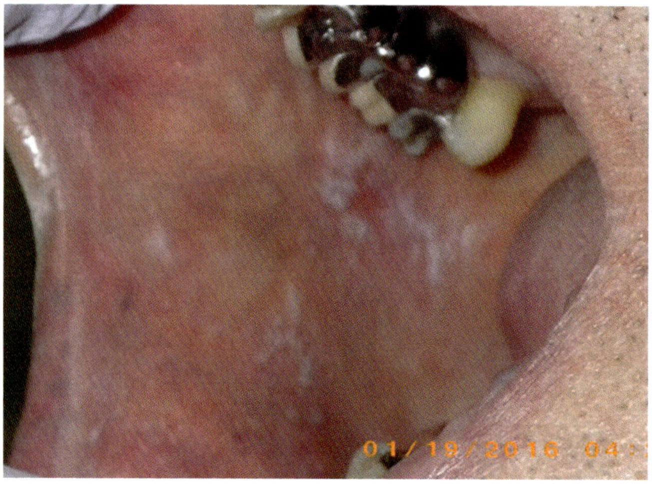

Fig. 12 Lichen planus.

General overview

The liver is vulnerable to an extensive variety of metabolic, toxic, microbial, circulatory, and neoplastic disease processes. The major primary diseases of the liver are viral hepatitis, alcoholic liver disease, nonalcoholic fatty liver disease (NAFLD), cirrhosis, and hepatocellular carcinoma.

NAFLD is a group of conditions that share the presence of a fatty liver and is the most common cause of cryptogenic cirrhosis (cirrhosis of unknown origin). Furthermore, it has become the most common cause of chronic liver disease in the United States, affecting more than 30% of the population.[76] NAFLD is strongly associated with obesity and other components of metabolic syndrome, which is possibly the reason for its high prevalence in the United States. It is estimated that more than 70% of obese individuals have some form of NAFLD.[76,79,80]

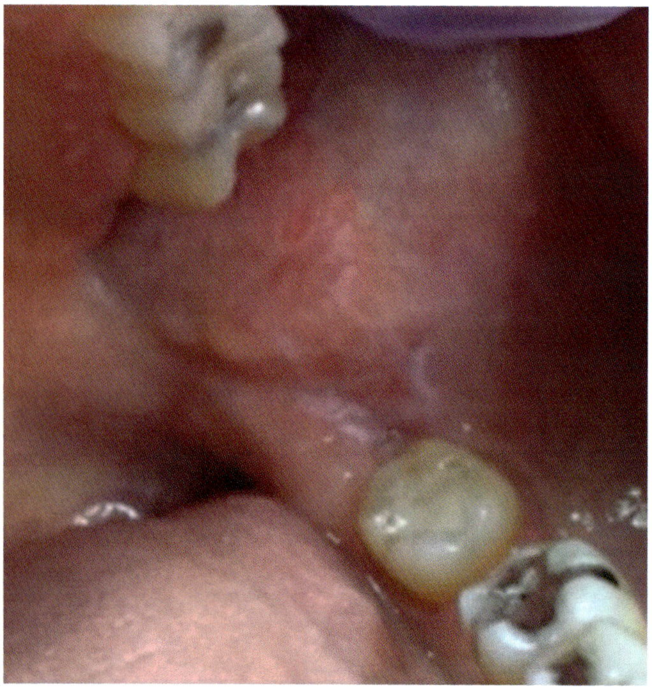

Fig. 13 Lichen planus.

Box 4. Liver functions

Metabolism or detoxification
- Metabolizes products of digestion
- Glucose regulation
- Vitamin storage
- Metabolizes drugs
  - Some of the common drugs used in dentistry (local anesthetics, analgesics, sedatives, antibiotics, antifungals)
  - Ethanol
- Breaks down bilirubin

Synthesis and secretion
- Components of clotting factors
- Cholesterol, triglyceride synthesis
- Bile production
- Other proteins and hormones

Storage and filtration of blood
- Acts as a blood reservoir
- Contains phagocytic cells
- Part of the reticuloendothelial system

Bleeding tendencies are a major problem in advanced liver disease. This is due to a deficiency of coagulation factors, especially the prothrombin group (factors II, VII, IX, and X), because these all rely on vitamin K as a precursor for production. Vitamin K is absorbed from the large intestine and stored in the liver, where it is converted into an enzymatic cofactor for the carboxylation of prothrombin complex proteins. Widespread hepatocellular destruction, as seen in cirrhosis, decreases the liver's storage and its ability to convert vitamin K, leading to deficiencies of the prothrombin-dependent coagulation factors.

In addition to these deficiencies, thrombocytopenia may be caused by splenomegaly secondary to portal hypertension and to bone marrow depression. The combination of hemorrhagic tendencies and severe portal hypertension (which causes thrombocytopenia as a consequence of sequestration of platelets in the spleen) sets the stage for episodes of GI bleeding, or ruptured esophageal varices. Most patients with advanced cirrhosis die of complications of hepatic coma, often precipitated by massive hemorrhage from esophageal varices or concurrent infection.[81–84]

Manifestations of liver disease

Jaundice

- Jaundice is a yellowing of the skin and eyes from excessive bilirubin in the blood.[73,77,81,84]
- Excess unconjugated bilirubin suggests decreased hepatic uptake, or decreased hepatic processing.
- Excess conjugated bilirubin can come from dysfunctional hepatocytes, slowing of bile flow from the liver, or obstruction of extrahepatic bile flow.
- The excess bilirubin in the skin causes pruritus (itching).

Portal hypertension

- Portal hypertension is an increased resistance to portal blood flow entering, leaving, or within the liver. The main causes for this restricted blood flow are cirrhosis, right-sided heart failure, fatty liver, and splenomegaly.

- Portal hypertension leads to the formation of collateral veins that bypass the liver. As a result, many of the toxins usually processed by the liver go directly into the blood stream. Some of these collateral vessels form at the base of the esophagus (esophageal varices), or in the stomach (gastric varices). These enlarged vessels are prone to rupturing, resulting in massive bleeding and often death.

Ascites

- Ascites is the accumulation of excess fluid in the peritoneal cavity due to high pressure in blood vessels of the liver and low levels of albumin (hypoalbuminemia). It is clinically detectable when at least 500 mL of fluid has accumulated.

Hepatic encephalopathy

- Hepatic encephalopathy is a spectrum of disturbances in consciousness, ranging from subtle behavioral abnormalities, to marked confusion and stupor, to deep coma and death. This can happen in hours or days in someone with acute liver failure, or more slowly in someone with chronic disease.
- It is associated with elevated levels of ammonia in the blood and central nervous system, promoting brain edema and impaired neural function. This is reversible if the underlying hepatic condition can be corrected.

Splenomegaly

- Portal hypertension often causes the spleen to enlarge because the pressure interferes with blood flow from the spleen into the portal blood vessels. The white blood cell count can decrease (increasing the risk of infections) and the platelet count can decrease (increasing the risk of bleeding).

Blood abnormalities

- Leukopenia and thrombocytopenia often accompany splenomegaly in advanced portal hypertension. This can lead to increased infection and increased bleeding.
- Clotting abnormalities due to malabsorption of vitamin K lead to the liver's decreased ability to synthesize several clotting factors.

Light stools or dark urine

- Bilirubin is normally excreted along with bile into the gut where it is broken down by bacteria, giving stool its characteristic color. In patients with hepatitis or cirrhosis, bilirubin cannot be moved through the liver or bile ducts rapidly enough and, instead, it builds up in the blood stream. If bilirubin is not properly excreted, the resulting stool is light in color.
- Dark brown but clear urine is a sign of a liver disorder such as acute viral hepatitis or cirrhosis, which causes excess bilirubin in the urine. Light stool and dark urine are generally consistent with jaundice.

Peripheral edema

- Albumin, a circulating protein synthesized in the liver, becomes deficient (hypoalbuminemia) causing reduced blood osmolarity. This in turn causes fluid to escape into the tissues and migrate to the lower extremities with gravity.

Abdominal pain

- Hepatomegaly, or an enlarged liver, is generally asymptomatic; however, an obviously enlarged liver can cause abdominal pain, discomfort, or feeling of fullness.
- Chronic abdominal pain can also be a symptom of hepatocellular carcinoma.

Oral manifestations and considerations

The following are common oral finding in patients with liver disease (Fig. 14).[73,83,85]

- Oral candidiasis or angular cheilitis: can be caused by immunotherapy following liver transplant to prevent rejection of the organ
- Atrophic glossitis: caused by anemia from malabsorption of vitamin B12, and iron
- Petechiae: small red dots generally seen on the palate, caused by thrombocytopenia
- Lichen planus: associated with hepatitis C (HCV) infection. Association can be partially explained by geographic effect and variances in study design, with genetic factors, age, and interferon-based treatments also playing a role. Numerous studies suggest that, in patients with established diagnosis of lichen planus (clinically and histologically), HCV infection should be ruled out.[86]
- Oral metastases of hepatocellular carcinoma primarily manifest as hemorrhagic expanding masses located in the premolar and mandible ramus area.

Protection

One of the most important considerations as a health care provider in the management of any patient is personal health and safety. Dentists need to follow standard precautions and wear protective gear, including gown, mask, eye protection, and gloves. Many cases of hepatitis B virus (HBV) and HCV are asymptomatic and go undetected. Patients may be unaware that they are carriers of HBV or HCV. Vaccination for HBV is available and is required for individuals who are at risk of exposure. Proper postexposure HBV protocol is important as well. The estimated risk of contracting HBV from a sharps injury is approximately 30%. If a vaccinated person has a needle stick, he or she needs to be tested for adequate antibody levels and, if needed, be given immunoglobulin and a booster. Nonvaccinated people would receive the HBV immunoglobulin. No postexposure protocol exists yet for HCV, but the individual should be followed for 6 months for HC antibodies and liver enzyme activity.[72]

Other considerations

- Before surgical procedures, patients with liver disease must have a careful evaluation of their capacity for

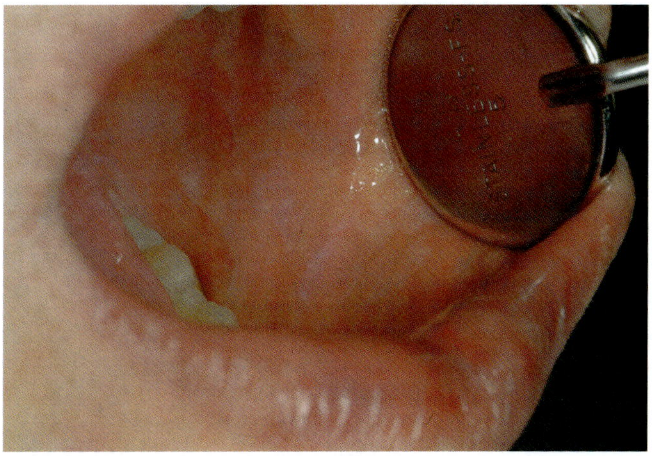

Fig. 14 Lichen planus in a patient with hepatitis C.

hemostasis, and testing should include, at minimum, a platelet count, and PT or INR tests. Platelet count should be above 50,000 and INR below 2.0 to 3.5 for surgical procedures, depending on the extent of surgery and the surgical proficiency of the clinician.

- Nonsurgical dental procedures may be safely performed in the higher INR ranges (below 4.0) and lower platelet counts. If laboratory values are not within an acceptable range, consult with the physician. The patient may need platelet transfusions to correct the thrombocytopenia and/or fresh frozen plasma (FFP) to correct the factor-related coagulopathy. Generally, 2 units of FFP will increase levels of all the clotting factors by 4% to 6%, and 6 units of platelets (60,000).
- Vitamin K injections the week before dental surgery may also be helpful. Intraoperative hemostatic agents, such as collagen matrix or absorbable gelatin sponge, should be used in extraction sites when hemostasis is impaired.

Dental drugs

Generally, normal therapeutic doses of drugs can be used for short periods of time except when liver function is severely compromised. When necessary, alternative drugs not metabolized in the liver can be selected or doses and intervals adjusted. Extreme caution should be used in prescribing medications that are metabolized in the liver for patients with severe liver disease. Table 1 presents a summary of the main drugs used in dentistry, potential issues, and recommendations.

Table 1 Dental drugs and recommendations

Local anesthetics	• Lidocaine and mepivacaine, limit maximum dosage to 300 mg • Prilocaine, limit to 400 mg max dosage • Articaine, safe, metabolized in plasma
Analgesics or pain control	• Aspirin, ibuprofen, and other nonsteroidal anti-inflammatory drugs (NSAIDs); use caution, NSAIDs increase the risk of GI bleeding and interfere with fluid balance • Acetaminophen; use caution, some studies advise to avoid acetaminophen but others state that is relatively safe if limited to<3.2 g/d for acute pain management • Narcotics, increase dose interval, short-term • Morphine, safe • Codeine, hydrocodone, and oxycodone, meperidine are conjugated in the liver and should be used at increased dose intervals and for short-term only
Sedatives or Anxiolytics	• Benzodiazepines, reduce dosage, increase intervals
Antibiotics	• Beta-lactam (penicillin, ampicillin, cephalexin, cefazolin, ceftriaxone), safe (renal excretion) • Metronidazole, severe interaction with alcohol and should be avoided if there is any chance that the patient may drink, metabolized in the liver • Clindamycin, aminoglycosides, tetracycline are all metabolized in the liver; use caution, reduce dosages, and increase intervals

Summary

Dentists play an important role in the early detection and multidisciplinary medical management of systemic conditions. Oral manifestations are encountered with high frequency in patients with GI diseases and are often the first clinical signs or symptoms of the condition. It is important to recognize prevalent medical and dental issues, as well as special needs of patients with GI problems. During differential diagnosis of these oral manifestations, side effects of drugs, nutritional deficiencies, infections, as well as other granulomatous diseases with oral involvement should be considered. The treatment of these lesions, when indicated, may consist of topical and systemic steroids, immunosuppressive drugs, antibiotics, and biological therapies in severe cases.

It is important to pay careful attention to oral hygiene, prescribe appropriate fluoride, and counsel patients about lifestyle modifications (nutrition, tobacco cessation). These measures managed by the practicing dentist should be incorporated in patient's treatment to help to improve the oral and systemic patient health.

Acknowledgment

I would like to thank Dr Michael A. Siegel, for his support and collaboration with editing this article.

References

1. U.S. Department of Health and Human Services. Oral Health in America: A Report of the Surgeon General. Rockville (MD): U.S. Department of Health and Human Services, National Institute of Dental and Craniofacial Research, National Institutes of Health; 2000.
2. Swinson B, Witherow H, Norris P, et al. Oral manifestations of systemic diseases. Hosp Med 2004;65(2):92–9.
3. Daley TD, Armstrong JE. Oral manifestations of gastrointestinal diseases. Can J Gastroenterol 2007;21(4):241–4.
4. Islam NM, Bhattacharyya I, Cohen DM. Common oral manifestations of systemic disease. Otolaryngol Clin North Am 2011;44(1): 161–82. vi.
5. Jurge S, Hegarty AM, Hodgson T. Orofacial manifestations of gastrointestinal disorders. Br J Hosp Med (Lond) 2014;75(9): 497–501.
6. Fumagalli LA, Gatti H, Armano C, et al. Oral Pathology unmasking gastrointestinal disease. J Dent Health Oral Disord Ther 2016;5(5): 00170.
7. Dundar A, Sengun A. Dental approach to erosive tooth wear in gastroesophageal reflux disease. Afr Health Sci 2014;14(2): 481–6.
8. Chi AC, Neville BW, Krayer JW, et al. Oral manifestations of systemic disease. Am Fam Physician 2010;82(11):1381–8.
9. Vinesh E, Masthan K, Kumar MS, et al. A clinicopathologic study of oral changes in gastroesophageal reflux disease, gastritis, and ulcerative colitis. J Contemp Dent Pract 2016;17(11):943–7.
10. Vakil N, van Zanten SV, Kahrilas P, et al. The Montreal definition and classification of gastroesophageal reflux disease: a global evidence-based consensus. Am J Gastroenterol 2006;101: 1900–20.
11. Roesch-Ramos L, Roesch-Dietlen F, Remes-Troche JM, et al. Dental erosion, an extraesophageal manifestation of gastroesophageal reflux disease. The experience of a center for digestive physiology in Southeastern Mexico. Rev Esp Enferm Dig 2014; 106(2):92–7.

12. El-Serag HB, Petersen NJ, Carter J, et al. Gastroesophageal reflux among different racial groups in the United States. Gastroenterology 2004;126:1692–9.
13. Herbella FAM, Sweet MP, Tedesco P, et al. Gastroesophageal reflux disease and obesity. Pathophysiology and implications for treatment. J Gastrointest Surg 2007;11(3):286–90.
14. Di Fede O, Di Liberto C, Occhipinti G, et al. Oral manifestations in patients with gastro-oesophageal reflux disease: a single-center case-control study. J Oral Pathol Med 2008;37(6): 336–40.
15. Malfertheiner P, Hallerbäck B. Clinical manifestations and complications of gastroesophageal reflux disease (GERD). Int J Clin Pract 2005;59(3):346–55.
16. Ranjitkar S, Smales RJ, Kaidonis JA. Oral manifestations of gastroesophageal reflux disease. J Gastroenterol Hepatol 2012; 27(1):21–7.
17. Farrokhi F, Vaezi MF. Extra-esophageal manifestations of gastroesophageal reflux. Oral Dis 2007;13:349–59.
18. Sonnenberg A, El-Serag HB. Clinical epidemiology and natural history of gastroesophageal reflux disease. Yale J Biol Med 1999; 72(2–3):81–92.
19. Richter JE. What's new in gastroesophageal reflux disease for 2014. Gastroenterol Clin North Am 2014;43(1):xiii–xiv.
20. Peery AF, Dellon ES, Lund J, et al. Burden of gastrointestinal disease in the United States: 2012 update. Gastroenterology 2012; 143(5):1179–87.e1–3.
21. Giannini EG, Zentilin P, Dulbecco P, et al. Management strategy for patients with gastroesophageal reflux disease: a comparison between empirical treatment with esomeprazole and endoscopy-oriented treatment. Am J Gastroenterol 2008;103(2):267–75.
22. Spechler S. Barrett's esophagus: the American perspective. Dig Dis 2013;31:10–6.
23. Sharma N, Ho KY. Risk factors for Barrett's oesophagus. Gastrointest Tumors 2016;3(2):103–8.
24. Duits LC, van der Wel MJ, Cotton CC, et al. Patients with Barrett's esophagus and confirmed persistent low-grade dysplasia at increased risk for progression to neoplasia. Gastroenterology 2017; 152(5):993–1001.e1.
25. Svoboda P, Dítě P, Klvaňa P, et al. Risk factors and progression predictors of Barrett's oesophagus to adenocarcinoma. Vnitr Lek 2014;60(5–6):467–73.
26. Brimhall B, Wani S. Current endoscopic approaches for the treatment of Barrett esophagus. J Clin Gastroenterol 2017; 51(1):2–11.
27. Qureshi I, Shende M, Luketich J. Surgical palliation for Barrett's esophagus cancer. Surg Oncol Clin N Am 2009;18:547–60.
28. Katz PO, Gerson LB, Vela MF. Guidelines for the diagnosis and management of gastroesophageal reflux disease. Am J Gastroenterol 2013;108:308.
29. De Groot NL, Burgerhart JS, Van De Meeberg PC, et al. Systematic review: the effects of conservative and surgical treatment for obesity on gastro-oesophageal reflux disease. Aliment Pharmacol Ther 2009;30(11–12):1091–102.
30. Ness-Jensen E, Hveem K, El-Serag H, et al. Lifestyle intervention in gastroesophageal reflux disease. Clin Gastroenterol Hepatol 2016; 14(2):175–82.e1–3.
31. Singh M, Lee J, Gupta N, et al. Weight loss can lead to resolution of gastroesophageal reflux disease symptoms: a prospective intervention trial. Obesity 2013;21(2):284–90.
32. Gawron AJ, French DD, Pandolfino JE, et al. Economic evaluations of gastroesophageal reflux disease medical management. Pharmacoeconomics 2014;32(8):745–58.
33. Chey WD, Mody RR, Wu EQ, et al. Treatment patterns and symptom control in patients with GERD: US community-based survey. Curr Med Res Opin 2009;25(8):1869–78.
34. Fass R, Sifrim D. Management of heartburn not responding to proton pump inhibitors. Gut 2009;58(2):295–309.
35. Preetha A, Sujatha D, Patil BA, et al. Oral manifestations in gastroesophageal reflux disease. Gen Dent 2015;63(3): e27–31.
36. Lankarani KB, Sivandzadeh GR, Hassanpour S. Oral manifestation in inflammatory bowel disease: a review. World J Gastroenterol 2013; 19(46):8571–9.
37. Vasovic M, Gajovic N, Brajkovic D, et al. The relationship between the immune system and oral manifestations of inflammatory bowel disease: a review. Cent Eur J Immunol 2016;41(3):302–10.
38. Jacobsen BA, Fallingborg J, Rasmussen HH, et al. Increase in incidence and prevalence of inflammatory bowel disease in northern Denmark: a population-based study, 1978-2002. Eur J Gastroenterol Hepatol 2006;18(6):601–6.
39. Loftus EV Jr. Update on the incidence and prevalence of inflammatory bowel disease in the United States. Gastroenterol Hepatol (N Y) 2016;12(11):704–7.
40. Baumgart DC, Sandborn WJ. Crohn's disease. Lancet 2012; 380(9853):1590–605.
41. Fatahzadeh M. Inflammatory bowel disease. Oral Surg Oral Med Oral Pathol Oral Radiol Endod 2009;108(5):e1–10.
42. Levine JS, Burakoff R. Extraintestinal manifestations of inflammatory bowel disease. Gastroenterol Hepatol (N Y) 2011;7(4): 235–41.
43. Lourenco SV, Hussein TP, Bologna SB, et al. Oral manifestations of inflammatory bowel disease: a review based on the observation of six cases. J Eur Acad Dermatol Venereol 2010;24(2):204–7.
44. Ghosh S, Shand A, Ferguson A. Ulcerative colitis. BMJ 2000; 320(7242):1119–23.
45. Langan RC, Gotsch PB, Krafczyk MA, et al. Ulcerative colitis: diagnosis and treatment. Am Fam Physician 2007;76(9):1323–30.
46. Ludwig D, Stange EF. Treatment of ulcerative colitis. Hepatogastroenterology 2000;47(31):83–9.
47. Aggarwal A, Sabol T, Vaziri H. Update on the use of biologic therapy in ulcerative colitis. Curr Treat Options Gastroenterol 2017;15(1): 155–67.
48. Elahi M, Telkabadi M, Samadi V, et al. Association of oral manifestations with ulcerative colitis. Gastroenterol Hepatol Bed Bench 2012;5(3):155–60.
49. Tan CX, Brand HS, de Boer NK, et al. Gastrointestinal diseases and their oro-dental manifestations: part 1: Crohn's disease. Br Dent J 2016;221(12):794–9.
50. Femiano F, Lanza A, Buonaiuto C, et al. Pyostomatitis vegetans: a review of the literature. Med Oral Patol Oral Cir Bucal 2009;14(3): E114–7.
51. Patil DT, Moss AC, Odze RD. Role of histologic inflammation in the natural history of ulcerative colitis. Gastrointest Endosc Clin N Am 2016;26(4):629–40.
52. Matias Fde A, Rosa DJ, Carvalho MT, et al. Piodermatite-pioestomatite vegetante: relato de caso e revisão de literatura. An Bras Dermatol 2011;86:137–40.
53. Ruiz-Roca JA, Berini-Aytés L, Gay-Escoda C. Pyostomatitis vegetans. Report of two cases and review of the literature. Oral Surg Oral Med Oral Pathol Oral Radiol Endod 2005;99(4):447–54.
54. Nico MMS, Hussein TP, Aoki V, et al. Pyostomatitis vegetans and its relation to inflammatory bowel disease, pyoderma gangrenosum, pyodermatitis vegetans, and pemphigus. J Oral Pathol Med 2012; 41:584–8.
55. Siegel MA, Jacobson JJ. Inflammatory bowel diseases and the oral cavity. Oral Surg Oral Med Oral Pathol Oral Radiol Endod 1999;87: 12–4.
56. Kreuter A, Wieland U. Oral hairy leukoplakia: a clinical indicator of immunosuppression. CMAJ 2011;183:932.
57. Noonan V, Woo SB, Kabani S. Pathology snapshot. Oral manifestations of Crohn's disease. J Mass Dent Soc 2015;64(1):41.
58. Podolsky DK. Inflammatory bowel disease. N Engl J Med 2002; 347(6):417–29.
59. Antunes H, Patraquim C, Baptista V, et al. Oral manifestations of Crohn's disease. BMJ case Rep 2015;2015 [pii: bcr2015212300].
60. Scheper HJ, Brand HS. Oral aspects of Crohn's disease. Int Dent J 2002;52(3):163–72.
61. Ghandour K, Issa M. Oral Crohn's disease with late intestinal manifestations. Oral Surg Oral Med Oral Pathol 1991;72(5): 565–7.

62. Harty S, Fleming P, Rowland M, et al. A prospective study of the oral manifestations of Crohn's disease. Clin Gastroenterol Hepatol 2005;3(9):886–91.
63. Lemberg DA, Day AS. Crohn disease and ulcerative colitis in children: an update for 2014. J Paediatr Child Health 2015;51(3): 266–70.
64. Litsas G. Crohn's disease of the mouth: report of a case. Eur J Paediatr Dent 2011;12(3):198–200.
65. Siegel MA, Hupp WS. Oral considerations in patients with gastrointestinal disorders. Chapter 7. In: Bayless TM, Diehl AM, editors. Advanced therapy in gastroenterology and liver disease. 5th edition. Burlington (ON): B.C. Decker, Inc; 2005. p. 43–8.
66. Han M, Fang H, Li QL, et al. Effectiveness of laser therapy in the management of recurrent aphthous stomatitis: a systematic review. Scientifica (Cairo) 2016;2016:9062430.
67. Stricker T, Braegger CP. Images in clinical medicine. Oral manifestations of Crohn's disease. N Engl J Med 2000;342(22): 1644.
68. Chavan M, Jain H, Diwan N, et al. Recurrent aphthous stomatitis: a review. J Oral Pathol Med 2012;41:577–83.
69. Lakatos L, Pandur T, David G, et al. Association of extraintestinal manifestations of inflammatory bowel disease in a province of western Hungary with disease phenotype: results of a 25-year follow-up study. World J Gastroenterol 2003;9:2300–7.
70. Trost LB, McDonnell JK. Important cutaneous manifestations of inflammatory bowel disease. Postgrad Med J 2005;81(959):580–5.
71. Siegel MA, Silverman SS, Sollecito TP, editors. Clinicians guide to the treatment of common oral lesions. 6th edition. Hamilton (ON): BC Decker; 2006. p. 57–61.
72. Michael G. Burket's oral medicine. 12th edition. 2015.
73. Patton L, Glick M, editors. Index in The ADA Practical Guide to Patients with Medical Conditions. 2nd edition. Hoboken (NJ): John Wiley & Sons, Inc; 2015.
74. Laranjeira N, Fonseca J, Meira T, et al. Oral mucosa lesions and oral symptoms in inflammatory bowel disease patients. Arq Gastroenterol 2015;52(2):105–10.
75. Zbar AP, Ben-Horin S, Beer-Gabel M, et al. Oral Crohn's disease: is it a separable disease from orofacial granulomatosis? A review. J Crohns Colitis 2012;6(2):135–42.
76. Kim WR, Brown RS, Terrault NA, et al. Burden of liver disease in the United States: summary of a workshop. Hepatology 2002;36(1): 227–42.
77. Glick M. Medical considerations for dental care of patients with alcohol-related liver disease. J Am Dent Assoc 1997;128(8): 61–70.
78. Byron RJ Jr, Osborne PD. Dental management of liver transplant patients. Gen dentistry 2005;53(1):66–9 [quiz: 70–2].
79. Wang FS, Fan JG, Zhang Z, et al. The global burden of liver disease: the major impact of China. Hepatology 2014;60(6): 2099–108.
80. Younossi ZM, Stepanova M, Afendy M, et al. Changes in the prevalence of the most common causes of chronic liver diseases in the United States from 1988 to 2008. Clin Gastroenterol Hepatol 2011; 9(6):524–30.e1.
81. Little JW, Falace DA, Miller CS, et al. Dental management of the medically compromised patient. 8th edition. St. Louis (MO): Mosby; 2013.
82. Helenius-Hietala J, Aberg F, Meurman JH, et al. Oral surgery in liver transplant candidates: a retrospective study on delayed bleeding and other complications. Oral Surg Oral Med Oral Pathol Oral Radiol 2016;121(5):490–5.
83. Carrozzo M, Scally K. Oral manifestations of hepatitis C virus infection. World J Gastroenterol 2014;20(24):7534–43.
84. Hong CH, Scobey MW, Napenas JJ, et al. Dental postoperative bleeding complications in patients with suspected and documented liver disease. Oral Dis 2012;18(7):661–6.
85. Guggenheimer J, Close JM, Eghtesad B, et al. Characteristics of oral abnormalities in liver transplant candidates. Int J Organ Transplant Med 2010;1(3):107–13.
86. Garcovich S, Garcovich M, Capizzi R, et al. Cutaneous manifestations of hepatitis C in the era of new antiviral agents. World J Hepatol 2015;7(27):2740–8.

Oral Manifestations of Immunodeficiencies and Transplantation Medicine

Elizabeth Waring, DMD*, Alessandro Villa, DDS, MPH, PhD

KEYWORDS

• Hematopoietic cell transplant • Solid organ transplant • Immunocompromised • Oral complications of transplant

KEY POINTS

- Patients who have received a stem cell or solid transplant are acutely and often chronically immunosuppressed.
- Signs and symptoms of immunosuppression can often present in the oral cavity.
- Oral manifestations of immunocompromised patients include mucositis, infections (viral, fungal, and bacteria), and increased risk of oral cancer.
- Early recognition and treatment of oral manifestations of immunodeficiencies secondary to stem cell or solid organ transplant improves quality of life of patients.

Introduction

Solid organ transplantation and hematopoietic cell transplantation (HCT) are becoming increasingly more popular treatments options for various diseases. Solid organs are transplanted from a donor to the body of a recipient to replace a missing or damaged organ. Solid organs that have been successfully transplanted include kidney, liver, heart, lung, pancreas, intestine, and thymus. HCT is the administration of hematopoietic progenitor cells used to reconstitute the bone marrow in hematologic disorders, including hemoglobinopathies, bone marrow failure syndromes, and several malignancies (eg, leukemias, lymphomas).

Oral complications after transplantation can be characterized as early (or acute) or late (or chronic). Early effects tend to develop during treatment and are mainly due to direct tissue toxicity. They usually last days to months and are self-limiting. Late effects occur months to years after treatment, are long-lasting and cause permanent tissue damage and significant morbidity. Several oral complications are secondary to immunosuppression and their presentation is similar to that seen in immunocompromised human immunodeficiency virus (HIV) patients.

Orofacial care providers (eg, dentists, oral medicine specialists, and oral surgeons) can play an important role in the cancer or transplant care team by recognizing and diagnosing oral complications. It is important to be able to recognize and treat these complications because some can contribute to increased morbidity and mortality.

Disclosure Statement: The authors have nothing to disclose.

Division of Oral Medicine and Dentistry, Brigham and Women's Hospital, 75 Francis Street, Boston, MA 02215, USA

* Corresponding author.

E-mail address: ewaring@partners.org

Atlas Oral Maxillofacial Surg Clin N Am 25 (2017) 105–111

http://dx.doi.org/10.1016/j.cxom.2017.04.003

Early effects

Mucositis

Mucositis is a common early complication of HCT, affecting 60% to 85% of patients. This is due to the conditioning regimen of high-dose chemotherapy administered before HCT. Mucositis occurs approximately 1 week after conditioning and clinically appears intraorally as diffuse painful ulcerations mainly affecting the nonkeratinized mucosa (buccal mucosa, soft palate, and lateral and ventral tongue) (Fig. 1). Mucositis can also affect the gastrointestinal tract (GI) causing many GI-related symptoms, including intestinal cramping and diarrhea. Patients at increased risk of mucositis are those who received total body irradiation as part of their conditioning regimen, have an unrelated donor, or are receiving methotrexate as graft versus host disease (GVHD) prophylaxis.

Because these patients are immunocompromised, mucositis can put the patient at risk for infection and bacteremia. Patients may require total parenteral nutrition due to oral pain and poor oral intake. Mucositis is also associated with increased length of hospital stay and cost of care.

Management strategies are mostly palliative and include systemic opioids and topical agents such as topical anesthetic, Caphosol (EUSA Pharma, Hemel Hempstead, United Kingdom), GelClair (Midatech Pharma US Inc, Raleigh, NC, USA), and MuGard (AMAG Pharmaceuticals, Waltham, MA, USA). Palifermin is a keratinocyte growth factor approved by the US Food and Drug Administration (FDA) for prevention of mucositis. Cryotherapy can also be useful in preventing mucositis secondary to fluorouracil (5-FU). Oral mucositis peaks between days +7 to +14 after HCT and resolves in the next week when normal hematopoiesis resumes.[1,2]

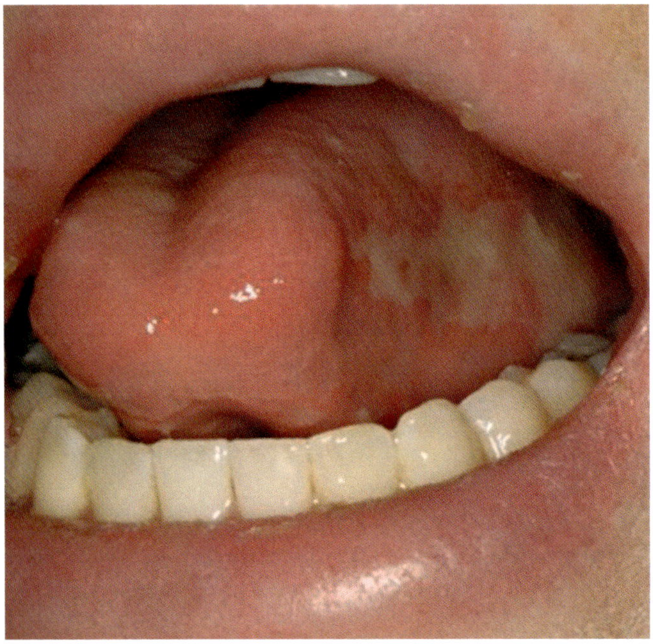

Fig. 1 Mucositis affecting the left tongue in a patient shortly after HCT before engraftment.

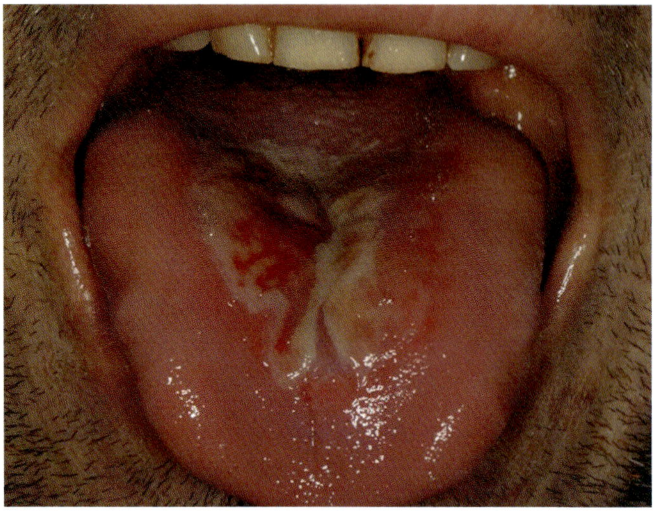

Fig. 2 HSV-related ulceration of the dorsal tongue in an immunocompromised patient.

Infection

Infections can be both an early and late complication of solid organ or HCT. Early infections typically occur within first 30 days of transplant and include fungal, viral, and bacterial infections. After this period, patients are at higher risk for opportunistic infections. Late infections include encapsulated organisms. The following section discusses the most common oral infections encountered in this patient population.

Viral

Human herpes virus

There are 8 viruses in the herpes family, which are pathogenic to humans, 6 of which can present clinically in the head and neck region.

Herpes simplex virus (HSV), including HSV-1 and 2, and human herpes virus (HHV), including HHV-1 and HHV-2, can present as a primary infection or as recrudescent of a latent infection. Primary herpetic gingivostomatitis presents acutely with painful coalescing ulcers, which can affect any oral mucosal surface and is often associated with systemic signs (eg, malaise, lymphadenopathy, and fever). Primary infections usually occur in children and young adults. Antiviral therapy can reduce viral shedding and shorten the duration of ulceration.

Recrudescent HSV usually presents as clustered coalescing ulcers on keratinized surfaces, such as the lips, in recurrent herpes labialis or gingival tissue, palatal mucosa, or dorsal tongue (Fig. 2). In immunocompromised patients (eg, individuals who undergo HCT), nonkeratinized tissue can also be involved and may present as single or multiple, larger (>0.5 cm) ulcers. Antiviral prophylaxis is common in immunocompromised patients but recrudescence of HSV can still occur. Due to this atypical presentation, the diagnosis can be challenging and lead to delay in treatment, putting the patient at risk for disseminated disease. Viral cultures of active lesions can be helpful in diagnosis but does not distinguish between viral shedding and recrudescence. Exfoliative cytology can also be performed, which can give a diagnosis within hours. Biopsy of the lesion can be useful in those cases that do not respond to therapy or in patients in whom the clinical diagnosis remains unclear. Treatment includes pain management, supportive care, and antiviral therapy.

Varicella-zoster virus (VZV; HHV-3) causes primary varicella and, as a recurrent infection, causes herpes zoster (shingles) in 10% to 20% of cases. Primary infections usually occur in childhood but have become uncommon due to the VZV vaccine, which was approved by the FDA in 1995. Primary infections are accompanied by flu-like symptoms and pruritic papular rash followed by vesicle formation.

Herpes zoster can cause small ulcers that are similar in appearance to oral HSV but are almost always unilateral and along 1 nerve dermatome. Herpes zoster affecting the skin presents as grouped vesicles or crusted lesions on an erythematous base. Viral culture can differentiate between an HSV or VZV infection. Herpes zoster infections require systemic antiviral therapy at greater doses than treatment of HSV infections.

Epstein-Barr virus (HHV-4) has been linked with many conditions, such as infectious mononucleosis; some cancers, including nasopharyngeal carcinoma; lymphoproliferative disorders; and oral hairy leukoplakia (OHL) (Fig. 3). OHL is a benign condition that presents as a white corrugated papule or plaque

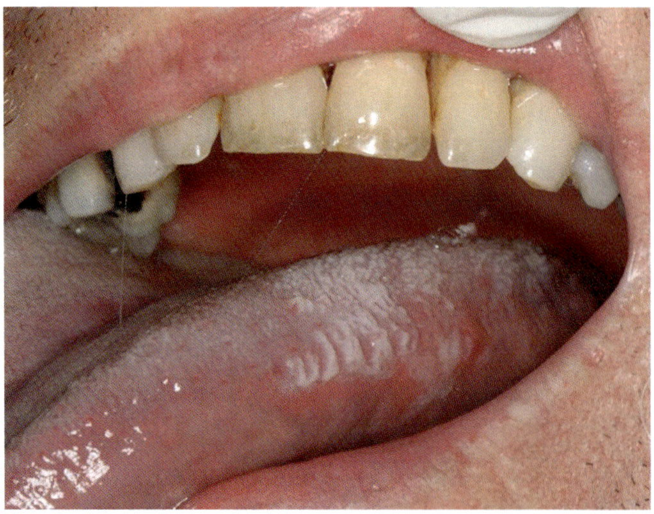

Fig. 3 White corrugated plaques of the left lateral tongue in an HIV patient with OHL.

on the lateral border of the tongue that does not wipe away. OHL occurs almost exclusively in immunocompromised patients, especially in the HIV with acquired immune deficiency syndrome (AIDS) population. Definitive diagnosis can be made by biopsy. OHL does not require treatment but usually responds well to antiviral therapy and antiretroviral therapy in HIV patients.

Cytomegalovirus (CMV; HHV-5) infects approximately half of adults by the age of 40 years but is generally not pathogenic in healthy individuals and remains latent in salivary glands, endothelial cells, and leukocytes. It is reactivated in the setting of profound immunosuppression. Intraorally, CMV presents as a nonspecific, painful solitary penetrating ulcer (usually >1 cm) (Fig. 4). Diagnosis usually requires biopsy because the virus is deep in the connective tissue and cultures may not come in contact with the virus. First-line therapy for CMV infection is ganciclovir or valganciclovir.

HHV-8 is the virus known to cause Kaposi sarcoma seen almost exclusively in patients with AIDS. Intraorally, Kaposi sarcoma presents as a red or purple vascular lesion most commonly on the gingiva and hard palate (Fig. 5). Biopsy and histopathological examination is required for the diagnosis. HHV-8 has also been associated with lymphoproliferative disorders, namely primary effusion lymphoma and Castleman disease.[3,4]

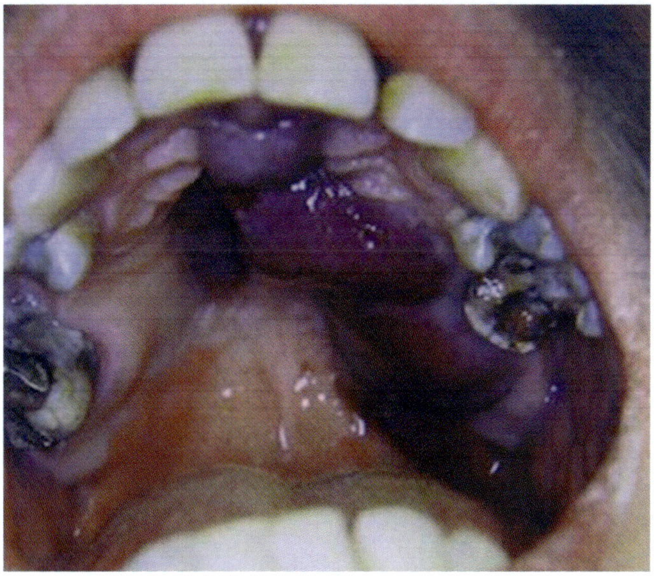

Fig. 5 Kaposi sarcoma affecting the left hard palate. (*Courtesy of* Sook-Bin Woo, DMD, MMSc, Harvard School of Dental Medicine, Boston, MA.)

Fungal

Candidiasis

Candida albicans is a commensal organism found in the oral flora of approximately 20% to 30% of individuals and does not cause disease but in immunocompromised patients can cause oropharyngeal candidiasis. Candidiasis can also occur in the immunocompetent host when the oral flora is altered (ie, hyposalivation, denture wearers, recent antibiotic therapy). Clinically, oral candidiasis has 4 different presentations: pseudomembranous, erythematous, hyperplastic candidiasis, and angular cheilitis. Symptoms may or may not be present but include generalized burning and discomfort. The most common form is pseudomembranous candidiasis, which appears as curdy white papules or plaques that can be wiped away leaving an erythematous and bleeding base (Fig. 6). Erythematous candidiasis appears as a red, atrophic lesion commonly encountered on the palate under dentures or dorsal tongue with atrophy of the filiform papillae. In rare cases, candidiasis can present as a hyperplastic white plaque that cannot be wiped away and is suggestive of leukoplakia. These lesions require biopsy for further investigation and diagnosis. Angular cheilitis presents at the oral commissures causing erythema and fissures (Fig. 7).

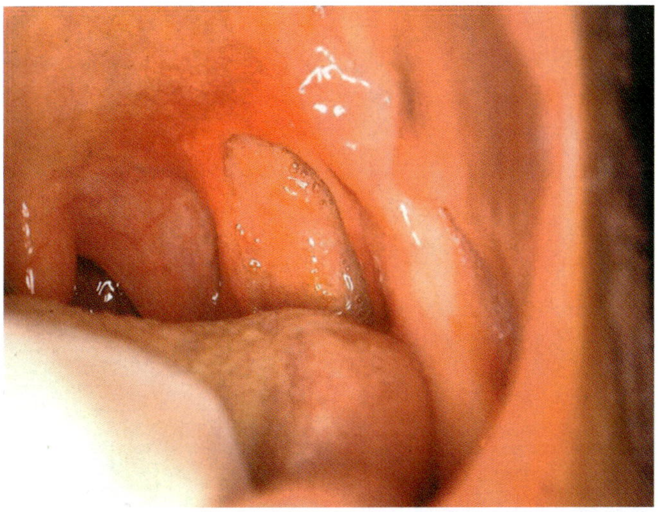

Fig. 4 CMV-related ulceration of the left tonsillar pillar. (*Courtesy of* Sook-Bin Woo, DMD, MMSc, Harvard School of Dental Medicine, Boston, MA.)

The diagnosis of oral candidiasis is often made by clinical presentation alone and treated empirically. Cytologic smear or fungal culture can also be used in cases in which the diagnosis is not clear or in cases in which empiric treatment fails. The mainstay of therapy includes topical or systemic antifungal agents.

Deep fungal infections

Deep fungal infections of the oral cavity may present in immunocompromised patients as deep, invasive, nonhealing ulcers often accompanied by dissemination. Causative organisms included opportunistic molds (*Aspergillus* and *Mucorales*) or endemic fungi (*Histoplasma capsulatum*). Mucormycosis occurs in patients with diabetes mellitus, malignancy, neutropenic patients, and post-transplant patients. Mucormycosis appears

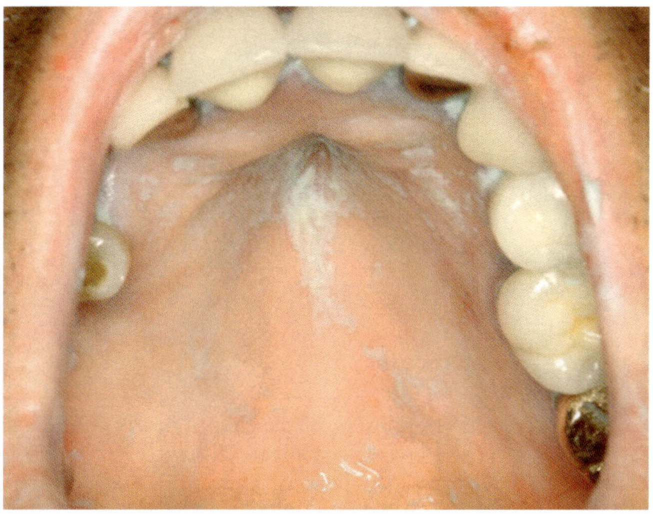

Fig. 6 Pseudomembranous candidiasis affecting the hard palate.

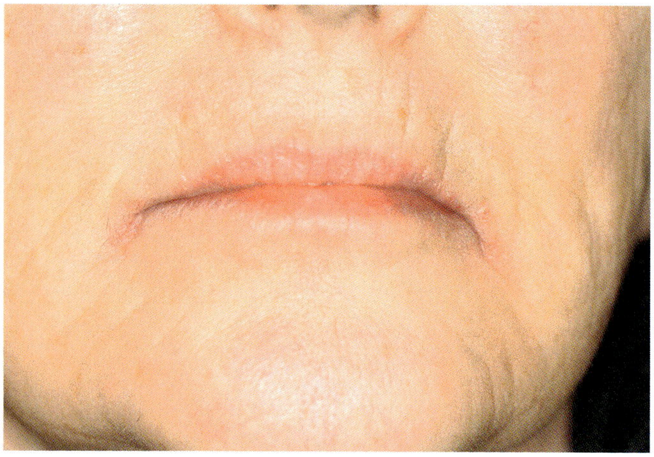

Fig. 7 Fissuring and erythema of the corners of the mouth in a patient with angular cheilitis.

intraorally as a black necrotic and/or fungating lesion. Mortality in HCT patients with mucormycosis is 65% to 90%. Aspergillosis (caused by *A fumigatus* or *A flavus*) occurs more often in patients with hematologic malignancies. Noninvasive aspergillosis in the immunocompetent host presents as fungal sinusitis (allergic or with established fungus ball, mycetoma). Invasive oral aspergillosis presents similarly to mucormycosis and has a fatality rate of 58%. A detailed social history is important in identifying possible exposures, such as occupation, hobbies, and current or previous residence or travel. Biopsy of the lesion is necessary for diagnosis. Treatment requires surgical debridement and systemic antifungal therapy.[3–7]

Bacterial

Bacterial infections in the oral cavity present most commonly as odontogenic infections. Odontogenic infections can have a periodontal or endodontic source. Due to immune suppression, many of the classic signs of infection, such as erythema, edema, pain, or purulence, may not be present making the diagnosis more difficult (Fig. 8). Imaging can be helpful when evaluating for an odontogenic infection. If an odontogenic infection is identified, systemic antibiotic therapy is indicated. If treatment requires a dental procedure, especially those in which bleeding is expected (ie, scaling, incision and drainage, or extraction), the patient's absolute neutrophil count (ANC) and platelet count should be checked before initiation of treatment, and the patient's main provider should be consulted.[3]

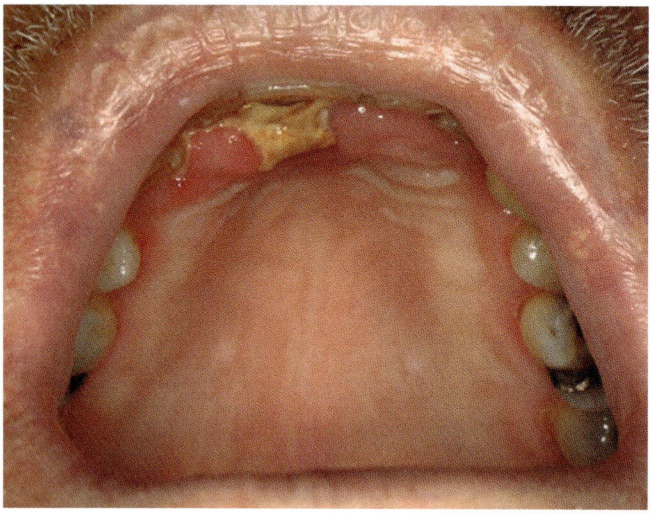

Fig. 8 HSV negative ulceration of the palatal gingiva of tooth #8 surrounded by diffuse erythema and edema due to acute exacerbation of periodontitis in a patient after HCT. The ulceration resolved after periodontal scaling. (*Photo courtesy of* Vidya Sankar, DDS from Harvard School of Dental Medicine, Boston, MA.)

Late effects

Malignancy

There is an increased risk of malignancy for both solid organ transplant and hematopoietic stem cell transplant (Fig. 9). This has been linked to prolonged immune suppression and oncogenic viral infections; and, for HCT patients, cancer therapy (ie, chemotherapy and radiation) and chronic GVHD (cGVHD). For HCT patients, the oral cavity has been reported as among the sites at most risk for cancer. An analysis of 28,874 patients who received allogeneic HCT showed an observed or expected ratio of 11.6 for oral squamous cell carcinoma and, for patients with oral cGVHD, a yearly examination by a specialist has been suggested. An analysis of 175,732 solid organ transplant recipients showed an observed or expected ratio of 2.6 for oral cavity and 16.9 for the lip. These patients should have a thorough oral cancer examination and any suspicious lesions should be biopsied to rule out dysplasia or malignancy.[8–12]

Graft versus host disease (lichenoid, xerostomia)

GVHD is a common complication following allogeneic HCT. It is the result of donor T cells not recognizing the recipient as self. This causes an inflammatory cascade and results in recipient tissue damage. The major risk factor for GVHD is human leukocyte antigen mismatch. GVHD can affect many organs, including skin, GI tract, liver, lungs, muscles, and oral cavity. GVHD can be categorized as either acute or chronic. Previously, this distinction was made based on the time after transplant; either before 100 days or after 100 days. Now, clinical features are used to discriminate between acute versus cGVHD.

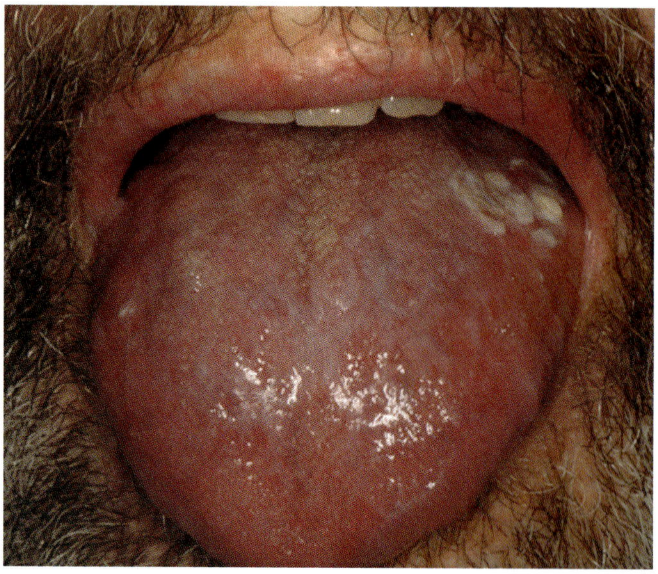

Fig. 9 Squamous cell carcinoma of the left dorsal tongue in a patient with cGVHD.

Oral acute GVHD is rare but presents as nonspecific, diffuse ulceration of the oral mucosa that affects the nonkeratinized and keratinized surfaces and often involves the lips (Fig. 10). Acute oral GVHD can present as the sole site of involvement but more often it occurs with other affected sites (ie, skin, liver, GI). HSV and mucositis should be ruled out before this diagnosis is made. Treatment of oral acute GVHD is similar to oral cGVHD, including topical and systemic immune suppression (see later discussion).

Oral cGVHD affects more than 70% of HCT patients and can affect the oral mucosa and salivary glands. Clinically, cGVHD presents as white reticulation commonly affecting the buccal mucosa and tongue, which is similar in appearance to oral lichen planus (Fig. 11). In more active cases, erythema and ulceration can also be present. Superficial mucoceles, mainly on the palate, can also be a sign of oral cGVHD. If symptoms are present, they typically include sensitivity to acidic, spicy, or crunchy foods, and also the mint often present in toothpaste and mouthwashes.

The salivary glands can also be affected by cGVHD, causing hyposalivation and xerostomia. Hyposalivation secondary to cGVHD puts the patient at higher risk for oral candidiasis and caries (Fig. 12).

Prophylaxis and treatment of GVHD is managed by use of topical and systemic immunosuppressants. The most common systemic medications include prednisone, tacrolimus, sirolimus, cyclosporine, and methotrexate. Topical therapy can be helpful for management of oral cGVHD. These medications include dexamethasone 5 mg/5 mL or compounded clobetasol 0.05% solution, fluocinonide 0.05% gel, clobetasol 0.05% gel, tacrolimus 0.03% or 0.1% ointment, and tacrolimus 0.5 mg/mL solution.[13,14]

Postinflammatory hypermelanosis

Oral postinflammatory hypermelanosis (PIH) is an increase in melanin deposition within the basal cells as part of an inflammatory reaction. HCT patients may present with oral PIH due to postchemotherapy mucositis and postradiation mucositis as part of the conditioning regimen or inflammation from cGVHD, similarly to oral lichen planus. PIH is more common in darker skin types. Clinically, PIH presents as diffuse pigmentation of the oral mucosa in the area of inflammation (Fig. 13). Treatment includes treating the source of inflammation and may take weeks to months to fade.[15]

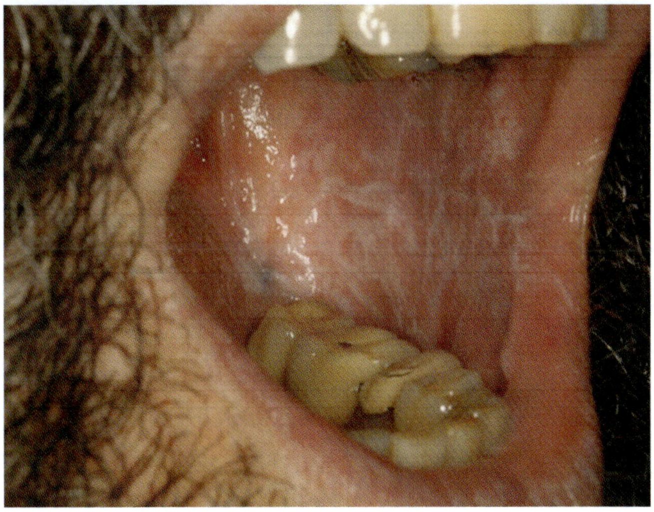

Fig. 11 cGVHD affecting the left buccal mucosa.

Neutropenic ulcer

In the setting of neutropenia ANC (less than 1500 neutrophils per microliter), patients may experience oral neutropenic ulcers. Oral neutropenic ulcers can appear on keratinized and nonkeratinized surfaces, and are generally painful (Fig. 14). Other causes of ulceration must be ruled out before this diagnosis can be made (ie, viral infection, deep fungal infection, and mucositis). Oral neutropenic ulcers may present in the early or late stages of transplantation or in other conditions that cause neutropenia, such as HIV/AIDS. Treatment includes identifying the cause of neutropenia and treatment of neutropenia when possible. This may include granulocyte colony-stimulating factor or alteration of antiretroviral therapy in HIV/AIDS patients. Topical or intralesional steroids can be helpful in treating the oral ulcerations.[16–18]

Drug-related effects

Drug-induced gingival hyperplasia

Patients who have received either a solid organ transplant or HCT are treated with immunosuppressive medications to

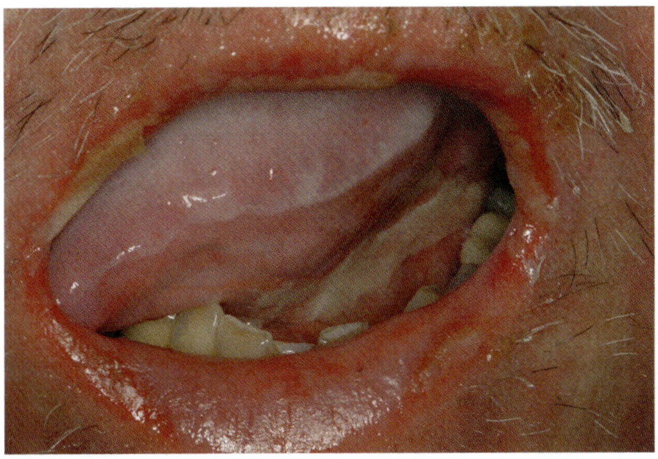

Fig. 10 Acute GVHD in a patient after HCT involving the lips, left ventral tongue, and left floor of mouth.

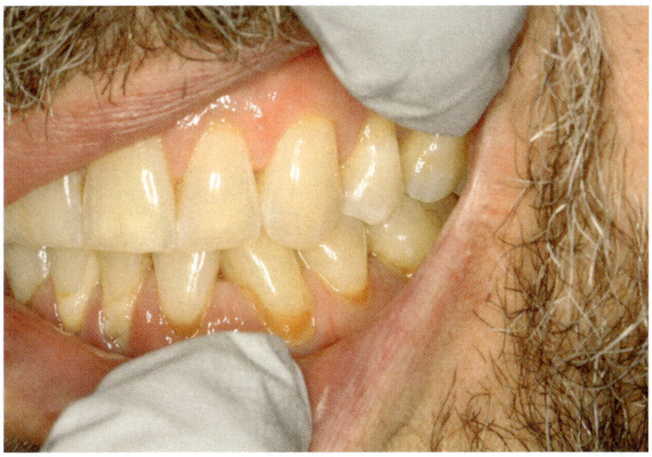

Fig. 12 Cervical caries in a patient with dry mouth due to GVHD affecting the salivary glands.

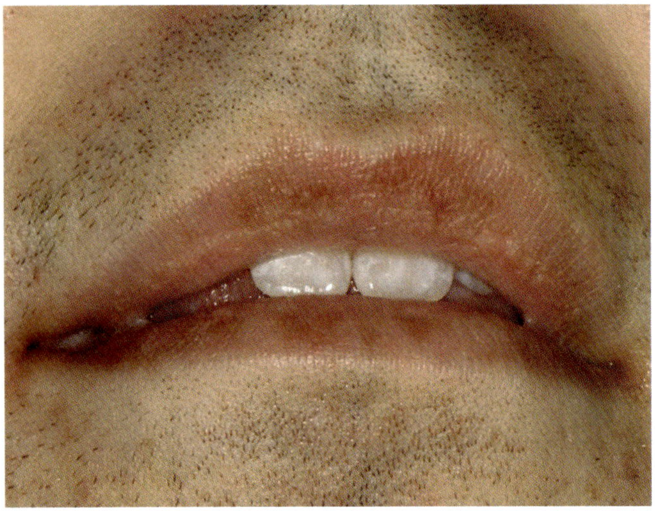

Fig. 13 Postinflammatory hyperpigmentation of the lips in a patient with cGVHD.

prevent and treat graft rejection or, for HCT patients, prevent and treat GVHD. Some of these medications can have unintended adverse effects that affect the oral cavity. One known adverse effect of cyclosporine is drug-induced gingival overgrowth (DIGO) with a prevalence of 20% to 76% for transplant patients. Cyclosporin inhibits normal collagen turnover causing a buildup of collagen in the gingival tissue. DIGO is clinically different from conventional gingivitis because it tends to be less erythematous and more fibrotic and nodular (Fig. 15). Dental plaque may play a role in overgrowth, so adequate hygiene is important for these patients and may reduce overgrowth. Excision of the hyperplastic gingiva can be performed. Ultimately, cyclosporine may have to be reduced or discontinued to resolve DIGO.[19]

Mammalian target of rapamycin inhibitor–associated stomatitis

Mammalian target of rapamycin (mTOR) inhibitors, such as sirolimus or everolimus, are commonly used in both solid organ and hematopoietic transplants for immunosuppression or prophylaxis for GVHD. One adverse effect that has been associated with mTOR inhibitors is mTOR inhibitor–associated stomatitis (mIAS). Clinically, mIAS presents as aphthous-like ulcers that are discrete, ovoid, superficial ulcers with gray-white pseudomembrane and surrounding erythematous halo mostly affecting nonkeratinized surfaces (Fig. 16). The median time to onset of mIAS is 10 days after beginning an mTOR inhibitor. These ulcers are painful and may require dose reduction or discontinuation of the mTOR inhibitor when they do not respond to treatment. Management of mIAS is usually with topical or intralesional steroid therapy. Refractory cases may require systemic steroid treatment.[20,21]

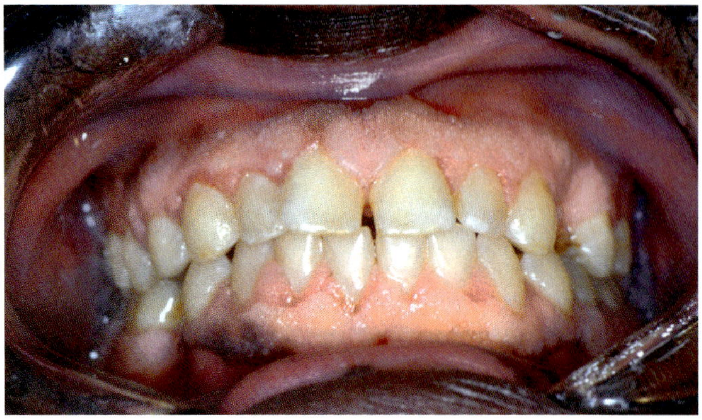

Fig. 15 Drug-induced gingival hyperplasia due to cyclosporine.

Other effects

A patient undergoing transplant may also experience orofacial pain secondary to teeth clenching and grinding. Specifically, they may develop myofascial pain, with or without secondary temporomandibular joint capsulitis. Other noninfectious causes of oral pain include dental hypersensitivity after conditioning regimen chemotherapy or preexisting gingival recession. Oral dysesthesia may be present in patients undergoing treatment with vascular endothelial growth factor receptor (VEGFR)-directed multitargeted tyrosine kinase inhibitors, which is characterized by numbness or tingling of the oral cavity, mainly the tongue.[22]

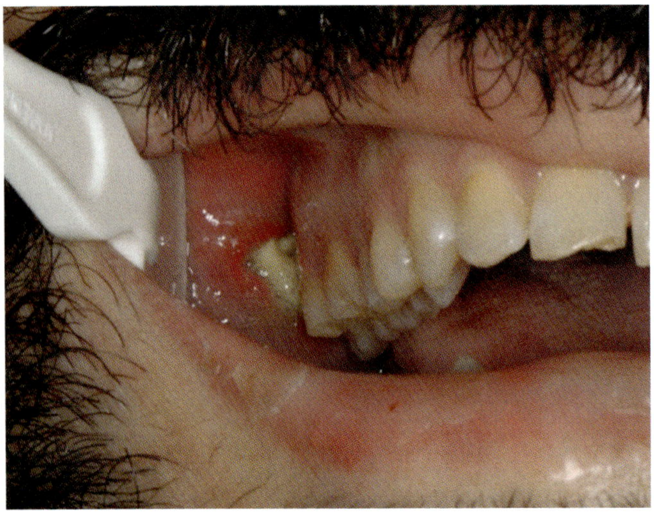

Fig. 14 Neutropenic ulcer of the right buccal mucosa.

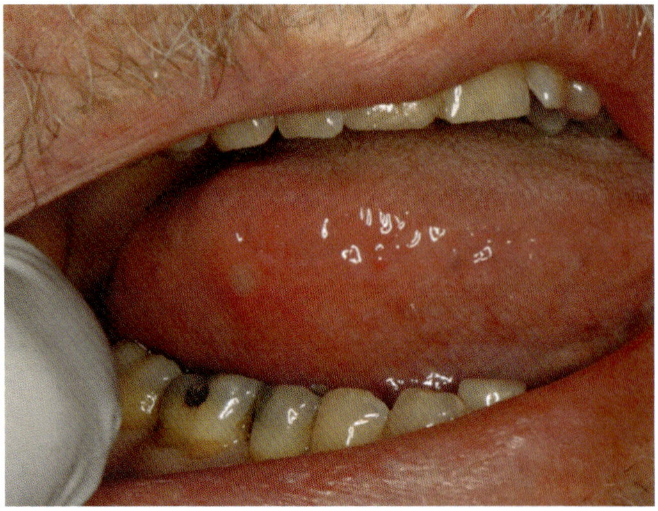

Fig. 16 Aphthous-like ulcer in a patient on sirolimus affecting the right lateral tongue.

References

1. Sonis ST. Pathobiology of oral mucositis: novel insights and opportunities. J Support Oncol 2007;5(9 Suppl 4):3–11.
2. Villa A, Sonis ST. Mucositis: pathobiology and management. Curr Opin Oncol 2015;27(3):159–64.
3. Lerman MA, Laudenbach J, Marty FM, et al. Management of oral infections in cancer patients. Dent Clin North Am 2008;52(1):129–53. ix.
4. Palmason S, Marty FM, Treister NS. How do we manage oral infections in allogeneic stem cell transplantation and other severely immunocompromised patients? Oral Maxillofac Surg Clin North Am 2011;23(4):579–99. vii.
5. Cho H, Lee KH, Colquhoun AN, et al. Invasive oral aspergillosis in a patient with acute myeloid leukaemia. Aust Dent J 2010;55(2):214–8.
6. Marques SA. Fungal infections of the mucous membrane. Dermatol Ther 2010;23(3):243–50.
7. Tejani S, Sultan A, Stojanov I, et al. Candidal carriage predicts candidiasis during topical immunosuppressive therapy: a preliminary retrospective cohort study. Oral Surg Oral Med Oral Pathol Oral Radiol 2016;122(4):448–54.
8. Curtis RE, Metayer C, Rizzo JD, et al. Impact of chronic GVHD therapy on the development of squamous-cell cancers after hematopoietic stem-cell transplantation: an international case-control study. Blood 2005;105(10):3802–11.
9. Engels EA, Pfeiffer RM, Fraumeni JF Jr, et al. Spectrum of cancer risk among US solid organ transplant recipients. JAMA 2011;306(17):1891–901.
10. Socie G, Rizzo JD. Second solid tumors: screening and management guidelines in long-term survivors after allogeneic stem cell transplantation. Semin Hematol 2012;49(1):4–9.
11. Mawardi H, Elad S, Correa ME, et al. Oral epithelial dysplasia and squamous cell carcinoma following allogeneic hematopoietic stem cell transplantation: clinical presentation and treatment outcomes. Bone Marrow Transplant 2011;46(6):884–91.
12. Rizzo JD, Curtis RE, Socie G, et al. Solid cancers after allogeneic hematopoietic cell transplantation. Blood 2009;113(5):1175–83.
13. Ion D, Stevenson K, Woo SB, et al. Characterization of oral involvement in acute graft-versus-host disease. Biol Blood Marrow Transplant 2014;20(11):1717–21.
14. Kuten-Shorrer M, Woo SB, Treister NS. Oral graft-versus-host disease. Dent Clin North Am 2014;58(2):351–68.
15. Woo SB. Oral pathology: a comprehensive atlas and text. Philadelphia: Saunders Elsevier; 2012.
16. Hasturk H, Tezcan I, Yel L, et al. A case of chronic severe neutropenia: oral findings and consequences of short-term granulocyte colony-stimulating factor treatment. Aust Dent J 1998;43(1):9–13.
17. Raber-Durlacher JE, Elad S, Barasch A. Oral mucositis. Oral Oncol 2010;46(6):452–6.
18. Reznik DA. Oral manifestations of HIV disease. Top HIV Med 2005;13(5):143–8.
19. Petti S, Polimeni A, Berloco PB, et al. Orofacial diseases in solid organ and hematopoietic stem cell transplant recipients. Oral Dis 2013;19(1):18–36.
20. Martins F, de Oliveira MA, Wang Q, et al. A review of oral toxicity associated with mTOR inhibitor therapy in cancer patients. Oral Oncol 2013;49(4):293–8.
21. Sonis S, Treister N, Chawla S, et al. Preliminary characterization of oral lesions associated with inhibitors of mammalian target of rapamycin in cancer patients. Cancer 2010;116(1):210–5.
22. Yuan A, Kurtz SL, Barysauskas CM, et al. Oral adverse events in cancer patients treated with VEGFR-directed multitargeted tyrosine kinase inhibitors. Oral Oncol 2015;51(11):1026–33.

Oral Manifestations of Autoimmune and Connective Tissue Disorders

Vidya Sankar, DMD, MHS [a,*], Marcel Noujeim, DDS, MS [b]

KEYWORDS

- Oral manifestations • Sjögren's syndrome • Rheumatoid arthritis • Pemphigus vulgaris
- Benign mucous membrane pemphigoid • Behçet disease • Sarcoidosis • Oral lichen planus

KEY POINTS

- Immune system malfunction is the underlying cause of symptoms in autoimmune, autoinflammatory and connective tissue disorders.
- Orofacial manifestations occur in these conditions either as a component of the disorder itself or as a consequence of the drugs used to treat the condition.
- The informed practitioner should be aware of the most common autoimmune, autoinflammatory and connective tissue disorders that present with oral manifestations.

Introduction

Blisters and vesicles are mucosal or skin reactions that involve dissection of intramucosal or epithelial cells. Within the group of blistering diseases, autoantibodies to integrins and adhesion molecules that maintain mucosal integrity may vary; however, clinically, it results in similar appearing lesions a differential diagnosis. Skin involvement may be found in several when compiling of these conditions with varying severity resulting in symptoms with a high morbidity, and rarely, mortality of the patient with the disease. The most common autoimmune/immune-mediated bullous diseases are presented. Our review is limited to those conditions presenting with oral manifestations: pemphigus vulgaris (PV), cicatricial pemphigoid or benign mucous membrane pemphigoid, lichen planus, and Behçet disease (BD). In the second half of this article, we review the most common connective tissue disorders that may present with oral manifestations that the well-informed oral health care provider may encounter in their patient population.

Autoimmune and autoinflammatory-related blistering and ulcerative diseases

Pemphigus vulgaris

Incidence, predilection, and genetics

Pemphigus disease (Table 1) is a rare and potentially life-threatening autoimmune blistering disease with an incidence of 0.1 to 0.5 in 100,000.[1] The most frequently occurring variant, PV represents about 70% to 80% of the cases and whose incidence varies from 0.76 to 16 cases per million per year depending on geographic location being studied. The disease is most commonly found in the Jewish population, particularly those of Ashkenazi origin, and Eastern countries such as Malaysia, China, and Japan, with a slight female predilection. Genetic association between HLA class II genes and observations of increased prevalence in certain ethnic groups illustrate a genetic predisposition. This, combined with exogenous factors (medications, viral infection, diet, etc.) and/or endogenous factors (stress) initiate autoimmune mechanisms leading to tissue damage.[2]

Clinical features

Clinically, PV almost always begins with multiple mucosal site involvement; frequently, those areas that are subjected to frictional trauma such as the gingiva, palate, buccal mucosa, and tongue (Fig. 1). Oral involvement can precede skin involvement by up to 1 year. Lesions begin as flaccid vesicles or bullae that rupture quickly, leaving behind painful shallow ulcerations that heal without scarring.

Diagnosis and histopathology

Histologic examination of perilesional or even normal-appearing mucosa shows a suprabasalar cleft leaving 1 to 2 layers of basal and suprabasal keratinocytes attached to the connective tissue papillae yielding a tombstonelike pattern (Fig. 2A). Round acantholytic (Tzanck) cells are often noted within the cleft. Antibodies against keratinocyte adhesion molecules (desmoglein [Dsg] 1 and 3, E-cadherin, desmoplakin, and alpha-9-acetylcholine) and desmosomes induce intraepithelial acantholysis resulting in blistering. Dsg 1 (primarily found in skin) and Dsg 3 (chiefly detected in mucosal epithelium) are the most important target antigens. Direct immunofluorescence (DIF) studies reveal binding of IgG, in the intracellular spaces between epithelial cells revealing a characteristic netlike pattern (see Fig. 2B). Recently, serum and salivary IgG

No disclosures.

[a] Division of Oral Medicine and Dentistry, Department of Surgery, Brigham and Women's Hospital, 1620 Tremont Street, Suite 3-028, Boston, MA 02120, USA
[b] Department of Comprehensive Dentistry, UT Health San Antonio, 7703 Floyd Curl Drive, San Antonio, TX 78229, USA
* Corresponding author.
E-mail address: vsankar@bwh.harvard.edu

Atlas Oral Maxillofacial Surg Clin N Am 25 (2017) 113–126

http://dx.doi.org/10.1016/j.cxom.2017.04.004

Table 1 Autoantibodies in autoimmune blistering diseases

	Autoantigens	DIF immunoreactants
Pemphigus groups		
Pemphigus vulgaris	Desmoglein 3 and 1	IgG, IgM, C3
Pemphigus foliaceus	Desmoglein 1	
Paraneoplastic pemphigus	Desmoglein 1, and 3, periplakin, desmoplakin	IgG, IgM, C3
Pemphigoid groups		
BulloSpemphigoid	BP-AG 1, plectin, $\alpha6\beta4$ integrin	
Pemphigoid gestationis	BP-AG 2	
Mucous membrane pemphigoid	Collagen XVII/BP180, BP230, laminin 332, $\alpha6\beta4$ integrin	IgG, C3, IgA, IgM

and IgA antibodies to Dsg 3 have been suggested as a diagnostic alternative to biopsy.[3]

Treatment considerations

Corticosteroids remain the most common treatment modality for this condition. When there are only oral lesions present, corticosteroids are applied topically in rinse or gel formulations. PV is a potentially life-threatening disease and, therefore, requires an early and more intensive therapeutic regimen than other autoimmune blistering diseases; if skin lesions are present, treatment consists of systemic steroids (pulse or continuous) and may be combined with adjuvant immunomodulatory or immunosuppressive medications, including azathioprine as first-line therapy. Other immunosuppressants may be considered if patients are unresponsive or experience significant side effects to first-line therapy (Table 2). More recently, anti–B-cell monoclonal antibodies have been used for the treatment of refractory cases with some success. Of these biologic agents, most is known about rituximab; however, other agents such as veltuzumab and ofatumumab either have been or are currently undergoing clinical trials. These agents seem to be well-tolerated with rare serious adverse events; however, patients are at increased risk

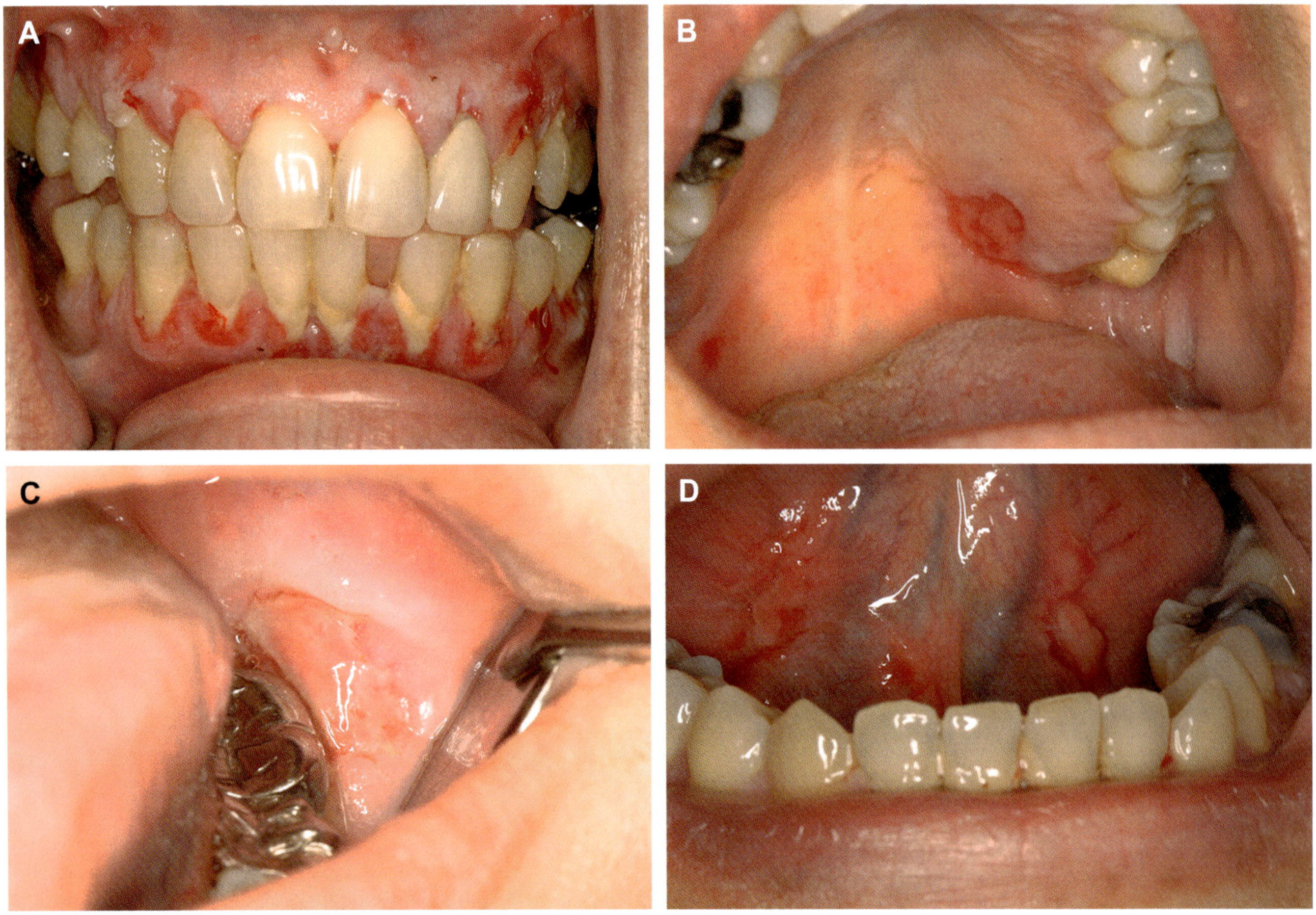

Fig. 1 Pemphigus vulgaris can affect the keratinized and nonkeratinized tissues of the oral cavity including the gingiva forming erosions often resembling desquamative gingivitis (*A*) hard palatal mucosa (*B*), buccal mucosa/vestibule, (*C*) and ventral tongue (*D*). When affecting the gingiva, patients may find it painful to brush their teeth effectively, causing plaque accumulation that exacerbates gingival inflammation and pain (*A*). (*Courtesy of* Michaell Huber, DDS, UT Health San Antonio, San Antonio, TX.)

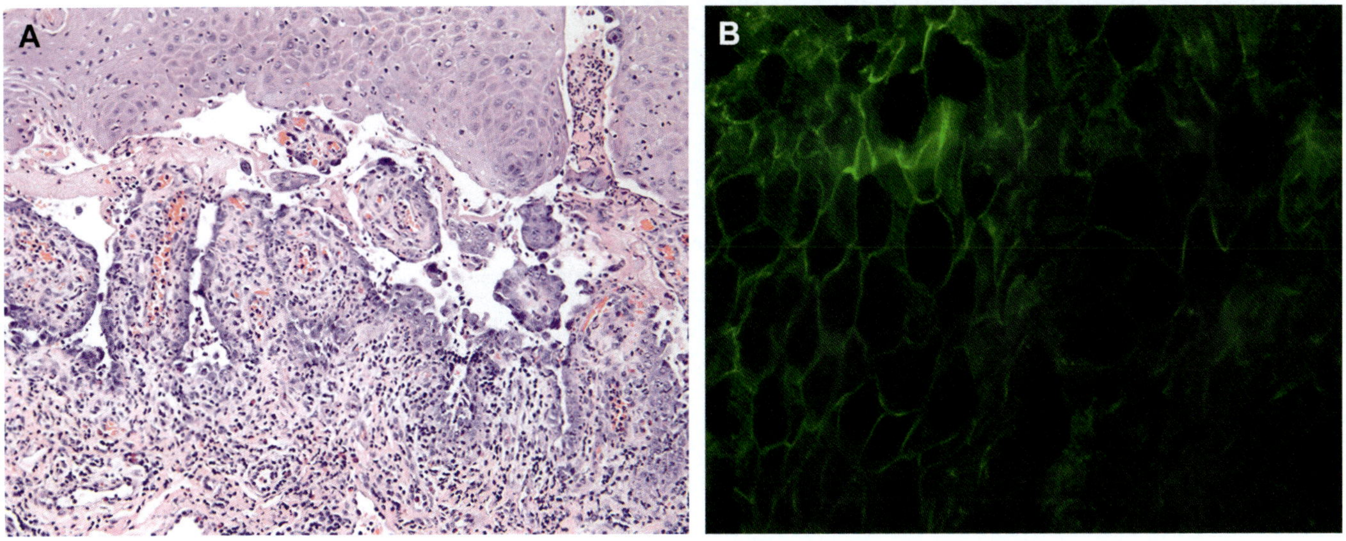

Fig. 2 Suprabasalar clefting of surface epithelium with a tombstone-like pattern of basal and parabasal cells (*A*). Direct immunofluorescence reveals tissue binding of IgG, in the intercellular spaces with a characteristic netlike pattern (*B*) (hematoxylin-eosin, original magnification ×200). (*Courtesy of* Sook-Bin Woo, DMD, MMSc, Harvard School of Dental Medicine, Boston, MA.)

Table 2 Medical management for autoimmune and autoinflammatory diseases

	Topical steroids	Intralesional steroids	Other topical agents	Systemic medications	Other
Pemphigus vulgaris		0.1 mL/cm^2 triamcinolone 10 mg/mL		Corticosteroids Azathioprine[a] MMF Methotrexate Cyclophosphamide Retuximab	Self-management: good oral hygiene
Mucous membrane pemphigoid			Tacrolimus	Dapsone[b] 50 mg/d up to 100–200—mg/d Tetracyclines Cyclosporine Pentoxifylline IVIG TNF-alpha inhibitors Retuximab	Low-level laser
Oral lichen planus	Fluocinonide Clobetasol propionate Betamethasone dipropionate		Tacrolimus Sirolimus Retinoic acid Vitamin A Isotretinoin Thalidomide Cyclosporine	Retinoic acid Vitamin A Etretinate Isotretinoin Griseofulvin Levamisole Dapsone Thalidomide TNF-alpha inhibitors MMF Curcumin Glycyrrhizin	Oral PUVA Low-level laser CO_2 laser Phototherapy Photodynamic therapy
Behçet disease				Colchicine Thalidomide Cyclosporine Dapsone Methotrexate Pentoxifylline TNF-alpha inhibitors Azathioprine	

Abbreviations: IVIG, intravenous immunoglobulin; MMF, mycophenolate mofetil; PUVA, psoralen ultraviolet A; TNF, tumor necrosis factor.

[a] Screen for thiopurine methyltransferase deficiency.

[b] Monitor for anemia.

of infection, relapse, and resistance. These agents may be very costly and, depending on the route of administration (infusions or injections vs per oral), may require more frequent medical office visits.[4]

Serum antibody concentrations using high-sensitivity ELISA to Dsg 3 and Dsg 1 (IgA and IgE subtype) seem to correlate with disease activity and clinical response, and may indicate potential relapse. Additionally, salivary IgG antibody titers to Dsg 3 has been shown to correlate with changes in disease severity. Monitoring disease severity using these serum and salivary markers may aid in determining systemic treatment options and treatment response.[5]

Mucous membrane pemphigoid

Incidence, predilection, and genetics

Pemphigoid disease (see Table 1) is a blistering disorder affecting the skin or mucosa at the level of the subepithelia or subepidermis. When the mucosal membranes are the primary site of involvement it is known as mucous membrane pemphigoid. The true prevalence rates in the United States are unknown; however, the estimated incidence is 1.16 and 0.87 cases per million per year in France and Germany, respectively.[6,7] The disease occurs more often in women than men (2:1) and is most often diagnosed in the sixth to eighth decades. The pathogenesis is heterogeneous in that several different antigens have been identified with the development of auto antibodies directed against several components at the mucosal—submucosal junction. About two-thirds of patients have autoantibodies targeting collagen XVII/BP180; about 25% of patients show reactivity to BP230, and about 20% of patients show antibodies to laminin 332.[2]

Clinical features

Mucous membrane pemphigoid predominantly affects the mucous membranes of the oral cavity (85%); however, other mucosal surfaces such as the ocular conjunctiva (65%) nasopharynx (20%—40%), anogenital (20%), larynx (5%—15%), and esophagus (5%—15%) can be affected less commonly.[8,9] Oral involvement may precede skin involvement by up to 1 year. Lesions will almost always begin with multiple intraoral mucosal site involvement, those areas that are subjected to frictional trauma such as the buccal mucosa, labial mucosa, palate, and gingiva frequently (Fig. 3A). In contrast with PV, vesicles or bullae may be more readily seen in the oral cavity owing to the location of tissue separation, albeit rarely (see Fig. 3B). It is not uncommon for ulceration to heal with scarring. Scarring of the conjunctiva could lead to adhesions (symblepharons), eyelid inversions (entropion), and/or corneal abrasion from eyelashes (trichiasis). Laryngeal involvement could potentially cause voice alterations and airway limitations in severe cases.[8,9]

Diagnosis and histopathology

The pathogenesis of mucous membrane pemphigoid is complex and has been found to be associated with several different antigens (see Table 1). Ultimately, autoantibodies are directed against components at the mucosal—connective tissue junction leading to separation between the surface epithelium and the underlying connective tissue, importantly with preservation of the basal cells (Fig. 4A). DIF of perilesional tissue demonstrate deposition of IgG and/or C3 and sometimes IgA in a linear bandlike pattern at the basement membrane zone (see Fig. 4B).

Treatment considerations

Topical treatments can effectively control mild to moderate disease of the oral cavity. Similar to PV, topical corticosteroids remain the most common treatment modality. If unsuccessful, a treatment algorithm developed as part of a systematic review then recommends systemic dapsone, tetracycline, sulphamethoxypyridazine and sulphapyridine, azathioprine, mycophenolate mofetil, and cyclophosphamide (see Table 2).[10] A recent case report yielded success with topical tacrolimus solution as an oral rinse or, with localized lesions, a series of repeated intralesional triamcinalone injections.[11,12] With systemic involvement, the primary outcome of therapy is reducing the possibility of irreversible scarring of the ocular, esophageal, genital, and laryngeal mucosa and preventing blindness, strictures, or airway obstruction depending on the areas of involvement. In severe cases intravenous immunoglobulin and prednisolone/cyclophosphamide combination, tumor necrosis factor (TNF)-alpha inhibitors or anti—CD-20 antibodies are treatment options.[1]

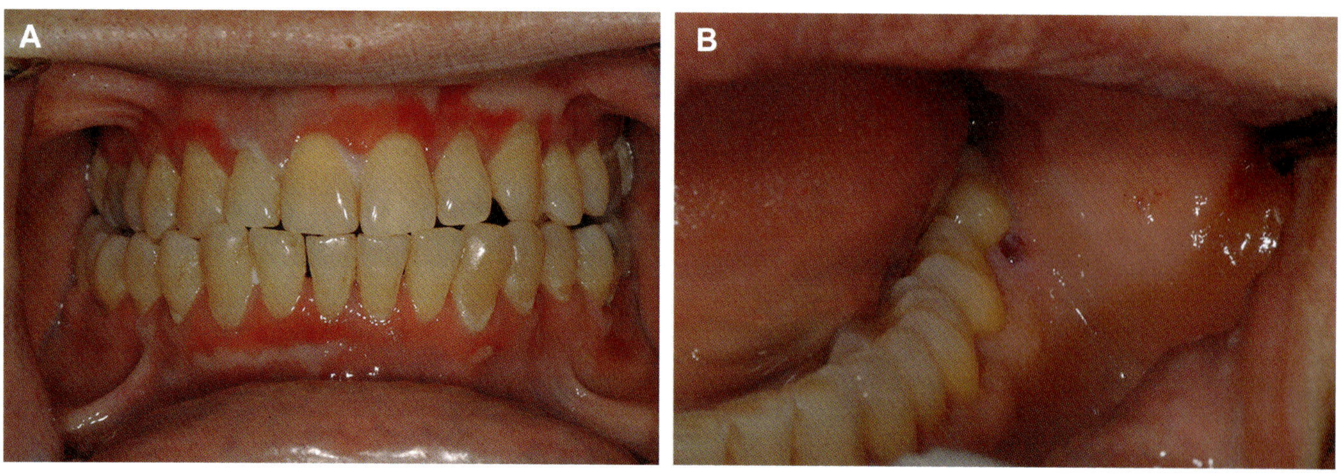

Fig. 3 Mucous membrane pemphigoid frequently presents with bright erythema of the gingiva referred to as desquamative gingivitis; note plaque accumulation because of pain on brushing (*A*). There is an intact vesicle on the buccal gingiva of the left mandibular third molar (*B*). (*Courtesy of* Michaell Huber, DDS, UT Health San Antonio, San Antonio, TX.)

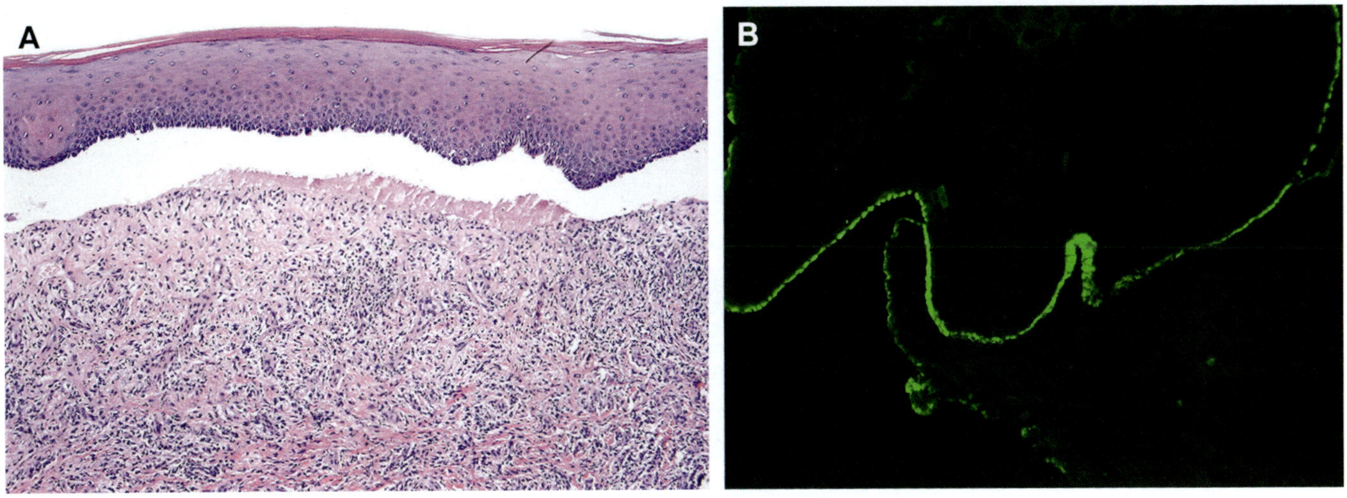

Fig. 4 Subbasalar clefting with preservation of basal cells and separation of the surface epithelium from the underlying connective tissue of mucous membrane pemphigoid (*A*; hematoxylin-eosin, original magnification ×100). Direct immunofluorescence reveals binding of IgG in a linear pattern at the basement membrane zone (*B*; hematoxylin-eosin, original magnification ×200). (*Courtesy of* Sook-Bin Woo, DMD, MMSc, Harvard School of Dental Medicine, Boston, MA.)

Oral lichen planus

Incidence, predilection, and genetics

Oral lichen planus (OLP) is a common mucosal inflammatory disorder affecting up to 2% of the population. The true prevalence of OLP is not known; however; depending on the particular population being examined, it has an estimated prevalence of 1.27%. The typical age of presentation is in the 40s and affects women more so than men.[13]

The etiology of OLP is uncertain, but it is thought to be an immune-related process triggered by an antigen(s) that alter basal keratinocytes making them susceptible to cell mediated immune response. $CD4^+$ T and $DC8^+$ T lymphocytes are activated and cytokines such as IL-2, interferon-gamma, and TNF are produced. Other cells such as dendritic cells, mastocyte cells, and macrophages may play a role in the pathologic processes. The triggering antigen is unknown; however, several reports have suggested a possible association between OLP and viral infections (herpes simplex, Epstein-Barr, cytomegalovirus, herpes simplex-6, human papilloma virus, and hepatitis C virus). Increased expression of heat shock protein suggests that it might be an autoantigen for the disorder but, because heat shock protein may also be expressed when exposed to several other exogenous agents, this may not necessarily be the actual trigger. It is believed that stressful situations may influence the development of the disease promoting dysregulation of immune functions and alterations in Th1/Th2 cytokines and a Th2 response. Additionally, IL-18, Il-4, Il-6, Il-10, interferon-gamma, matrix metalloproteinases, and TNF-alpha seem to have some influence on the susceptibility and progression of OLP. HLA-DR-1 has been associated with cutaneous LP but not OLP, and HLA-DR6 has been linked with hepatitis C virus—associated OLP. More studies are needed to determine if there is a possible genetic link in different geographic areas.[14]

Clinical features

Typically, patients present with complaints of pain and burning in the mouth owing to the presence of erosions and shallow ulcerations, exacerbated by eating spicy or acidic foods. Forty percent of patients may have both oral and cutaneous involvement, cutaneous lesions alone in 35%, and mucosal lesions alone in 25% of affected individuals.[15] OLP has 4 distinct clinical presentations: reticular, erosive, plaque-like, and bullous. Each can occur individually; however, patients frequently have a combination of any of these patterns. Reticular OLP is the most common and is usually asymptomatic. Lesions typically present with bilateral buccal mucosa involvement followed by the buccal vestibule, tongue, and gingiva (Fig. 5).

Diagnosis and histopathology

Although the histologic features of the disease may vary depending on the clinical presentation, the site of the biopsy, stage of evolution or devolution of disease, or whether the lesion has been previously treated, the main features associated with the disease are hyperorthokeratosis or hyperparakeratosis, acanthosis or atrophy, saw-tooth pattern of the rete ridges in the hyperplastic forms or loss of rete ridges in the atrophic/erosive forms, degeneration of the basal cell layer, and a variable band of T lymphocytes in the subepithelial connective tissue (Fig. 6). DIF studies may show a ragged band of fibrinogen along the basement membrane with IgM labeling colloid bodies.

Treatment considerations

There is no cure for the condition, most likely because the cause is unknown. Treatment goals are focused on alleviating symptoms by hastening the healing of erosions and ulcerations and, if possible, increasing the periods of disease remission. As in the other blistering conditions discussed, topical corticosteroids are the first-line treatment modality. Topical macrolide immunosuppressants, including calcineurin inhibitors, cyclosporine, rapamycin, and tetracycline, have used with varying degrees of success. Systemic steroids as well as other immunosuppressants are used in recalcitrant cases. Several other pharmacologic and nonpharmacologic interventions show potential (see Table 2).

Behçet disease

BD is a rare systemic vasculitis characterized by recurrent oral, ocular, and genital involvement. Cardiovascular, neurologic,

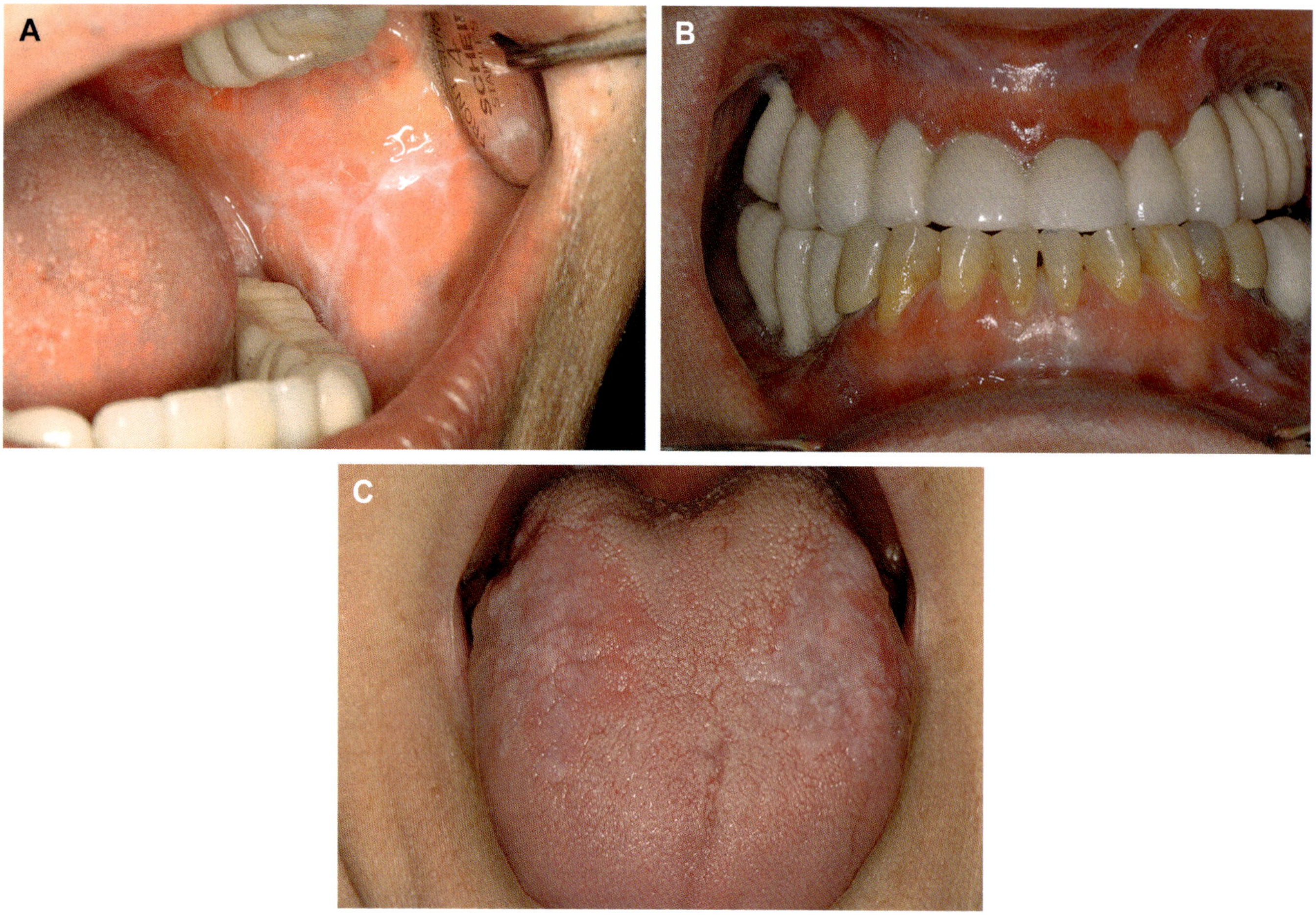

Fig. 5 Oral lichen planus most commonly present in the classic reticular form on the buccal mucosa, which is typically asymptomatic (*A*) or as gingival erythema/erosion, also known as desquamative gingivitis (*B*) or plaques (*C*). ([*A, C*] *Courtesy of* Sook-Bin Woo, DMD, MMSc, Harvard School of Dental Medicine, Boston, MA.)

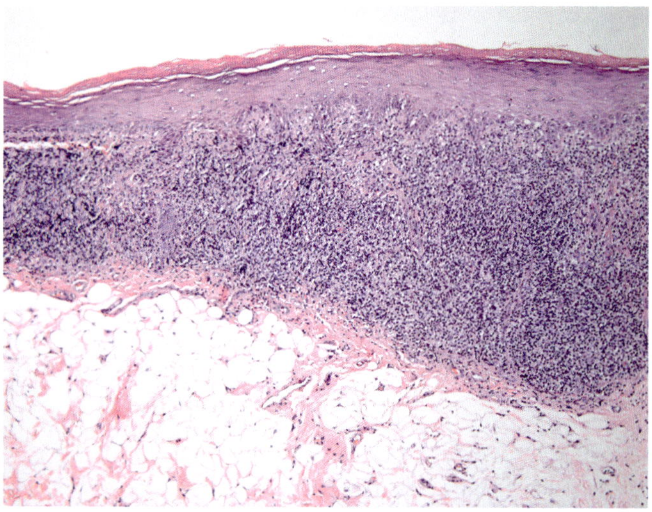

Fig. 6 This case of lichen planus from the buccal mucosa exhibits hyperkeratosis, epithelial atrophy, degeneration of the basal cell layer and a dense band of lymphocytes at the epithelium–connective tissue interface (hematoxylin-eosin, original magnification ×100). (*Courtesy of* Sook-Bin Woo, DMD, MMSc, Harvard School of Dental Medicine, Boston, MA.)

and gastrointestinal involvement is associated with worsened prognosis. Oral ulcerations are the earliest manifestation of the disease and will affect almost all patients at some point during the course of the disease. The pathophysiology is characterized by hyperfunction of neutrophils in the absence of infection with resultant increase in superoxide production, enhanced chemotaxis, and excessive production of lysosomal enzymes leading to tissue injury. The resultant autoimmune response induces vascular injuries and superimposed hypercoagulation that may be due in part to activated endothelial cells and activated platelets.

Incidence, predilection, and genetics

Worldwide, the prevalence of BD ranges between 0.1 per 1000 to 1 per 10,000. Turkey is reported to have the highest prevalence (80–420/100,000) followed by Japan, Korea, and other Asian countries. In the United States, the prevalence ranges from 0.12 to 0.33 per 100,000. In Western Asia, it affects males more than females; however, in Japan and Korea, females are affected more commonly. The etiology is broadly thought to be a T-cell–mediated inflammatory response in genetically susceptible individuals. Geographic distribution, familial aggregation and an association with HLA class I antigens (HLA-B51) has been observed. The age of onset is usually between the third and fourth decade with more severe disease manifestations in those diagnosed at a younger age.[16,17]

Clinical features

Recurrent, aphthous-like ulcerations (minor, major, or herpetiform) are the earliest features of the disease and are the main criteria for diagnosis (Fig. 7). Genital ulcers usually occur on the scrotum and penis in men and on the vulva in women. They are painful and morphologically similar to the oral ulcers, but are usually larger, deeper, and heal with scarring. Ocular lesions occur in the uvea and retina and symptoms include blurred vision, eye pain, photophobia, lacrimation, floaters, and periglobal hyperemia. Severe retinal disease can lead to bilateral decrease in visual acuity. Erythema nodosum, pseudofolliculitis, and acneiform nodules on the back, face, and neck, especially along the hairline, are common cutaneous manifestations. Joint involvement, including monoarthritis or polyarthritis (knees, wrists, ankles, and elbows), develops in about one-half of patients. Gastrointestinal involvement causes abdominal pain, diarrhea, melena, and sometimes perforation, but oral ulceration is usually considered separately from the gastrointestinal involvement. Gastrointestinal involvement may often be misdiagnosed as irritable bowel disease, ulcerative colitis, or Crohn's disease.[17] Neurologic involvement occurs infrequently but is associated with a poor prognosis. Manifestations include headache syndromes, meningoencephalitis, ophthalmoparesis, cranial neuropathy, intracranial hypertension, and aneurysms. Cardiovascular manifestations include thrombophlebitis, deep vein thrombosis, occlusions, aneurysms, pericarditis, myocarditis, and endocarditis. Severe cardiovascular involvement in large vessels resulting in sudden death by aneurysm rupture or thrombosis have been reported in up to 9.8% of patients.[16]

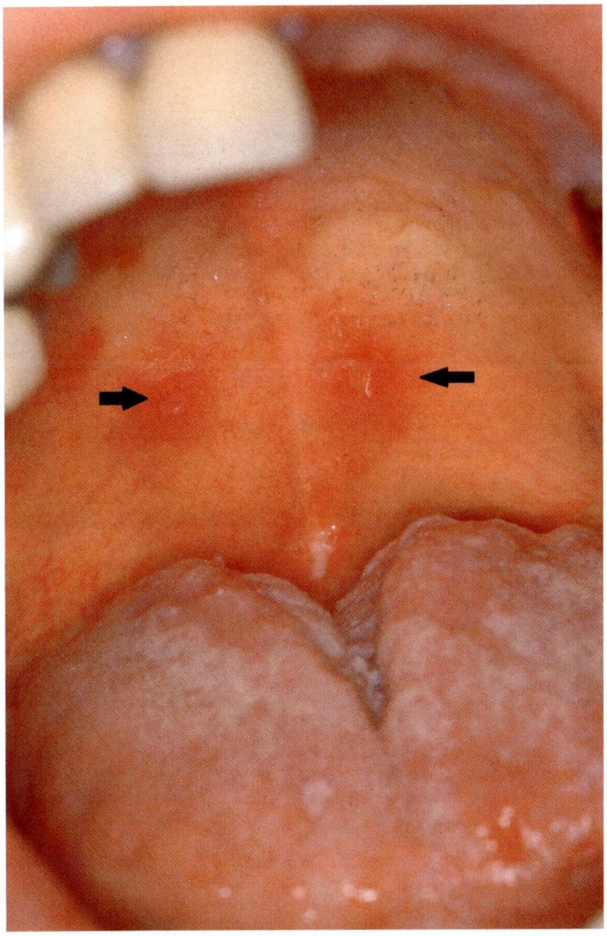

Fig. 7 Shallow ulcers (*arrows*) of the soft palate in a patient with Behçet disease along with a superimposed candidal overgrowth on the tongue from topical oral steroid use.

Diagnosis and histopathology

Owing to the lack of a single diagnostic test for the disease, a diagnosis of BD is made based on clinical findings. The current criteria consist of oral ulcerations plus any 2 of the following: recurrent genital ulcers, eye lesions (uveitis or retinal vasculitis), skin lesions (erythema nodosum, pseudofolliculitis, papulopustular lesions, acneiform nodules), and a positive pathergy test.[18,19] The histopathologic features of BD is characterized by leukocytoclastic vasculitis with intramural invasion by neutrophils, into small blood vessels. However, most cases show only nonspecific findings of ulceration with acute and chronic inflammation.

Treatment considerations

As in all of the conditions listed herein, treatment is geared toward symptom relief of mucosal lesions with topical corticosteroids. Another treatment strategy is decreasing systemic inflammation, particularly important when other organ systems are involved. For these, or if topical therapies are ineffective, disease-modifying antirheumatic drugs are used including colchicine and systemic steroids (see Table 2). Because inflammatory mechanisms as well B-cell factors are activated, biological drugs such as infliximab, adalimumab, daclizumab, and tocilizumab are being used with increasing frequency.

Connective tissue diseases

Systemic lupus erythematosus

Systemic lupus erythematosus is a complex, systemic, autoimmune disorder with multiorgan involvement. Oral lesions have been reported, on balance, in 54%[20] of patients and are considered one of the distinguishing features that aid in diagnosing the condition.

Incidence, predilection, and genetics

In US population-based studies, the incidence is 5.5 per 100, 000 per year and the prevalence was 72.8 per 100,000.[21] The condition is more prevalent in persons of African American or African Caribbean descent. It affects females more frequently than males ranging from 2 to 8:1 depending on the population being studied. Systemic lupus erythematosus is a multifactorial disease with evidence of genetic susceptibility, environmental effects, and disturbances in both innate and adaptive immunity manifest by disturbances in apoptotic cell clearance, cytokines, B-cell immunity, and T-cell signaling. Early apoptotic cells express cell surface proteins, such as phosphatidyl serine, that prompt circulating immune cells to engulf these cells and attract macrophages and dendritic cells. Failure of phagocytes to remove apoptotic material efficiently leads to fragments of nuclear particles being captured by antigen presenting cells, and through interactions with T and B cells, ultimately to the development of antinuclear antibodies.

Clinical features

Oral lesions may be found in systemic or cutaneous lupus and have been detected in up to 80% of patients with lupus depending on the population being studied[22] (Fig. 8A). On balance and confirmed by Khatabi and colleagues,[20] 54.3% of 188 patients had oral lesions. The most common lesions found were oral ulceration, erythematous erosions, and lichenoid lesions (see Fig. 8B). Lesions are seen most commonly on the buccal mucosa (22.3%) and lip (12.2%). Oral lesions may also be seen in up to 24% of patients with discoid lupus. Multiple organ systems can be affected to varying degrees resulting in lupus nephritis, central nervous system lupus, and antiphospholipid syndrome (resulting in venous or arterial thrombosis).

Diagnosis and histopathology

The oral lesions demonstrate features similar to lichen planus: hyperkeratosis, alternating atrophy, thickening of the spinous cell layer, degeneration of the basal cell layer, and subepithelial lymphocytic infiltration. However, patchy deposits of a periodic acid-Schiff–positive material in the basement membrane zone, subepithelial edema, and the inflammatory infiltrate occurring in a perivascular orientation may also be present. DIF shows IGM, IgG, and/or C3 deposition in a shaggy or granular band at the basement membrane (often referred to as a positive lupus band test).

Differential diagnosis

As mentioned in the Histopathology section, the oral lesions of lupus resemble those of OLP. As such, attention must be given to other presenting signs and symptoms such as joint pains, swelling, neurologic signs and symptoms, and kidney dysfunction to aid with proper diagnosis.

Treatment considerations

As with many of the diseases discussed in this article that manifest with oral ulcerations or erosions, improved oral hygiene is associated with a reduction in the extent and severity of oral ulcerations. Topical corticosteroids are the first line of treatment for oral lesions. Systemic immune modulating drugs may also play a role in limiting oral involvement and are used to treat patients with more severe features of the disease.

One important factor to keep in mind is that oral lesions are side effects of some antirheumatic drugs such as hydroxyurea, mycophenolate mofetil, and methotrexate (erosions/ulcers) (Fig. 9A–C) or hydroxychloroquine, gold salts, penicillamine, sulfasalazine, allopurinol and biologics (obinutuzumab, infliximab, adalimumab, etanercept, abatacept; [lichenoid mucosal changes]) or pigmentations (tetracycline, hydroxychloroquine cyclophosphamide). Certain medications used to treat pain may also be associated with oral lesions (see Rheumatoid arthritis).

Salivary dysfunction is associated with several connective tissue diseases (see Sjögren syndrome) and patients on immunomodulators are more susceptible to secondary candidal and viral infections and/or symptoms of oral burning.

Sjögren syndrome

Sjögren syndrome is an increasingly common chronic inflammatory immune mediated disease. It is categorized as either

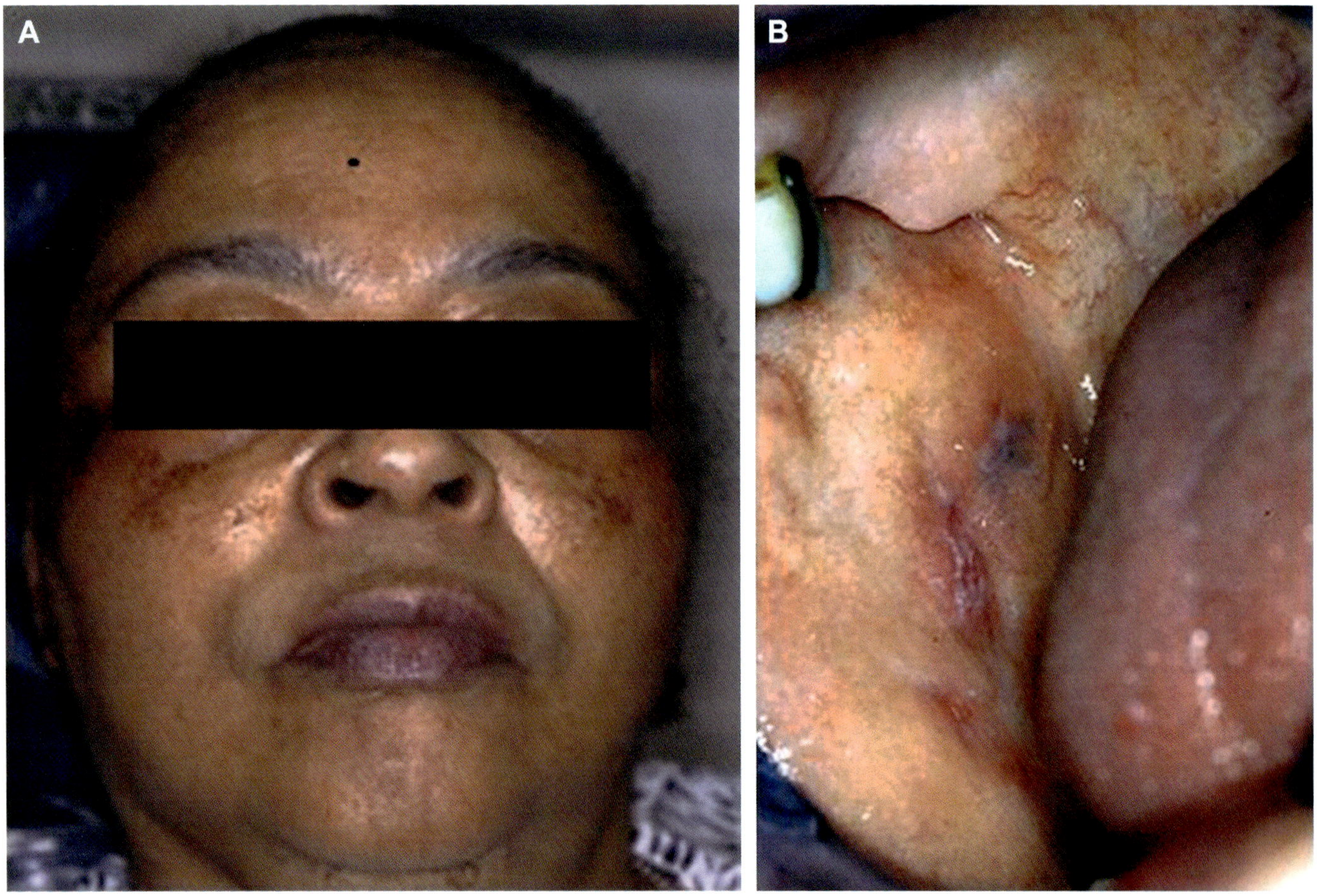

Fig. 8 Classic butterfly rash on the malar process, bilaterally, in this patient with systemic lupus erythematosus (*A*). Intraorally, lesions appear as mixed red/white erosions with subtle reticulations (lichenoid) (*B*).

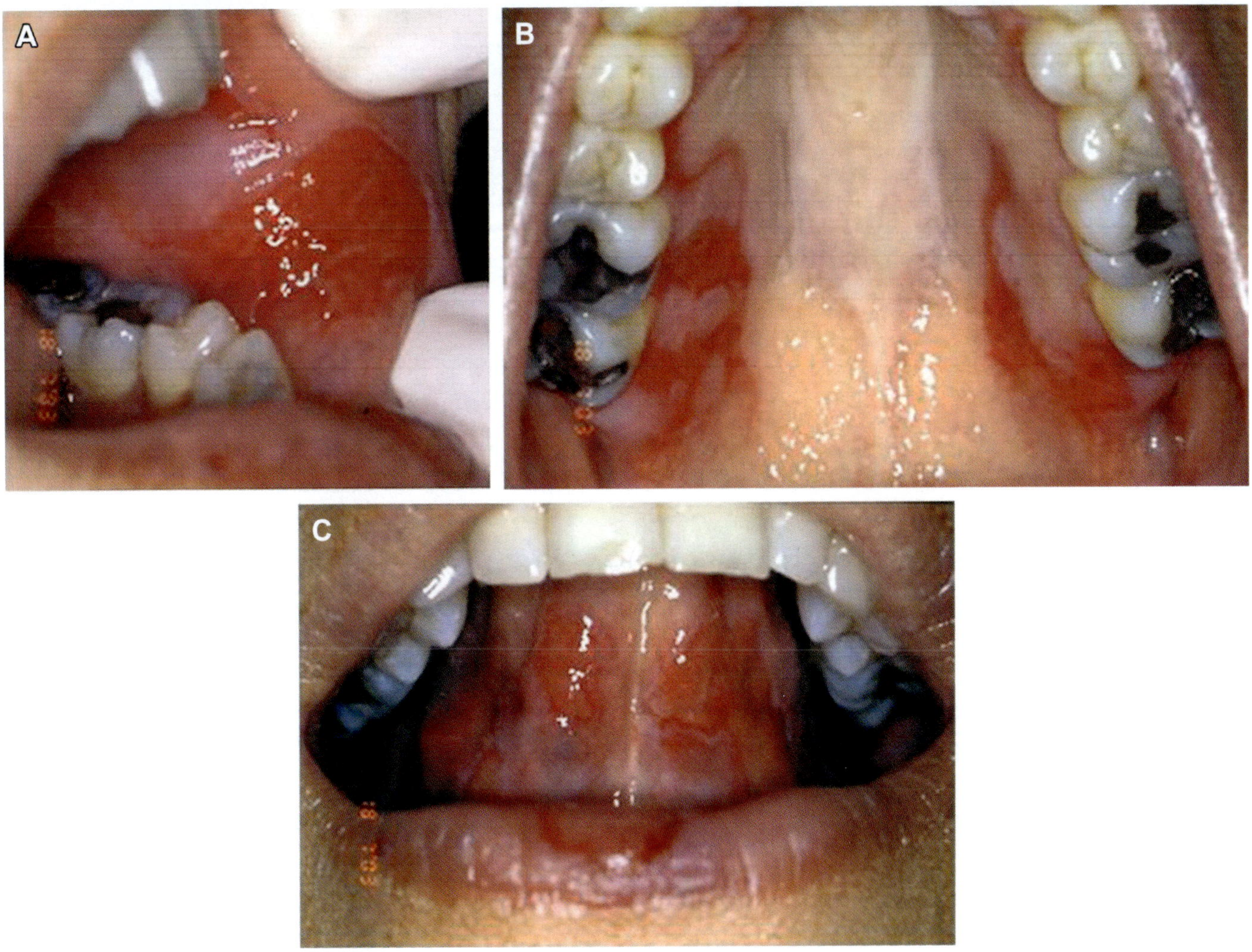

Fig. 9 Methotrexate-induced oral erosions and shallow ulcers on the hard palatal mucosa (*A*) and ventral tongue and lower lip (*B*) in this patient being treated for systemic lupus erythematosus.

primary or secondary Sjögren syndrome if occurring in an individual with another rheumatic disease. The lack of disease response to biologic agents indicates that this condition is associated with complex and diverse immune mechanisms that may explain the varied clinical expression. The disease process involves autoantibody production and chronic lymphocytic infiltration of exocrine glands, as well as multiple body organ systems manifesting as xerostomia, dry eyes, fatigue, vasculitis, neuropathy, arthralgias, kidney disorders, and lung disease. Approximately 5% of patients develop a non-Hodgkin's lymphoma that form within extranodal sites. The disease carries with it an increased direct health care–related cost burden and diminished quality of life.

Incidence, predilection, and genetics

Primary Sjögren syndrome is among the most prevalent rheumatic disorders, affecting up to 3.1 million Americans, approximately doubling in secondary Sjögren syndrome.[23] It has a wide gender predilection affecting women more than men in a 10:1 ratio.[24] The pathogenesis of Sjögren syndrome is multifactorial; both genetic and nongenetic factors are involved in disease susceptibility and initiation of disease process. There is dysregulation of the epithelial cells resulting in an autoimmune response and disease progression. Compelling evidence suggests that several biologic processes can be involved in Sjögren syndrome and contribute to the establishment of salivary gland pathology. Those pathways of activation belong both to the innate and acquired immune systems, such as interferon activation, defective T-regulatory activity, increased number and function of helper T cell and excessive costimulation. Lymphoneogenesis with germinal center formation and clonal expansion of malignant B cells is ascribed to the aberrant B-cell activation that characterized a subset of patients with high serum level of autoantibodies, systemic manifestations, and a high risk of lymphoma development.[25] First-degree relatives of patients with Sjögren syndrome have a risk ratio of 12.37 of developing the disease as compared with general population.

Clinical features

Sjögren syndrome causes destruction and dysfunction of the moisture-producing glands, most commonly the lacrimal and salivary glands, resulting in dry eyes and xerostomia. Lack of saliva and thickened saliva may result in taste alterations (either increased or decreased) affecting patients' ability to eat certain foods or lack of desire to eat, difficulty chewing and swallowing certain foods, burning mouth complaints, mucosal irritation and associated mouth pain, and/or dietary changes related to sensitivity to spicy, hot, or acidic foods. Depending on the extent of salivary gland impairment, swallowing and speech difficulties as well as an inability to create an adequate seal under full dentures may occur. Oral infections such as caries, salivary gland infections, and candidiasis are common.

Salivary gland infections present with complaints of pain, swelling (particularly after meals), induration, and increased warmth of the skin overlying the gland. Patients can develop a benign intermittent enlargement of the major salivary glands, which may be bilateral or unilateral. Owing to the increased relative risk for development of lymphoma, it is important to differentiate between benign salivary gland enlargement (Fig. 10A, B), salivary gland infection and lymphoma (see Fig. 10C). Lymphomas present as a unilateral progressive enlargement. Patients may have associated constitutional signs, such as fever, malaise, fatigue, and unexplained weight loss. A good history along with inquiry on accompanying signs and symptoms (fever, unexplained weight loss, pain within the gland, etc.) are essential to aid in determining the appropriate follow-up.

Diagnosis and histopathology

Minor salivary gland biopsy and serology still represent key tools for the identification of patients affected by Sjögren syndrome. Histologically, salivary gland (or lacrimal gland tissue) is examined for the presence of aggregates of 50 or more lymphocytes in a periductal distribution called a focus (Fig. 11). The number of foci per 4 mm^2 of tissue is evaluated and this represents the focus score. Through the years, several different classification criteria have been used to categorize patients. Currently, the new classification criteria by the European League American College of Rheumatology and the European League Against Rheumatism weigh items, giving 3 points to a minor salivary gland biopsy focus score of 1 or more, 3 points to the positivity for anti-Ro/SSA antibodies, and 1 point to a Schirmer's test of 5 mm or less in 5 minutes, an ocular staining score greater than or equal to 5, and to a salivary flow rate of 0.1 mL/min or less. A cutoff of 4 points is required to classify a patient as having Sjögren syndrome.[26]

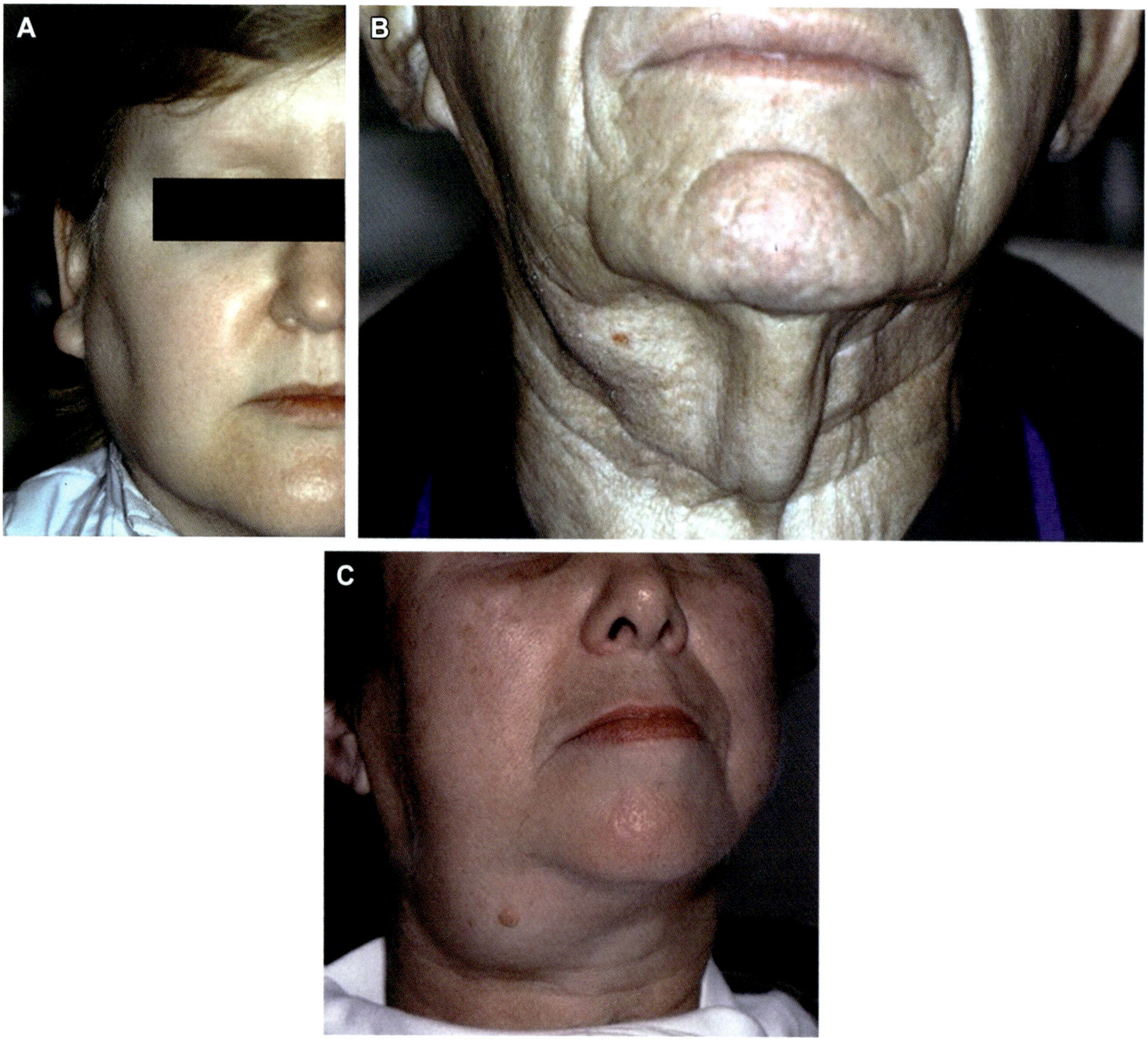

Fig. 10 Parotid (*A*) and submandibular (*B*) gland enlargement in patients with Sjögren syndrome. There was progressive enlargement of the submandibular region in a patient who subsequently developed non-Hodgkin's lymphoma secondary to Sjögren syndrome (*C*).

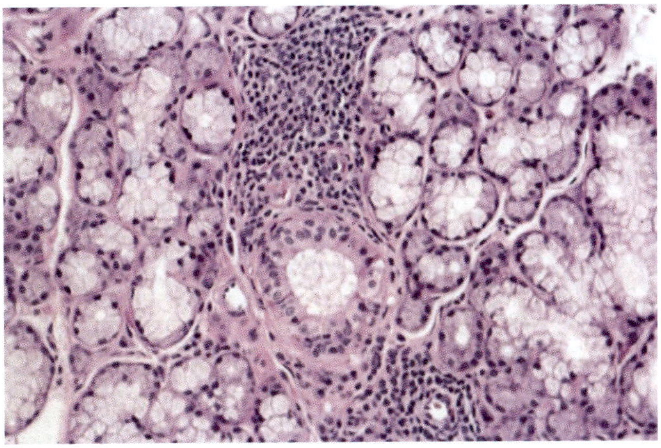

Fig. 11 Periductal lymphocytic foci (>50 lymphocytes) in this minor salivary gland biopsy of a patient with Sjögren syndrome (hematoxylin-eosin, original magnification ×200).

Differential diagnosis

There are multiple systemic illnesses that can present with dry mouth symptoms, including diabetes mellitus, AIDS, and thyroid dysfunction. Additionally, the side effects of medications used to treat systemic conditions such as allergies, depression, Parkinson's disease, and hypertension may result in xerostomia or reduced salivary flow rates. Indeed, the most common cause of xerostomia is a side effect of systemic medications. Several hundreds of prescriptions medications are associated with diminished salivary flow rates and/or xerostomia. Therefore, it is imperative that medications be ruled out as the cause of their oral dryness.

Treatment considerations

Most treatments for this condition have been those aimed at symptom relief, caries prevention, and the treatment of microbial infections. For those individuals more severely affected, systemic steroids as well as other disease-modifying antirheumatic drugs may be indicated. There are several clinical trials currently being conducted using biologic agents targeting cell receptors and cytokines that play a role in the pathogenesis of the disease. We refer the readers to recent publications for more information on treatment guidelines for systemic manifestations of the disease as well as caries management.[27,28]

Rheumatoid arthritis

Rheumatoid arthritis (RA) is a common systemic autoimmune disorder primarily involving the joints, but may also have extraarticular manifestations, such as rheumatoid nodules, pulmonary involvement, or vasculitis. Although specific oral lesions are not seen in this condition, patient may present with temporomandibular (TM) joint erosions with associated TM myofacial pain. With progressive joint degeneration, patients may develop malocclusion.

Incidence, predilection, and genetics

RA has an incidence of 0.5% to 1.0% with some Native American populations having a higher prevalence. Family members are at a 3 to 5 times greater risk of developing the condition implicating genetic factors in the pathogenesis. The HLA system (particularly HLA-DRB1) remains the dominant influence, strongly implicating peptide (and self-peptide) binding as well as other genetic loci. Epigenetics contribute to pathogenesis, probably by integrating environmental (smoking and/or infectious) agents and genetic effects.[29]

Clinical features

TM abnormalities have been reported in 67.6% of RA patients.[30] Myofacial pain was found in 64.8%, combined myofacial and TM joint pain in 18.5%, and joint involvement alone in 7.4% of patients.[31] Radiographic evaluation of the TM joint manifest very few changes that can be considered unique to RA. A variety of other TM conditions, mainly degenerative joint disease, show similar changes. Generally, the radiographic abnormalities are morphologic changes in the condyle head, glenoid cavity, and articular eminence, with surface erosion noted early on affecting the anterior and medial surfaces of the condyle, small cystlike areas presenting as punched out lesions on the anterior and superior surfaces of the condylar head beneath the fibrocartilage, osteophyte formation (during remission phases) beneath the lytic areas (not necessarily on the condyle surface itself), flattening of the anterosuperior aspect of the head of the condyle and posterior aspect of the articular eminence, sclerosis (either independently or with lytic changes), and bilateral condylysis in extreme cases. Other mandibular changes may include anterior positioning of the condyle in the fossa, diminished the vertical height of the ramus with increased gonial angle as a result of a diminished vertical height of the condyle, and in rare cases radiologic evidence of ankyloses (Fig. 12). Although true ankylosis with bony union between joint components does occur in some cases of RA, this finding does not seem to be found in the TM joint, except in very rare circumstances. Patients with RA almost always have adequate mouth opening, and consequently are able to maintain joint mobility; however, as malocclusion progresses, patients may develop an anterior open bite clinically (Fig. 13).

Treatment considerations

Medications used to treat pain may be associated with oral ulcerations (ibuprofen, rofecoxib, naproxen) or lichenoid mucosal changes (naproxin, oxicam) or erythematous papular lesions (acetaminophen). Certain biologics used to slow progression of joint damage or induce remission have been associated with lichenoid hypersensitivity reactions in the oral cavity as well (infliximab, obinutuzumab, adalimumab, etanercept, and abatacept).

Sarcoidosis

Sarcoidosis is a systemic disease characterized by a multisystem noncaseating granulomatous inflammation primarily in the lung, heart, brain, eyes, and skin. Within the head and neck, salivary gland involvement is the most common manifestation and infrequently, intraoral soft tissue lesions may also be encountered. The disease manifestations, severity, and long-term prognoses vary widely among affected individuals. Up to 5% of patient with sarcoidosis die from complications of the disease.[32]

Incidence, predilection, and genetics

The annual incidence of the disease varies from 5 per 100,000 in whites to 39 per 100,000 in African Americans, with an

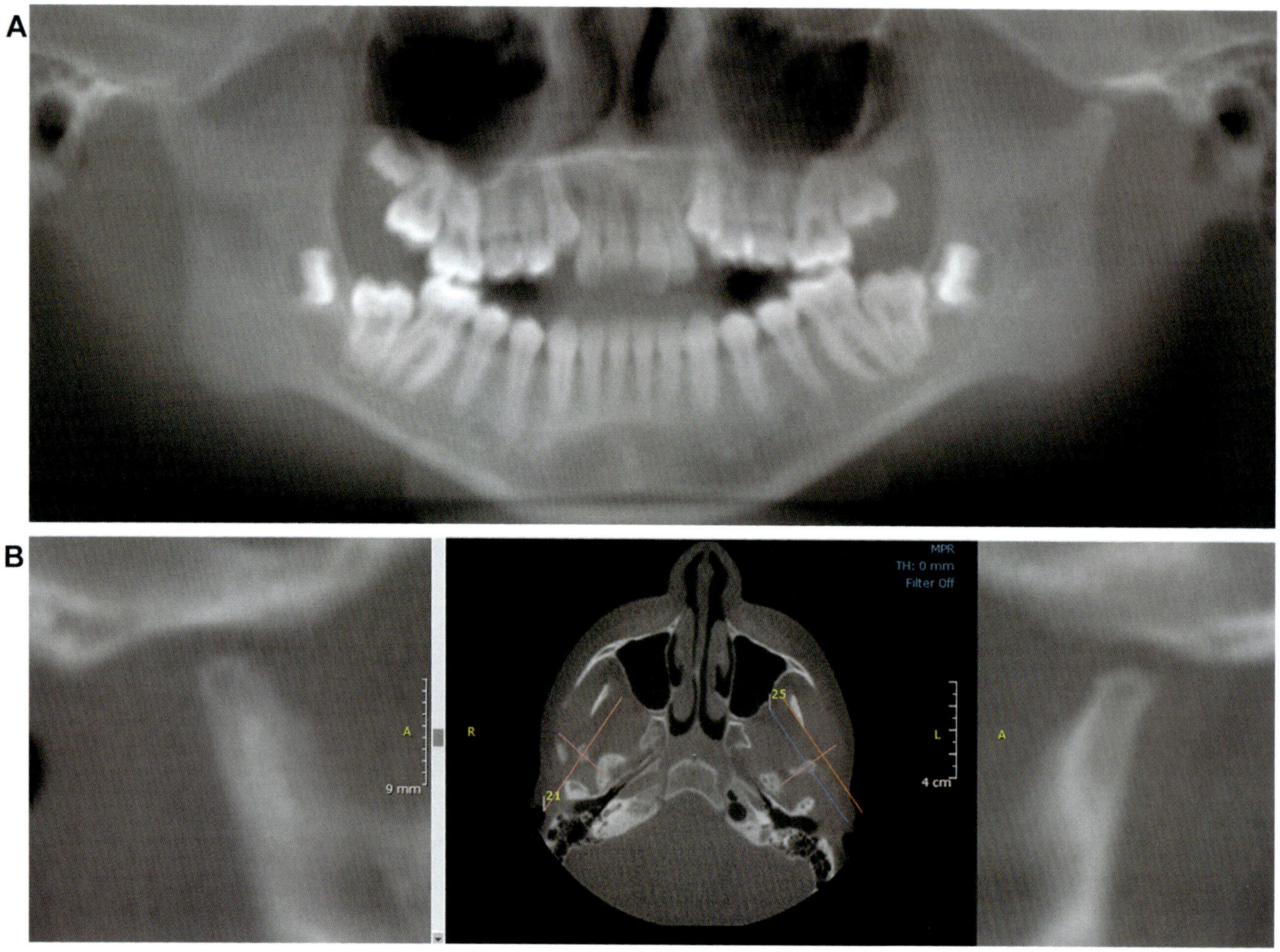

Fig. 12 Cone beam computed tomography images of the temporomandibular joints showing degenerative changes in a patient with rheumatoid arthritis.

overall prevalence estimated to be 15 per 100,000 in the United States.[33]

By recent reports, prevalence rates have increased 2-fold within the past 15 years. In Columbus, Ohio, the overall prevalence of sarcoidosis increased steadily from 164 per 100,000 in 1995 to 330 per 100,000 in 2010, a finding not fully explained by changes in the distribution of the patient population with respect to race or gender or changes in regional referral patterns.[34]

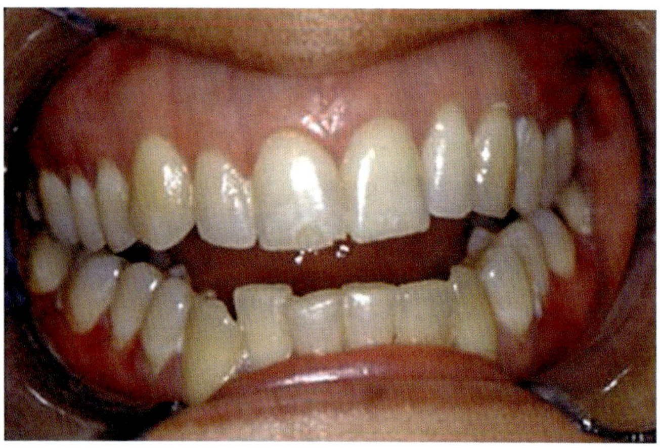

Fig. 13 Malocclusion and progressively worsening anterior open bite in a patient with rheumatoid arthritis.

The exact cause of sarcoidosis is unknown, but it is thought to be an exaggerated immune response to unknown environmental antigens in genetically susceptible individuals. Exposure to musty odors, insecticides, or to metal-processing industries are risk factors for the disease. Interestingly, a high incidence of sarcoidosis was reported in fire fighters and other responders after the attacks on the World Trade Center in 2001. Sarcoidosis is familial in 3.6% to 9.6% of cases, affecting siblings more often than parents, suggesting a recessive inheritance mode with incomplete penetrance. Monozygotic twins are at 80-times increased risk in acquiring the disease, lending support to the idea that genetic factors might account for two-thirds of disease susceptibility.[35]

Clinical features

Sarcoidosis is most commonly diagnosed in the third-fifth decades with a strong female gender bias. Mortality is significantly higher among African Americans and women for unknown reasons.[36] Symptoms include nonspecific complaints, ranging from fatigue and depression, "asthma symptoms" (wheezing, persistent cough), to arthritis and muscle pain or weakness. Clinically, patients may present with lymphadenopathy, erythema nodosum, and localized skin (Fig. 14) or eye lesions.

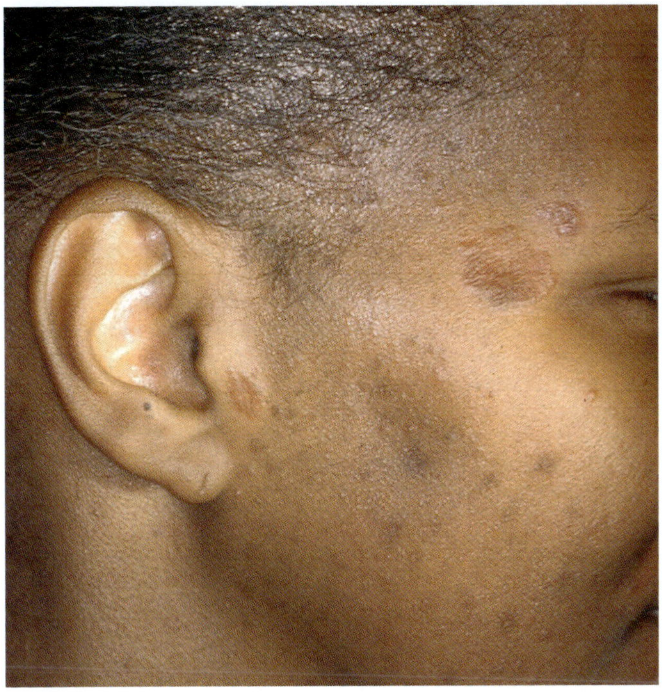

Fig. 14 Slightly raised brown papules and plaques of the periorbital skin and the pinna of the ear in a patient with sarcoidosis.

In the maxillofacial region, the salivary glands are the most frequently involved sites resulting in xerostomic complaints or presenting clinically as unilateral or bilateral parotid swelling, similar to that found in Sjögren syndrome. Oral lesions associated with sarcoidosis are considered to be rare with an unknown prevalence. Most cases of oral sarcoidosis present as single or multiple nodules or ulceration(s) of the longue, lips, palate, and gingiva; asymptomatic swelling of the involved mucosa; or mobility of the teeth owing to rapid alveolar bone loss. Lacrimal gland involvement occurs in up to 10% of patients. Symptoms include dry eye complaints and clinically presents as palpable masses, eyelid swelling, ptosis, or even globe displacement. Cranial nerve involvement can be seen in up to 50% of patients. Facial nerve (cranial nerve VII) involvement presents clinically as facial nerve palsy.[37]

Diagnosis and histopathology
There is no specific diagnostic test for sarcoidosis, diagnosis is made if patients fulfill 3 criteria: (1) clinical and radiologic presentation, such as symptoms (persistent cough, fatigue), signs (erythema nodosum, pulmonary function tests, chest radiograph, hematology [anemia, lymphocytopenia, elevated erythrocyte sedimentation rate], biochemical tests [angiotensin-converting enzyme levels, increased liver enzymes, hypercalcemia]), (2) evidence of noncaseating granulomas, and (3) no other evidence of alternative diseases. Biopsy shows noncaseating granulomas. Biopsy samples of minor salivary glands is useful when previous samples have failed, or when no other target is easily accessible.

Differential diagnosis
The differential diagnosis of the oral ulcerations would include Wegener granulomatosis, Crohn's disease, tuberculosis, histoplasmosis, and syphilis. In cases of nonspecific generalized soft tissue enlargement, orofacial granulomatosis may be difficult to distinguish from sarcoidosis. The neurologic involvement may lead one to consider Bell palsy, Ramsay Hunt syndrome, or perineural spread of malignancy and/or trigeminal neuralgia. Salivary gland enlargement either acute or chronic would include bacterial or viral sialadenitis. Xerostomia, ocular dryness, skin dryness, and fatigue would necessitate ruling out Sjögren syndrome disease. Heerfordt syndrome refers to a usually self-limiting presentation of sarcoidosis manifesting as uveitis, parotitis, fevers, and facial nerve palsy.[35]

Treatment considerations
There is no definitive cure at this time; however, systemic corticosteroids remain the standard treatment. Because long-term systemic steroids show little effect other disease-modifying antirheumatic drugs such as methotrexate, azathioprine, lefunomide, cyclophosphamide, and mycophenolate may be used as well as cytokine modulators such as pentoxifylline, thalidomide, and TNF-alpha antagonists (see Table 2).

References

1. Sticherling M, Erfurt-Berge C. Autoimmune blistering diseases of the skin. Autoimmun Rev 2012;11(3):226–30.
2. Mustafa MB, Porter SR, Smoller BR, et al. Oral mucosal manifestations of autoimmune skin diseases. Autoimmun Rev 2015;14(10): 930–51.
3. Ali S, Kelly C, Challacombe SJ, et al. Salivary IgA and IgG antibodies to bullous pemphigoid 180 noncollagenous domain 16a as diagnostic biomarkers in mucous membrane pemphigoid. Br J Dermatol 2016;174(5):1022–9.
4. Huang A, Madan RK, Levitt J. Future therapies for pemphigus vulgaris: rituximab and beyond. J Am Acad Dermatol 2016;74(4): 746–53.
5. Ali S, Kelly C, Challacombe SJ, et al. Serum and salivary IgG and IgA antibodies to desmoglein 3 in mucosal pemphigus vulgaris. Br J Dermatol 2016;175(1):113–21.
6. Bernard P, Vaillant L, Labeille B, et al. Incidence and distribution of subepidermal autoimmune bullous skin diseases in three French regions. Bullous Diseases French Study Group. Arch Dermatol 1995; 131(1):48–52.
7. Bertram F, Brocker E-B, Zillikens D, et al. Prospective analysis of the incidence of autoimmune bullous disorders in Lower Franconia, Germany. J Dtsch Dermatol Ges 2009;7(5):434–40.
8. Chan LS. Ocular and oral mucous membrane pemphigoid (cicatricial pemphigoid). Clin Dermatol 2012;30(1):34–7.
9. Thorne JE, Anhalt GJ, Jabs DA. Mucous membrane pemphigoid and pseudopemphigoid. Ophthalmology 2004;111(1):45–52.
10. Taylor J, McMillan R, Shephard M, et al. World Workshop on Oral Medicine VI: a systematic review of the treatment of mucous membrane pemphigoid. Oral Surg Oral Med Oral Pathol Oral Radiol 2015;120(2):161–171.e20.
11. Al-Shehhi F, Balakirski G, Baratli J, et al. Localized oral mucous membrane pemphigoid: successful topical treatment with 1% tacrolimus solution as steroid-sparing therapy. J Eur Acad Dermatol Venereol 2016;31(3):e176–8.
12. Kalinska-Bienias A, Kalowska M, Kwiek B, et al. Efficacy and safety of perilesional/intralesional triamcinolone injections in oral mucous membrane pemphigoid. Br J Dermatol 2016;174(2): 436–8.
13. McCartan BE, Healy CM. The reported prevalence of oral lichen planus: a review and critique. J Oral Pathol Med 2008;37(8): 447–53.
14. Payeras MR, Cherubini K, Figueiredo MA, et al. Oral lichen planus: focus on etiopathogenesis. Arch Oral Biol 2013;58(9):1057–69.
15. DeRossi SS, Ciarrocca KN. Lichen planus, lichenoid drug reactions, and lichenoid mucositis. Dent Clin North Am 2005;49(1): 77–89. viii.

16. Zeidan MJ, Saadoun D, Garrido M, et al. Behcet's disease physiopathology: a contemporary review. Auto Immun Highlights 2016; 7(1):4.
17. Sakane T, Takeno M, Suzuki N, et al. Behcet's disease. N Engl J Med 1999;341(17):1284–91.
18. Criteria for diagnosis of Behcet's disease. International study group for Behcet's disease. Lancet 1990;335(8697):1078–80.
19. Davatchi F, Assaad-Khalil S, Calamia KT, et al. The International Criteria for Behçet's Disease (ICBD): a collaborative study of 27 countries on the sensitivity and specificity of the new criteria. J Eur Acad Dermatol Venereol 2014;28(3):338–47.
20. Khatibi M, Shakoorpour AH, Jahromi ZM, et al. The prevalence of oral mucosal lesions and related factors in 188 patients with systemic lupus erythematosus. Lupus 2012;21(12):1312–5.
21. Somers EC, Marder W, Cagnoli P, et al. Population-based incidence and prevalence of systemic lupus erythematosus: the Michigan Lupus Epidemiology and Surveillance program. Arthritis Rheumatol 2014;66(2):369–78.
22. Brennan MT, Valerin MA, Napenas JJ, et al. Oral manifestations of patients with lupus erythematosus. Dent Clin North Am 2005;49(1): 127–41. ix.
23. Helmick CG, Felson DT, Lawrence RC, et al. Estimates of the prevalence of arthritis and other rheumatic conditions in the United States. Part I. Arthritis Rheum 2008;58(1):15–25.
24. Ramos-Casals M, Brito-Zeron P, Kostov B, et al. Google-driven search for big data in autoimmune geoepidemiology: analysis of 394,827 patients with systemic autoimmune diseases. Autoimmun Rev 2015;14(8):670–9.
25. Campos J, Hillen MR, Barone F. Salivary gland pathology in Sjogren's syndrome. Rheum Dis Clin North Am 2016;42(3):473–83.
26. Shiboski CH, Shiboski SC, Seror R, et al. 2016 American College of Rheumatology/European League against Rheumatism classification criteria for primary Sjogren's syndrome: a consensus and data-driven methodology involving three international patient cohorts. Ann Rheum Dis 2017;76(1):9–16.
27. Carsons SE, Vivino FB, Parke A, et al. Treatment guidelines for rheumatologic manifestations of Sjogren's: use of biologics, management of fatigue and inflammatory musculoskeletal pain. Arthritis Care Res (Hoboken) July 2016;69(4):517–27.
28. Zero DT, Brennan MT, Daniels TE, et al. Clinical practice guidelines for oral management of Sjogren disease: dental caries prevention. J Am Dent Assoc 2016;147(4):295–305.
29. Smolen JS, Aletaha D, McInnes IB. Rheumatoid arthritis. Lancet 2016;388(10055):2023–38.
30. Yamakawa M, Ansai T, Kasai S, et al. Dentition status and temporomandibular joint disorders in patients with rheumatoid arthritis. Cranio 2002;20(3):165–71.
31. Kurtoglu C, Kurkcu M, Sertdemir Y, et al. Temporomandibular disorders in patients with rheumatoid arthritis: a clinical study. Niger J Clin Pract 2016;19(6):715–20.
32. Gerke AK. Morbidity and mortality in sarcoidosis. Curr Opin Pulm Med 2014;20(5):472–8.
33. Orphanet report series. Prevalence of rare diseases: Bibliographic data. November 2016, Number 1. Available at: http://www.orpha.net/orphacom/cahiers/docs/GB/Prevalence_of_rare_diseases_by_alphabetical_list.pdf. Accessed May 24, 2017.
34. Erdal BS, Clymer BD, Yildiz VO, et al. Unexpectedly high prevalence of sarcoidosis in a representative U.S. Metropolitan population. Respir Med 2012;106(6):893–9.
35. Valeyre D, Prasse A, Nunes H, et al. Sarcoidosis. Lancet 2014; 383(9923):1155–67.
36. NHLBI workshop on sarcoidosis. Leveraging scientific advancements to understand sarcoidosis variability and improve outcomes. August 31st – September 1st 2015. Available at: https://www.nhlbi.nih.gov/research/reports/nhlbi-workshop-sarcoidosis-%E2%80%9Cleveraging-scientific-advancements-understand-sarcoidosis-variability. Accessed May 24, 2017.
37. Shah R, Roberson GH, Cure JK. Correlation of MR imaging findings and clinical manifestations in neurosarcoidosis. AJNR Am J Neuroradiol 2009;30(5):953–61.

Drug-Induced Oral Complications

Kentaro Ikeda, DDS, MPH, FDS RCSEd [a,b,*]

KEYWORDS

• Drug-induced • Adverse reaction • Oral complications • Angioedema • Erythema multiforme • Gingival hyperplasia • Biologics • Antitumor necrosis factor

KEY POINTS

- Because of an aging population and rapid development of new medications, dentistry and medicine will likely face a significant increase in patients with drug related reactions.
- Patient history and physical examination are the most essential components of diagnosing drug-induced oral complications.
- Although treatment options vary depending on clinical diagnosis, a multidisciplinary approach is often required.

Drug-induced oral complications

According to US Census Bureau, the projected population aged 65 and over in 2050 will almost double the estimated projection in 2012.[1] As a result of this aging population, emerging medicine, and the rapid development of new medications, dentistry and medicine will likely face a significant increase in patients with drug-related reactions. Several common drug-induced oral complications are discussed in this article. When patients with possible drug-induced oral complications present, thorough medication and social histories are mandatory, including prescription medication, over-the-counter medication, dietary habit, and oral and cosmetic products.

This article focuses on drug-induced complications that directly affect oral mucosa. Hard tissue involvement such as medication-related osteonecrosis of the jaw (MRONJ) and neurologic involvement such as taste alteration or burning mouth syndrome (BMS) are not discussed in this article. Moreover, the complications discussed in this article are due to idiosyncratic reactions. Therefore, exaggerated reactions of expected pharmacologic actions such as excessive bleeding associated with anticoagulant medications are not discussed in this article.

Drug-induced angioedema

Brief description

Angioedema is a diffuse edematous swelling of the subcutaneous and submucosal connective tissue that may affect anywhere in the body, often manifests in the head and neck, and may lead to life-threatening airway obstruction.[2,3]

There are numerous medications that can cause angioedema including NSAIDs (nonsteroidal anti-inflammatory drugs) and antibiotics that are commonly used in dental settings. Many of these are immunoglobulin E (IgE)-mediated hypersensitivities that lead to mast cell degradation.[3,4]

Another common medication that has unique causal mechanism for angioedema is ACEI (angiotensin-converting enzyme inhibitor). It is caused by the inhibition of enzymatic breakdown of tissue bradykinin, causing bradykinin levels to increase.[4] It can occur rapidly or on delayed bases even years after introduction of an ACEI.[4]

Incidence, predilection

Prevalence rates of NSAID-induced angioedema range from 0.1% to 0.3%, which is partly because of the large size of the exposed (at risk) population.[5]

ACEI-associated angioedema affects up to 2% of patients using this medication class and is responsible for 30% of cases presenting to emergency departments.[6]

A recent large epidemiologic study showed an association between ACEI-related angioedema and patients older 65 years, seasonal allergies, a history of drug rash, sensitization to certain food components, and pollen season, but failed to show female predilection or association with smoking that was previously suggested.[7]

Clinical features

Angioedema is characterized by the relatively rapid onset of soft, nontender tissue swelling (Fig. 1). Most common sites are face, hands, feet, and trunk.[8] Although pain is unusual, itching is common.[3,4]

Differential diagnosis

By far, the most essential component required for the diagnosis is history and physical examination. The diagnosis of

Disclosures: No relationship with a commercial company.

[a] Department of Diagnostics and Biological Sciences, University of Colorado School of Dental Medicine, 13065 East 17th Avenue, Mail Stop F844, Aurora, CO 80045, USA

[b] Department of Family Medicine, University of Colorado School of Medicine, 12631 East 17th Avenue, Aurora, CO 80045, USA

* Department of Diagnostics and Biological Sciences, University of Colorado School of Dental Medicine, 13065 East 17th Avenue, Mail Stop F844, Aurora, CO 80045.

E-mail address: kentaro.ikeda@ucdenver.edu

Atlas Oral Maxillofacial Surg Clin N Am 25 (2017) 127-132

http://dx.doi.org/10.1016/j.cxom.2017.04.005

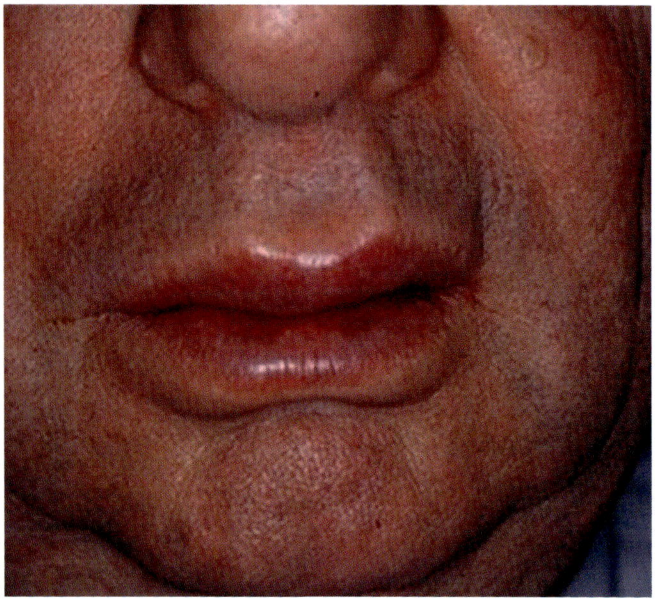

Fig. 1 Angioedema of the lips. (*Courtesy of* Dr John D. McDowell, Department of Diagnostics and Biological Sciences, University of Colorado School of Dental Medicine, Aurora, CO.)

drug-induced angioedema is often made based upon the patient's clinical presentation in conjunction with the history.[3,4] There are no unique histopathologic features of drug-induced angioedema. Dietary diaries and antigenic testing may be indicated when a patient is exposed to possible multiple antigens.[3,4] Complement tests (C1-INH) may be indicated if relations to antigenic exposure cannot be determined.[3,4,6]

Treatment considerations

The primary approach for managing drug-induced angioedema is discontinuation of the offending medication and supportive measures for airway protection.[3,6,9] For IgE-mediated drug-induced angioedema, antihistamines and corticosteroids may be effective.[3,6] For ACEI-Induced angioedema, antihistamines and corticosteroids are often ineffective, because these do not target the underlying mechanism of the ACEI-induced angioedema. Fresh frozen plasma (FFP), C1 inhibitor, Ecallantide, and Icatibant have been reported to be effective treatments in several cases.[9,10] However, there are no definitive data to prove this efficacy.[9,10]

Erythema multiforme

Brief description

Erythema multiforme (EM) represents a group of acute immune-mediated disorders that can affect the skin and mucous membranes.[11] Historically, EM has been classified into 2 groups, EM major (EMM) or EM minor (EMm). Numerous reported cases of EM manifesting in oral mucosa without skin lesion have resulted in a third group being named oral EM by several authors.[11–13] Previously, HSV (herpes simplex virus) was suggested to be the most common cause.[14] However, a recent large case series in oral EM, the largest in the last 2 decades, suggests that medications may be the leading trigger of EM.[11]

Essentially any medication or even food additives can cause EM. Most commonly reported causative medications include NSAIDs and antibiotics.[11–16] Yet, the list of the medications associated with the induction of EM continues to expand and includes new categories of drugs such as biologics.[11,16] It has been also reported that drug-induced EM typically affects oral mucosa.[11–13] Therefore, oral health care providers may face drug-induced EM more than EM triggered by other causes regardless of the commonality.

Incidence, predilection

Current literature regarding the epidemiology of EM remains scarce and controversial, largely due to a lack of universal diagnostic criteria and possible under-reporting of mild cases.[11] There is no gender predilection.[11–15] EM frequently affects young adults, but the age of reported cases ranges widely, from infancy to 80 plus years of age.[11–15,17] The oral cavity is the most frequently involved mucosal site, with a frequency that is varied, ranging from 25% to more than 70%.[3,11–18]

Clinical features

Oral manifestations may be varied, ranging from diffuse oral erythema to multifocal superficial ulcerations. Vesicles/bullae may be present at the initial stage of the disease.[3,11,18] Any area of the mouth may be involved, with the lip, labial mucosa, buccal mucosa, tongue, floor of the mouth, and soft palate being the most common sites.[3,11]

The oral mucosal ulcerations are usually irregular and large with necrotic tissue tags (Fig. 2). In most cases, lip lesions are observed that show hemorrhagic crusting of the lips (Fig. 3). Oral lesions may be an initial manifestation of EM before skin involvement.[11–13] The pain from oral lesions may compromise daily functions such as speech, eating, and fluid intake.

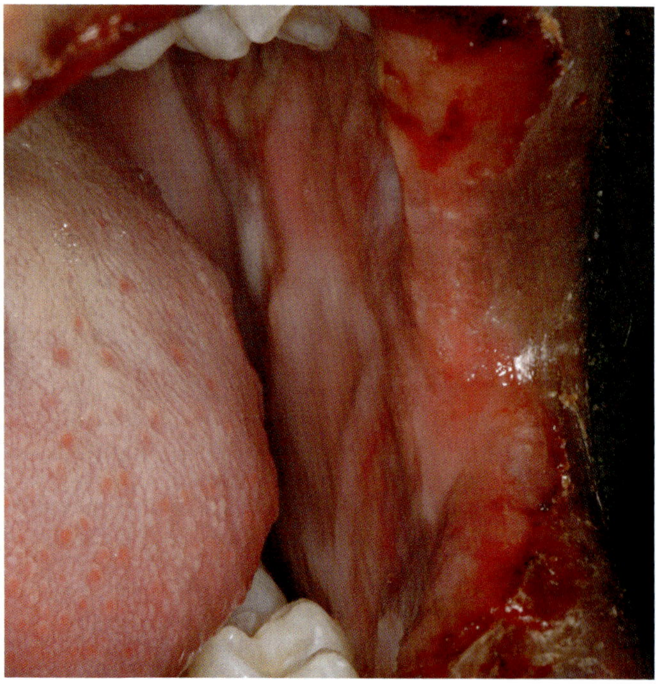

Fig. 2 EM affecting buccal mucosa, lips, and labial mucosa.

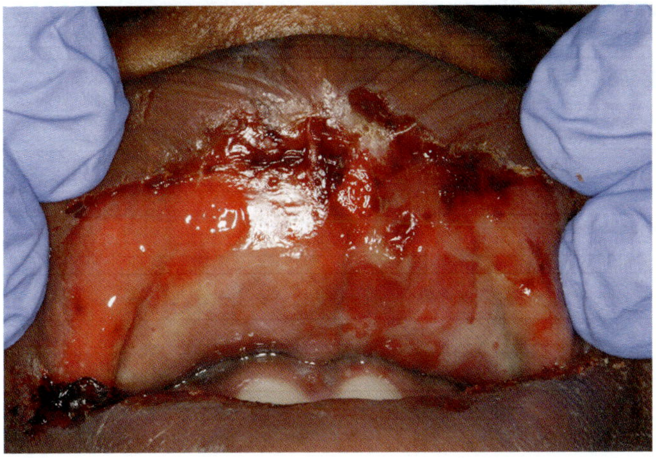

Fig. 3 Hemorrhagic crusting of the lips in a patient with EM.

Differential diagnosis

The diagnosis of drug-induced EM is often made based upon the patient's clinical presentation in conjunction with the patient history.[3,11–15,18] Because drug-induced EM often present without skin lesions, exclusion of other vesiculobullous disorders may be necessary for the diagnosis. Direct immunofluorescence (DIF) may be useful only to exclude the other vesiculobullous disorders. If offending agent cannot be determined by history, polymerase chain reaction (PCR) assay of HSV association may be suggestive.[11,18]

Histopathology

The histopathology is characteristic, but not specific. Immunopathologic features are also nonspecific.[3] Subepithelial or intraepithelial vesiculation may be seen in association with necrotic basal keratinocytes. A mixed inflammatory infiltrate is generally present, consisting of lymphocytes, neutrophils, and often eosinophils.[3]

Treatment considerations

If a causative drug is identified or suspected, then it should be discontinued immediately. Primary management is supportive therapy with appropriate food and fluid intake. Treatment may include topical anesthetics, analgesics, and protectant. Although there is little or no scientific evidence to show the efficacy of any medications, many medications have been described as treatment options. Topical or systemic steroids have been used widely.[3,14,15,18] Other medications include dapsone, azathioprine, hydroxychloroquine, and mycophenolate mofetil.[14,15,18]

Drug-induced gingival hyperplasia

Brief description

Drug-induced gingival hyperplasia (GH) refers to an abnormal growth of the gingival tissues secondary to use of a systemic medication.[19] Despite many medications having been reported as causal, 3 classes of drugs, CCBs (calcium channel blockers), anticonvulsants, and immunosuppressants, are associated as the most common causative agents.[3,19–23] A strong association has been noted only with phenytoin, nifedipine, and cyclosporine, although other agents, especially in CCBs such as diltiazem, verapamil, and amlodipine, are reported in the literature.[3,19–21]

Incidence, predilection

Prevalence of drug-induced GH varies widely. Approximately 50% of patients taking phenytoin, 30% to 50% of patients taking nifedipine, and 25% of patients taking cyclosporine are reported to be affected.[3,19–21] Because of commonality in the use of each medication (anticonvulsants used in children, CCBs in middle-aged and older patients, and cyclosporine in a broad age range of patients), commonly affected age groups correlate with which medication has been prescribed.[3,19,20] There is no sex or race predilection.[3,20]

Clinical features

After 1 to 3 months of the causative medication use, the enlargements originate in the interdental papillae (Fig. 4) and spread across the tooth surfaces.[3,19,24] Most common affected sites are anterior facial gingiva.[3,19,20] The GH can cover a portion or all of tooth crowns of an affected area (Fig. 5). The GH extension lingually or covering much of the crowns of teeth can lead to functional speech and mastication difficulties. Because some of the causative agents are used commonly in young adults, esthetic appearance may be a major concern for many patients.

Differential diagnosis

The diagnosis of drug-induced GH is often made based upon the patient's clinical presentation in conjunction with the patient history. Because there are number of reported cases associated with medications besides the common ones mentioned in this article, clinicians should not disregard any new medication that a patient recently started as being a possible cause.[22,23]

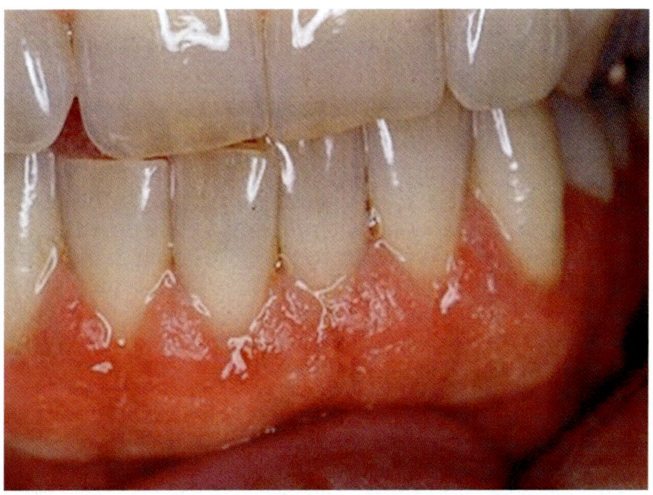

Fig. 4 Early stage of gingival hyperplasia originating from interdental papillae. (*Courtesy of* Dr John D. McDowell, Department of Diagnostics and Biological Sciences, University of Colorado School of Dental Medicine, Aurora, CO.)

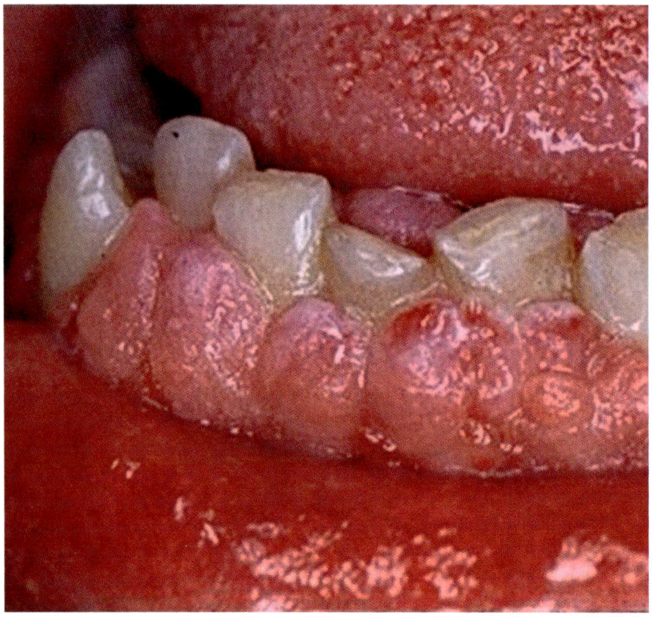

Fig. 5 Advanced stage of gingival hyperplasia covering much of crowns of lower anterior teeth. (*Courtesy of* Dr John D. McDowell, Department of Diagnostics and Biological Sciences, University of Colorado School of Dental Medicine, Aurora, CO.)

If no offending agent is detectable through the history, hyperplastic gingivitis (usually associated with pregnancy, puberty, or diabetes) and gingival fibromatosis (children) should be on the list of differential diagnoses. If bleeding is present and other systemic signs suggest other conditions that cause gingivostomatitis, including leukemia, primary herpes, or vesiculobullous disorders, those conditions should be ruled out.

Histopathology

The overlying surface epithelium may demonstrate elongation of the rete ridges, with long extensions into the underlying stroma. The lamina propria exhibits an increased amount of fibrous connective tissue that demonstrates a normal density of fibroblasts.[19] No histologic features are specific to drug-related gingival hyperplasia.

Treatment considerations

Discontinuation of the offending medication often results in cessation of progression, and possibly some regression.[3,19–23] Substitution of 1 medication for another in the same class may be beneficial.[3,19] A multidisciplinary approach should be taken in treatment, including discussing the process with patient's primary care physician, along with assessment of possible discontinuation or alteration to the offending agent. If the drug cannot be alternated, efficient oral hygiene for plaque control and frequent professional cleaning are very important to control the severity of GH.[3,19,24,25] Azithromycin has been shown to improve GH (especially for cyclosporine-induced GH).[3,19,25] Other treatment options that have been reported include metronidazole and roxithromycin therapy; however, these have been studied less than azithromycin.[3,19,25–27] Surgical removal of the excess tissues may be a treatment of choice, especially if the patient suffers from a functional difficulty or if esthetic appearance is a major concern for the patient.[3,19]

Newer evolving medications, biologics

Brief description

In the past several decades, there has been a significant increase in the use of biologics to treat chronic disease including autoimmune disorders such as rheumatoid arthritis (RA), inflammatory bowel disease (IBD), psoriasis, and ankylosing spondylitis.[28–32] Biologics or biopharmaceuticals are drugs extracted or semi-synthesized from a biological source. Discussion in this article focuses on genetically engineered newer biologics such as monoclonal antibodies and fusion protein drugs. Commonly used biologics for chronic disease include antitumor necrosis factor (anti-TNF) antibody and various interleukin inhibitors. The development of biologics has been rapid, and their use is expanding; as a result, the number patients using these agents is increasing.[28–33] Thus, oral health care providers will likely manage more patients taking biologics in the future, and they should be aware of potential adverse reactions in the oral cavity.

Incidence/clinical features

Increased cutaneous infection and drug eruptions have been reported and are well described.[33,34] However, the effect on oral mucosa has been considerably less documented. There are multiple literature reports of increased oral candidiasis as well as colonization of *Candida* species in this group of patients.[35–37] There is controversy related to any increased risk of malignancy. One meta-analysis showed that patients are at about a fourfold increased risk of developing cancers when treated with high-dose anti-TNF antibody compared with a placebo.[38] One large cohort study found no increased risk of malignancy.[39] Another meta-analysis found an increased risk of developing only nonmelanoma skin cancers.[40] There are some case reports that suggests an association between anti- TNF and malignancy or premalignant lesions.[41–43] Drug eruptions involving oral mucosa vary and may manifest as a lichenoid reaction, vesicle/bullae, or ulcer (Fig. 6).[44,45]

Differential diagnosis

The possibility of an association between biological agents and oral disease should be considered if the onset of the oral

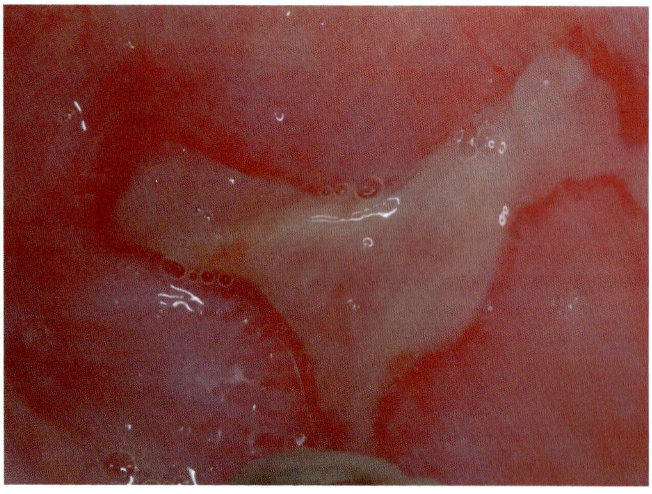

Fig. 6 Ulcer on left buccal mucosa that was caused by anti-TNF agent.

disease and the initiation of these agents were concurrent. The diagnosis should be made based upon the patient's clinical presentation in conjunction with patient history.

Treatment considerations

Because many patients take biologics because other therapies have been ineffective, it may be difficult to discontinue or alter the use of these agents. A multidisciplinary approach is important in identifying a possible alternative to the offending agent. Disease severity and tolerability of the oral complications, as well as the manageability of the complications with supportive therapy, should be taken into the consideration. If the discontinuation or alteration of the offending agent is not a viable option, supportive therapy should be considered.

Acknowledgments

The author thanks Dr John D. McDowell, who provided insight, expertise, and clinical pictures that greatly assisted this article. The author thanks Dr Robert Greer and Dr Brad J. Potter for comments that greatly improved the article.

References

1. Ortman JM, Velkoff VA, Hogan H. An aging nation: the older population in the United States, current population reports, P25–1140. Washington, DC: U.S. Census Bureau; 2014. Available at: https://www.census.gov/prod/2014pubs/p25-1140.pdf.
2. Al-Khudari S, Loochtan MJ, Peterson E, et al. Management of angiotensin-converting enzyme inhibitor-induced angioedema. Laryngoscope 2011;121:2327–34.
3. Neville BW, Damm DD, Allen CM, et al. Oral and maxillofacial pathology. 4th edition. St Louis (MO): Elsevier; 2015.
4. Nguyen V, Simon L, Jaqua E. Allergic dermatoses. Prim Care Clin Off Pract 2016;43(3):433–49.
5. Sanchez-Borges M, Capriles-Hulett A, Caballero-Fonseca F. NSAID-induced urticaria and angioedema: a reappraisal of its clinical management. Am J Clin Dermatol 2002;3(9):599–607.
6. Kaplan A, Greaves M. Angioedema. J Am Acad Dermatol 2005;53: 373–88.
7. Mahmoudpour SH, Baranova EV, Souverein PC, et alPREDICTION-ADR consortium. Determinants of angiotensin-converting enzyme inhibitor (ACEI) intolerance and angioedema in the UK clinical practice research datalink. Br J Clin Pharmacol 2016;82(6): 1647–59.
8. Zuraw B. Hereditary angioedema. N Engl J Med 2008;359:1027–36.
9. Scalese MJ, Reinaker TS. Pharmacologic management of angioedema induced by angiotensin-converting enzyme inhibitors. Am J Health Syst Pharm 2016;73(12):873–9.
10. Bova M, Guilarte M, Sala-Cunill A, et al. Treatment of ACEI-related angioedema with icatibant: a case series. Intern Emerg Med 2015; 10(3):345–50.
11. Celentano A, Tovaru S, Yap T, et al. Oral erythema multiforme: trends and clinical findings of a large retrospective European case series. Oral Surg Oral Med Oral Pathol Oral Radiol 2015;120(6): 707–16.
12. Shah SN, Chauhan GR, Manjunatha BS, et al. Drug induced erythema multiforme: two case series with review of literature. J Clin Diagn Res 2014;8(9):ZH01–4.
13. Joseph TI, Vargheese G, George D, et al. Drug induced oral erythema multiforme: a rare and less recognized variant of erythema multiforme. J Oral Maxillofac Pathol 2012;16(1):145–8.
14. Sokumbi O, Wetter DA. Clinical features, diagnosis, and treatment of erythema multiforme: a review for the practicing dermatologist. Int J Dermatol 2012;51(8):889–902.
15. Wetter DA, Davis MDP. Recurrent erythema multiforme: clinical characteristics, etiologic associations, and treatment in a series of 48 patients at Mayo Clinic, 2000 to 2007. J Am Acad Dermatol 2010; 62:45–53.
16. Lee MK, Kwon WJ, Cho EB, et al. Imatinib mesylate-induced erythema multiforme: recurrence after rechallenge with 200 mg/day imatinib. Ann Dermatol 2015;27(5):641–3.
17. Tan ZH, Thoon KC, Koh MJ. Case series of three infants with erythema multiforme following hepatitis B vaccination. Pediatr Neonatal 2016;57(1):72–5.
18. Samim F, Auluck A, Zed C, et al. Erythema multiforme: a review of epidemiology, pathogenesis, clinical features, and treatment. Dent Clin North Am 2013;57(4):583–96.
19. Scully C, Bagan JV. Adverse drug reactions in the orofacial region. Crit Rev Oral Biol Med 2004;15:221–39.
20. Kaur G, Verhamme KM, Dieleman JP, et al. Association between calcium channel blockers and gingival hyperplasia. J Clin Periodontol 2010;37(7):625–30.
21. Bhatia V, Mittal A, Parida AK, et al. Amlodipine induced gingival hyperplasia: a rare entity. Int J Cardiol 2007;122(3):e23–4.
22. Salman A, Tekin B, Koca S, et al. Another adverse effect of vemurafenib: gingival hyperplasia. J Dermatol 2016;43(6): 706–7.
23. Mangold AR, Bryce A, Sekulic A. Vemurafenib-associated gingival hyperplasia in patient with metastatic melanoma. J Am Acad Dermatol 2014;71(5):e205–6.
24. Aral CA, Dilber E, Aral K, et al. Management of cyclosporine and nifedipine-induced gingival hyperplasia. J Clin Diagn Res 2015; 9(12):ZD12–5.
25. Dongari-Bagtzoglou AResearch, Science and Therapy CommitteeAmerican Academy of Periodontology. Drug-associated gingival enlargement. J Periodontol 2004;75(10):1424–31.
26. Ramalho VL, Ramalho HJ, Cipullo JP, et al. Comparison of azithromycin and oral hygiene program in the treatment of cyclosporine-induced gingival hyperplasia. Ren Fail 2007;29(3): 265–70.
27. Conde SA, Aarestrup FM, Vieira BJ, et al. Roxithromycin reduces cyclosporine-induced gingival hyperplasia in renal transplant patients. Transplant Proc 2008;40(5):1435–8.
28. Mutlu GM, Mutlu EA, Bellmeyer A, et al. Pulmonary adverse events of anti-tumor necrosis factor-alpha antibody therapy. Am J Med 2006;119(8):639–46.
29. Feldmann M, Charles P, Taylor P, et al. Biological insights from clinical trials with anti-TNF therapy. Springer Semin Immunopathol 1998;20:211–28.
30. Geale K, Henriksson M, Schmitt-Egenolf M. Evaluating equality in psoriasis healthcare: a cohort study of the impact of age on prescription of biologics. Br J Dermatol 2016;174(3):579–87.
31. Romero-Jimenez RM, Escudero-Vilaplana V, Baniandres Rodriguez O, et al. Efficiency of biological therapies in patients with moderate to severe psoriasis: impact of a pharmacotherapeutic protocol. J Dermatolog Treat 2016;27(3):198–202.
32. Mease PJ. Do biologic-treated psoriatic arthritis patients with spondylitis respond differently with or without concomitant methotrexate from patients without spondylitis? J Rheumatol 2016;43(3):471–3.
33. Hagen JW, Magro CM, Crowson AN. Emerging adverse cutaneous drug reactions. Dermatol Clin 2012;30(4):695–730. vii.
34. Flendrie M, Vissers WH, Creemers MC, et al. Dermatological conditions during TNF-alpha-blocking therapy in patients with rheumatoid arthritis: a prospective study. Arthritis Res Ther 2005;7(3): R666–76.
35. Moen K, Kvalvik AG, Hellem S, et al. The long-term effect of anti TNF-alpha treatment on temporomandibular joints, oral mucosa, and salivary flow in patients with active rheumatoid arthritis: a pilot study. Oral Surg Oral Med Oral Pathol Oral Radiol Endod 2005;100: 433–40.
36. Corazza M, Zauli S, Ricci M, et al. Does anti-tumour necrosis factor-alpha increase oral candida colonization? A case–control study in psoriatic patients. Acta Derm Venereol 2013;93(3):352–3.

37. Kaur N, Mahl TC. Pneumocystis carinii pneumonia with oral candidiasis after infliximab therapy for Crohn's disease. Dig Dis Sci 2004;49:1458–60.
38. Bongartz T, Sutton AJ, Sweeting MJ, et al. Anti-TNF antibody therapy in rheumatoid arthritis and the risk of serious infections and malignancies: systematic review and meta-analysis of rare harmful effects in randomized controlled trials. JAMA 2006;295:2275–85.
39. Raaschou P, Simard JF, Neovius M, et alAnti-Rheumatic Therapy in Sweden Study Group. Does cancer that occurs during or after anti-tumor necrosis factor therapy have a worse prognosis? A national assessment of overall and site-specific cancer survival in rheumatoid arthritis patients treated with biologic agents. Arthritis Rheum 2011;63:1812–22.
40. Mariette X, Matucci-Cerinic M, Pavelka K, et al. Malignancies associated with tumour necrosis factor inhibitors in registries and prospective observational studies: a systematic review and meta-analysis. Ann Rheum Dis 2011;70:1895–904.
41. Rahman N, Healy C, Flint SR, et al. Cautionary note: a possible association between oral squamous cell carcinoma and tumor necrosis factor antagonists; need for oral screening. J Clin Rheumatol 2010;16(4):197–9.
42. Chainani-Wu N, Chang C, Gross AJ, et al. Oropharyngeal carcinoma arising after methotrexate and etanercept therapy for rheumatoid arthritis. Oral Surg Oral Med Oral Pathol Oral Radiol 2014;117(3): e261–3.
43. Leao JC, Duarte A, Gueiros LA, et al. Severe oral epithelial dysplasia in a patient receiving adalimumab therapy. J Oral Pathol Med 2005;34(7):447–8.
44. Boussemart L, Jacobelli S, Batteux F, et al. Autoimmune bullous skin diseases occurring under anti-tumor necrosis factor therapy: two case reports. Dermatology 2010;221(3):201–5.
45. De Simone C, Caldarola G, D'Agostino M, et al. Lichenoid reaction induced by adalimumab. J Eur Acad Dermatol Venereol 2008;22(5): 626–7.

Oral Complications of Nonsurgical Cancer Therapies

Sharon Elad, DMD, MSc [a,*], Yehuda Zadik, DMD, MHA [b,c], Noam Yarom, DMD [d,e]

KEYWORDS

• Mucositis • Osteonecrosis • Medication related osteonecrosis of the jaws • Cancer • Immunosuppression • Chemotherapy • Radiotherapy • Hematopoietic stem cell transplantation

KEY POINTS

- There are a variety of nonsurgical cancer treatment modalities, such as chemotherapy, radiotherapy, hematopoietic stem cell transplantation, and targeted therapy.
- Each modality uses various protocols, medications, and techniques, and therefore a wide range of oral complications occur.
- The complications may be specific to the mouth, affecting the oral mucosa, salivary glands, dentition and gingivae; the complications may also affect the musculoskeletal system or sensory system.
- Complications may be non—tissue specific, such as bleeding, infection, secondary malignancy, and developmental disturbances.
- The range and severity of oral complications highlight the importance of appropriate management to optimize oral function, quality of life, and well-being.

Introduction

The aim of this article is to review the oral complications of nonsurgical cancer therapy. Novel treatments and advances in existing treatments come with a new set of side effects and complications, particularly in the radiation oncology and immunotherapy fields. This section will cover the oral complications following nonsurgical treatment modalities: chemotherapy, radiotherapy (RT), chemoradiotherapy, hematopoietic stem cell transplantation (HSCT), and targeted therapy.

Table 1 lists oral complications, organized according to the tissue affected. The text expands on most of these complications and when applicable refers to detailed reviews. The clinical photos show the plethora of oral complications.

Disclosures: S. Elad is the Medical Expert of the BUM5 study, sponsored by Falk Pharma, GmbH; Y. Zadik is a co-investigator in the BUM5 study, sponsored by Falk Pharma, GmbH; N. Yarom is a site Principal Investigator for the BRONJ study, sponsored by Micromedic Technologies Ltd, Israel.

[a] Department of Oral Medicine, Eastman Institute for Oral Health, University of Rochester Medical Center, 625 Elmwood Avenue, Rochester, NY 14620, USA

[b] Oral Medicine Clinic for Hematologic and Oncologic Patients, Department of Oral Medicine, Sedation and Maxillofacial Imaging, Hebrew University-Hadassah School of Dental Medicine, PO Box 91120, Jerusalem 9112102, Israel

[c] Department of Oral Medicine, Oral and Maxillofacial Center, Medical Corps, Israel Defense Forces, Military PO Box 02149, Tel Hashomer, Israel

[d] Oral Medicine Unit, Sheba Medical Center, Tel Hashomer, Israel

[e] Department of Oral Pathology and Oral Medicine, School of Dental Medicine, Tel Aviv University, Tel Aviv, Israel

* Corresponding author.

E-mail address: selad@urmc.rochester.edu

Oral mucosal complications

Mucositis

- The toxicity of chemotherapy, RT or combination affecting the oral mucosa, causing inflammation and tissue damage is termed oral mucositis. Clinically, it manifests as painful erythema and ulcerations.
- The incidence of oral mucositis varies according to treatment modality. For chemotherapy-associated mucositis, the cytotoxic agents used and the intensity of the regimen are among the main factors that determine the severity of the mucositis. In HSCT and hematologic malignancies, neutropenia is an additional risk factor. In head and neck cancer treated with RT the field of oral mucosa receiving weekly cumulative doses of approximately 10 Gy is at the greatest risk for lesions of mucositis. The use of concomitant chemoradiotherapy increases the risk for mucositis, as does the introduction of targeted therapy.[1] The wide range of mucosal responses to the same cancer treatment regimens have not been explained,[2,3] and the role genetics plays in these oral manifestations has recently gained attention.[4]
- The clinical features include localized or generalized denudation of the oral mucosa; frank ulcers on the nonkeratinized mucosa covered with fibrinous pseudomembranes are also seen (Fig. 1). The pain may be so severe that oral intake is impaired, cancer treatment is interfered with, opioid use increases, hospitalization is prolonged, and quality of life is reduced. Furthermore, oral mucositis may increase the risk of systemic spread of infection.[5]
- The differential diagnosis includes infection and drug eruptions. Local trauma from sharp anatomic structures or restorative materials may further irritate the injured

Atlas Oral Maxillofacial Surg Clin N Am 25 (2017) 133-147

http://dx.doi.org/10.1016/j.cxom.2017.04.006

Table 1 Oral complications associated with nonsurgical cancer therapy

Category	Tissue	Oral complication	Early presentation	Late presentation
Tissue-specific manifestations	Mucosa	Mucositis	+	+
		Anemia-related mucosal changes: atrophy and burning, paleness	+	−
		Neutropenic ulcer	+	−
		Lichenoid, erythema, and ulcers (cGVHD)	−	+
		Pyogenic granuloma	−	+
		Targeted therapy–associated stomatitis	+	+
		Targeted therapy–associated lichenoid	+	+
		Chemotherapy-associated pigmentation	−	+
		Targeted therapy–associated pigmentation	−	+
	Salivary glands	Salivary hypofunction	+	+
		Sialoadenitis	+	+
		Mucocele (cGVHD)	−	+
	Musculoskeletal complications	Osteoradionecrosis	−	+
		Drug-induced osteonecrosis of the jaw	−	+
		Impaired mastication	+	+
		Swallowing disorders	+	+
		Speech disorders	+	+
		Fibrosis + scarring + trismus (limited neck and shoulder mobility)	−	+
		Loss of elasticity, reduced range of motion and limited mouth opening (scleroderma-like GVHD)	−	−
	Sensory disturbances	Dysgeusia	+	+
		Neuropathy – dental/orofacial	−	+
		Tooth hypersensitivity	−	+
	Teeth and gingivae	Increased dental demineralization and caries	−	+
		Pulp necrosis/obliteration (cGVHD)	−	+
		Gingival enlargement	−	+
		Desquamative gingivitis (cGVHD)	−	+
		Acute periodontal infections	+	+
		Preexisting chronic periodontal infections	+	+
Non–tissue specific manifestations	Bleeding	Thrombocytopenia	+	+
		DIC	+	+
	Infection	Viral	+	+
		Bacterial	+	+
		Fungal	+	+
	Malignancy	Squamous cell carcinoma	−	+
		Posttransplant lymphoproliferative disorder	−	+
		Postradiation sarcoma	−	+
	Developmental	Developmental disturbances of teeth and craniofacial growth in pediatric patients	−	+

Abbreviations: cGVHD, chronic graft-versus-host disease; DIC, disseminated intravascular coagulation.

mucosa. Additional differential diagnoses depend on the cancer treatment modality. For chemotherapy-associated oral mucositis, the clinician should consider for differential diagnosis neutropenic ulcers. For HSCT-associated mucositis the differential diagnosis of the ulcerations may be neutropenic ulcers or acute graft-versus-host disease (GVHD). For RT-associated mucositis, if the findings are localized to the surgical site, postoperative complications should be suspected as differential diagnosis.

- Evidence-based clinical practice guidelines for the management of mucositis were developed by Multinational Association of Supportive Care in Cancer/International Society of Oral Oncology (MASCC/ISOO).[6] The most recent edition suggests treatments as outlined on Table 2. The MASCC/ISOO guidelines are being updated at this time.
- Chronic forms of oral mucositis were described after RT. Two subtypes were suggested: (1) persistent type, when the lesions do not heal within 3 months after the completion of the RT and (2) recurrent type, when new discrete ulcers wax and wane after the completion of RT.[7]

Neutropenic ulcer

- Neutropenic patients may present with ulceration of the nonkeratinized mucosa, with no obvious infectious cause or correlation to cytotoxic therapy.
- The incidence is unknown because most of the literature is based on case reports or small case series.
- Clinically, the ulceration may be surrounded by a diffuse area of erythema (Fig. 2). The ulcerative lesions vary in shape and size, ranging from irregular elliptical shapes to extensive amorphous lesions. The ulcerations may be deep and occur simultaneously in multiple sites. The

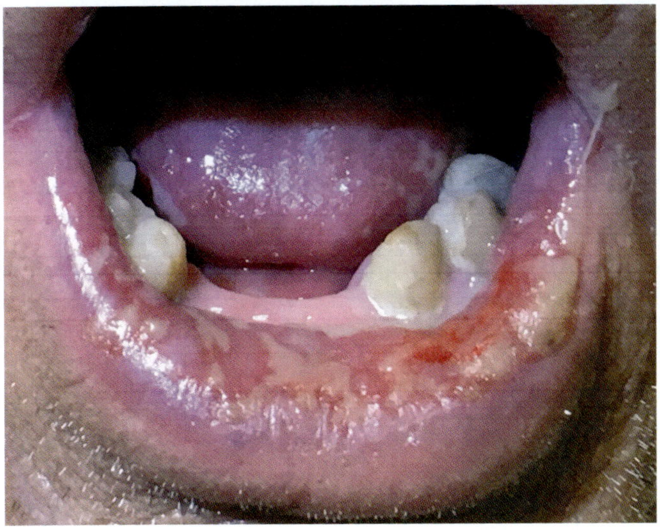

Fig. 1 Oral mucositis.

lesions may recur during repeated neutropenic periods, and tend to heal spontaneously when neutrophil counts return to normal range.[8]

- The primary differential diagnosis is infection, recurrent aphthous ulcers, ischemic complication of the leukemic infiltrate, or drug eruption.
- The treatment approach includes palliation of pain, prevention of secondary infection, and accelerating the recovery of the neutrophil count with growth factors, such as granulocyte macrophage colony stimulating factor.[9]

Lichenoid, erythema, and ulcers (chronic graft-versus-host-disease)

- Graft versus host disease (GVHD) is a complication of allogeneic HSCT that is triggered by the discrepancy between the self and the graft, leading to a reaction of the donor cells against the host organs. In the chronic form of GVHD the mouth is commonly affected and the oral mucosa typically presents lichenoid changes, erythema, or ulceration (Fig. 3). Other oral manifestations of cGVHD will be discussed below.

Pyogenic granuloma

- Pyogenic granuloma is a benign solitary polypoid soft lesion formed by highly vascularized granulation and fibrous tissue, often caused by trauma. This lesion has been reported in patients with oral chronic GVHD (cGVHD), and it seems that either the chronic inflammation of the mucosa or the treatment of GVHD with calcineurin inhibitors contribute to the development of the lesion.[10,11]

Targeted therapy–associated stomatitis

- The term stomatitis in relation to targeted therapy is frequently used to describe aphthouslike lesions. The early reports associated mammalian target of rapamycin inhibitors with this type of oral ulceration: sirolimus (Rapamune), everolimus (Afinitor), and temsirolimus (Torisel). Tyrosine kinase inhibitors, specifically sunitinib (Sutent), sorafenib (Nexavar), and pazopanib (Votrien), were reported to cause mucositis or stomatitis, but it is unclear if the presentation is aphthouslike.[12] Additional medications with similar mechanisms of action, involving the epidermal growth factor receptor, may cause the same oral adverse reaction.
- The incidence is dose related and varies by medication. For mammalian target of rapamycin inhibitors, the prevalence of any mucositis was reported as 2% to 73%, and the prevalence of severe mucositis was up to 21%.[13,14]
- The common clinical presentation is elliptical ulcerations, covered by a yellowish pseudomembrane, with an erythematous periphery (Fig. 4). The lesions may appear simultaneously in multiple sites. Similar to the major type of aphthous ulcers, in target therapy associated stomatitis the ulcerations may exceed 10 mm in size, with a less well-defined shape. Similar to the herpetiform type of aphthous ulcers, clustered distribution of lesions was also reported in targeted therapy associated stomatitis. Often the lesions are painful and impair quality of life.[15]
- Targeted therapy–associated aphthouslike stomatitis responds well to topical, oral, intralesional, and/or systemic steroids. This efficacy contrasts the lack of response to steroidal treatment in oral mucositis associated with chemotherapy or RT. If the symptoms are severe, dose reduction of the causative therapy may be needed. Furthermore, during episodes of severe stomatitis, it is important to maintain good hydration and oral intake. Patients are encouraged to have good oral hygiene to reduce the bacterial inoculum in the oral cavity.

Targeted therapy–associated lichenoid

- Nivolumab (anti–PD-1 antibody) and pembrolizumab (anti–PD-L1 antibodies) were reported to induce oral lesions with a lichenoid appearance. Nivolumab (Opdivo) is currently indicated for non–small cell lung cancer, metastatic melanoma, advanced renal cell carcinoma, squamous cell carcinoma of the head and neck, and for certain patients with Hodgkin disease. Pembrolizumab (Kytruda) is indicated for the same malignancies, except Hodgkin disease. The triggering of T-cell activation by these medications may explain the lichenoid reactions.
- As the use of these medications increases, the lichenoid adverse effect will become more noticeable and reported more often.
- The typical lichenoid presentation includes white reticulation and papules on multiple mucosal surfaces. The lesions may be symptomatic.
- Treatment is directed at relieving symptoms and minimizing the erosive/ulcerative component. The specific treatments for lichen planus are detailed in this issue (see Paolo G. Arduino's article, "Oral Complications of Dermatologic Disorders"). Considering the similarity to lichen planus, and the definition of lichen planus as a potentially malignant disorder, periodic reevaluation of the oral tissues is recommended.

Chemotherapy-associated hyperpigmentation

- Multiple cytotoxic medications were suggested to cause hyperpigmentation.
- Examples for such agents include doxorubicin, busulfan, cyclophosphamide, 5-fluorouracil, bleomycin, daunorubicin (daunomycin), and hydroxyurea.[16]
- This is usually a grayish or brownish pigmentation, involving multiple sites.

Targeted therapy–associated hyperpigmentation

- Imatinib (Gleevec) was reported in the literature in association with melanosis of the hard palate. Imatinib is a

Table 2 Summary of Multinational Association of Supportive Care in Cancer/International Society of Oral Oncology management guidelines for oral mucositis per treatment modality

	CT	RT	RT-CT	HSCT
Recommendations in favor				
Prevention of oral mucositis				
30 min of oral cryotherapy in patients receiving bolus 5-fluorouracil chemotherapy	X[a]	—	—	—
Recombinant human keratinocyte growth factor-1 (KGF-1/palifermin) at a dose of 60 μg/kg/d for 3 d before conditioning treatment and for 3 d posttransplantation in patients receiving high-dose chemotherapy and total body irradiation, followed by autologous stem cell transplantation, for a hematologic malignancy	—	—	—	X[a]
Low-level laser therapy (wavelength at 650 nm, power of 40 mW, and each square centimeter treated with the required time to a tissue energy dose of 2 J/cm^2) in patients receiving HSCT conditioned with high-dose chemotherapy, with or without total body irradiation	—	—	—	X[a]
Benzydamine mouthwash to prevent oral mucositis in patients with head and neck cancer receiving moderate dose radiation therapy (≤50 Gy), without concomitant chemotherapy	—	X[a]	—	—
Treatment of pain from oral mucositis				
Patient-controlled analgesia with morphine in patients undergoing HSCT	—	—	—	X
Suggestions in favor				
Prevention of oral mucositis				
Oral care protocols be used in all age groups and across all cancer treatment modalities	X	X	X	X
Oral cryotherapy in patients receiving high-dose melphalan, with or without total body irradiation, as conditioning for HSCT	—	—	—	X[a]
Low-level laser therapy (wavelength around 632.8 nm) in patients undergoing radiotherapy, without concomitant chemotherapy, for head and neck cancer	—	X[a]	—	—
Systemic zinc supplements administered orally may be of benefit in oral cancer patients receiving radiation therapy or chemoradiation	—	X	X	—
Treatment of pain from oral mucositis				
Transdermal fentanyl may be effective in patients receiving conventional or high-dose chemotherapy, with or without total body irradiation	—	—	—	X
0.2% morphine mouthwash may be effective in patients receiving chemoradiation for head and neck cancer	—	—	X	—
0.5% doxepin mouthwash may be effective	X	X	X	X

Recommendations and suggestions against use of certain agents for oral mucositis can be found on the full version of the Multinational Association of Supportive Care in Cancer/International Society of Oral Oncology guidelines.

Abbreviations: CT, chemotherapy; CT-RT, combined chemotherapy and radiotherapy; HSCT, hematopoietic stem cell transplantation; RT, radiotherapy.

[a] Applicable to a specific setting in this patient population.

Adapted from Lalla RV, Bowen J, Barasch A, et al. MASCC/ISOO clinical practice guidelines for the management of mucositis secondary to cancer therapy. Cancer 2014;120(10):1453–61; with permission.

tyrosine kinase inhibitor indicated for the treatment of a series of hematologic malignancies and gastrointestinal stromal tumors.

- There are only a handful of case reports about this rare complication.
- Clinically, the hyperpigmenation is localized to the hard palate, and is painless without swelling.[17] Occasionally, there is also hyperpigmentation on the tip of the nose or the ear lobes.
- This is a paradoxic adverse event because imatinib reportedly induced hypopigmentation manifesting as generalized skin lightening. The mechanism of the hyperpigmentation is unclear.
- The differential diagnosis includes racial pigmentation, melanoma, pigmentation owing to other medications, and adrenal gland disorders.[18] In patients after HSCT, the hyperpigmentation may be a result of oral cGVHD. Other oral pigmented lesions or systemic diseases manifesting in oral pigmented lesions are less likely owing to the diffuseness, location, and extensiveness of the lesions.
- No interventions are needed once the diagnosis has been confirmed and imatinib use can continue.

Salivary gland complications

Salivary gland hypofunction

- Salivary gland hypofunction and the subjective dry mouth sensation (xerostomia) are common adverse effects of cancer treatment. Salivary gland hypofunction is a decrease in salivary secretion, and is considered pathologic when secretion is 0.1 mL/min or less for unstimulated whole salivary flow and 0.5 mL/min or less for stimulated whole salivary flow.[19]

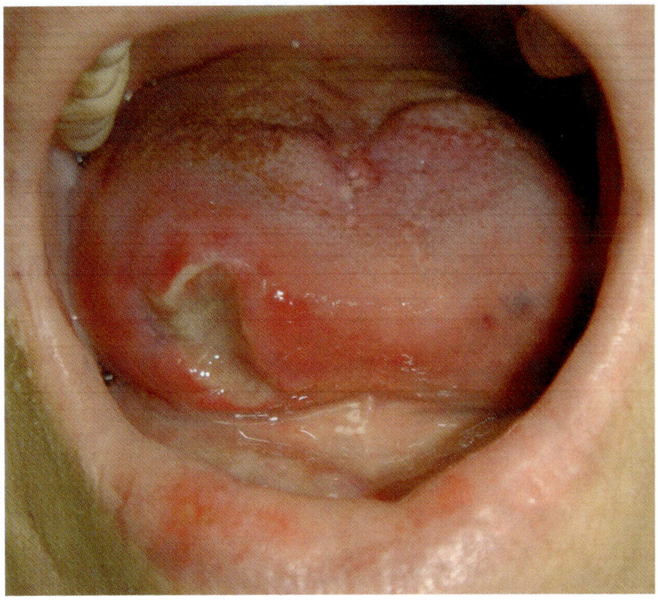

Fig. 2 Neutropenic ulcer.

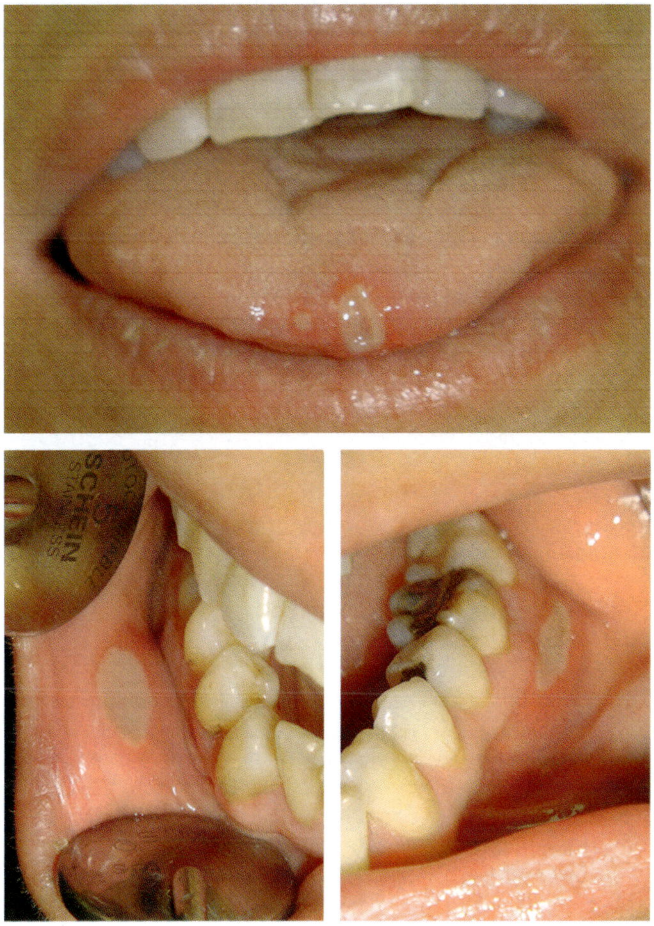

Fig. 4 Mammalian target of rapamycin inhibitor stomatitis, simultaneous ulcerations.

- The prevalence of salivary gland hypofunction varies according to the type of cancer treatment. For patients undergoing conventional RT for head and neck cancer, the important determinant is the cumulative radiation dose to the gland tissue. Therefore, techniques that spare the salivary glands from the ionizing beam are expected to reduce the prevalence of salivary gland hypofunction. The prevalence of xerostomia increases dramatically to 81% during RT, and remains within the 70% to 91% range at 2 years after RT.[19] It is thought that for intensity-modulated RT and proton beam RT the prevalence is lower. The prevalence of xerostomia for patients treated with chemotherapy for non–head and neck cancers was reported to be up to 59%,[20] and usually resolves within 6 to 12 months. In patients undergoing HSCT, salivary secretion is substantially reduced during conditioning and gradually recovers after transplantation. When total body irradiation is delivered as part of the conditioning regimen, the recovery is delayed and incomplete,[21] with a reported prevalence of 30%.[22] HSCT patients may develop dry mouth as a late complication of cGVHD.
- An evidence-based treatment approach was developed by the MASCC/ISOO for head and neck cancer patients. The main recommendations included parotid-sparing intensity-modulated RT to minimize salivary gland hypofunction and xerostomia, pilocarpine after RT to improve the xerostomia, and the use of oral mucosal lubricants and saliva substitutes for short-term improvement of symptoms. Likewise, the MASCC/ISOO panel suggested using acupuncture to stimulate salivary gland secretion and alleviate xerostomia, and potentially surgical intervention to transfer the submandibular salivary gland.[23] The American Academy of Oral Medicine Clinical Practice statement for the management of cancer therapy-induced salivary gland hypofunction and xerostomia included additional specifications (Box 1)[24]

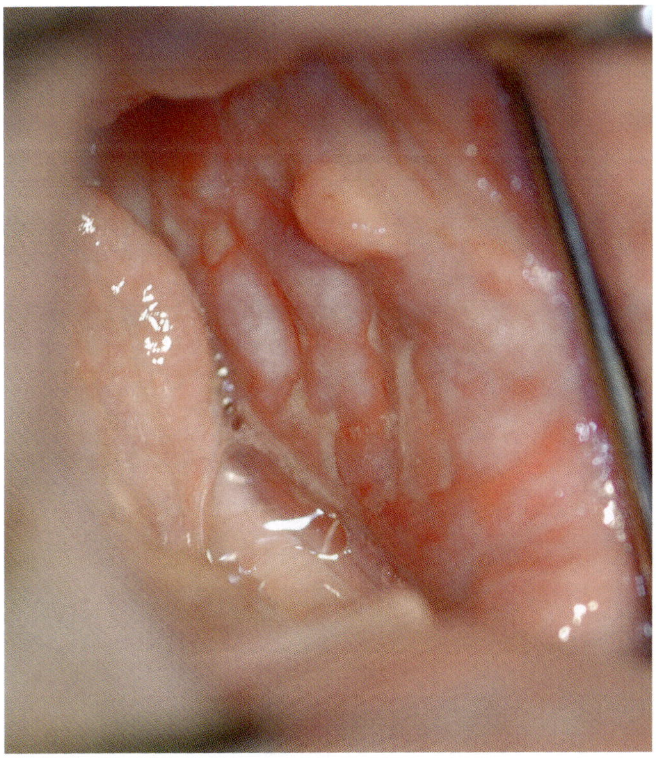

Fig. 3 Chronic graft-versus-host disease in the buccal mucosa showing white color changes, erythema, and ulceration.

Box 1. American Academy of Oral Medicine recommendations for clinical management of cancer therapy-induced salivary gland hypofunction and xerostomia

A. Ongoing monitoring to evaluate disease progression and/or effect of clinical management initiatives.
B. Stimulation of residual salivary activity by chewing and taste (eg, sugar-free chewing gum, lozenges, or mints) may be effective.
C. Pharmacologic stimulation of residual salivary activity by pilocarpine or cevimeline may be effective. However, these medications can cause significant adverse effects and are not currently approved in all countries for treatment of xerostomia.
D. Sipping water or the use of saliva substitutes (mouthwash, spray, or gel) may moisturize the oral cavity and alleviate xerostomia.
E. Bland rinses such as 0.9% saline or sodium bicarbonate solution (1 teaspoon salt and 1 teaspoon baking soda in 1 L of water) hydrate the oral cavity, alleviate xerostomia, and neutralize oral pH.
F. Acidic products should be avoided for stimulation of saliva secretion in dentate patients unless specially prepared for alleviating xerostomia.
G. Patients should be carefully instructed on how to benefit from the appropriate use of water, bland rinses, and saliva substitutes. Saliva substitutes should be used for 1 to 2 weeks before evaluating treatment efficacy.
H. Acupuncture or mild electrostimulation of the salivary glands may alleviate xerostomia in some patients.

From AAOM clinical practice statement: subject: clinical management of cancer therapy-induced salivary gland hypofunction and xerostomia. Oral Surg Oral Med Oral Pathol Oral Radiol 2016;122(3):310–2; with permission.

Sialoadenitis

- Sialoadenitis is an inflammation of the salivary glands. Often the salivary gland becomes painful and swollen, and the overlying skin becomes erythematous and warm. Constitutional signs such as fever may develop. In cancer patients, the reduced salivary flow increases the risk of a retrograde bacterial infection. This complication seems to be more common in thyroid cancer patients treated with radioactive iodine radioablation. The iodine has an affinity for the salivary glands and its accumulation in the gland increases the risk of injury.
- Treatment is usually with antibiotics, palliation, and appropriate hydration. Mechanical and gustatory stimulation of the salivary flow increases the washing effect and may be beneficial.

Mucocele

- Mucoceles occur when saliva accumulates in the submucosa. These cystlike raised lesions are typically located at the orifices of the minor salivary glands, in the soft palate, lower vestibulum, and buccal mucosa. Mucoceles are common in patients with cGVHD and may develop after RT.[25]

Musculoskeletal complications

Osteoradionecrosis

- Osteoradionecrosis (ORN), first described in 1922, is one of the most serious long-term complications of radiotherapy to the head and neck region.[26] ORN is associated with pain, morbidity, and diminished quality of life.
- The mean weighted prevalence of ORN in patients treated with conventional RT, intensity-modulated RT, and brachytherapy are 7.4%, 5.2%, and 5.3%, respectively.[27] An increased risk for ORN was reported with radiation dosages above 60 Gy, previous cancer resection, advanced dental disease, and postradiation dental extractions.[27]
- The hallmark of ORN is an exposed necrotic jawbone accompanied by erythema and swelling of the adjacent mucosa (Fig. 5). In advanced stages, submandibular cutaneous fistulae may appear and a pathologic fracture might develop.[27,28]
- To establish the diagnosis of ORN, dental infection should be excluded. Taking into account that RT was delivered owing to oral malignancy, recurrent or second primary cancer should also be excluded. Although described almost a century ago, there is still no definitive treatment for ORN. In early stages, conservative treatment (eg, antibiotics, tocopherol/pentoxifylline/clodronate, and sequestrectomy) may be considered. There is still no clear evidence for the role of hyperbaric oxygen in the management of ORN and economic/logistic issues need to be considered.[29]

Medication-related osteonecrosis of the jaw

- Medication-related osteonecrosis of the jaw (MRONJ) secondary to the use of certain drug classes was first described in 2003. Antiresoptive drugs (eg, bisphosphonates, denusomab) are most frequently associated with osteonecrosis of the jaw, whereas only sporadic cases associated with antiangiogenic agents (eg, bevacizumab, sunitinib, sorafenib) have been published.[30]
- The risk for MRONJ increases with the duration of treatment with the relevant medications. Old age, diabetes

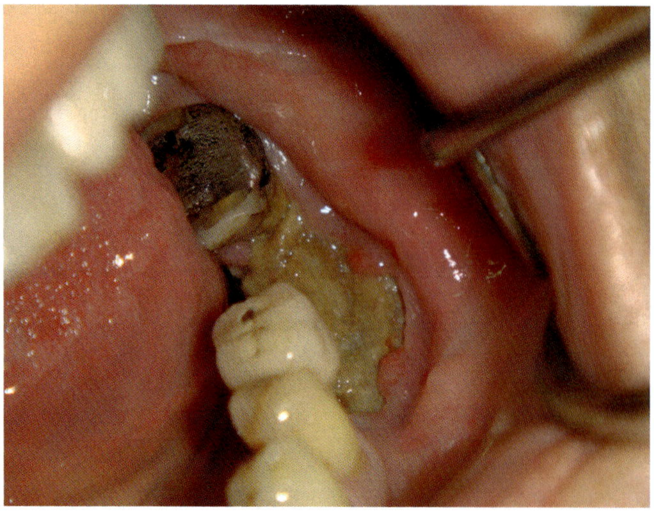

Fig. 5 Osteoradionecrosis.

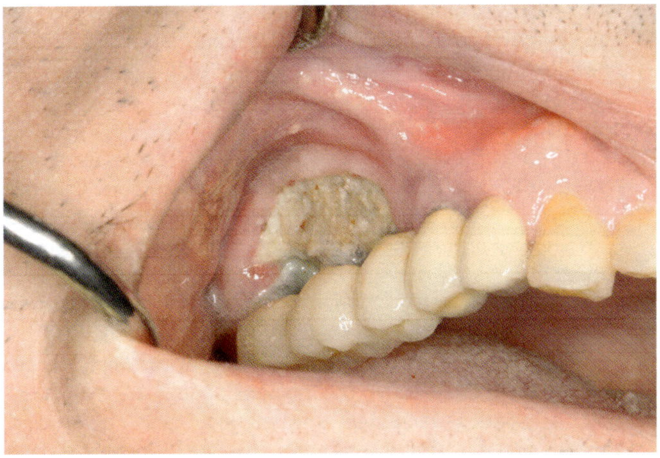

Fig. 6 Medication-related osteonecrosis of the jaw: clinical presentation.

mellitus, smoking, and dentoalveolar procedures may increase the risk for MRONJ.[31]

- The 2 populations at risk for MRONJ are cancer patients and osteoporosis patients. The cumulative incidence of MRONJ among cancer patients is relatively high (range, 0.7%–6.7%). However, the incidence of MRONJ after tooth extraction increases dramatically (range, 1.6%–14.8% for cancer patients).[31]
- To establish the diagnosis of MRONJ, exposed bone or bone that can be probed through an intraoral or extraoral fistula should be evident. Other clinical features include purulent discharge, erythema, swelling, and pain (Figs. 6 and 7). In some cases, osteonecrosis of the jaw might progress and involve adjacent structures and cause oro–antral communication, mental neuropathy, and even pathologic fracture.[32,33]
- In most cases, the diagnosis of MRONJ is straightforward; however, dental infections should always be ruled out. In cancer patients treated with bisphosphonate or denosumab for bone metastases or multiple myeloma, local extension of their underlying disease must be considered.
- Treatment should be tailored individually according symptom severity, the patient's medical status, and life expectancy. In most centers, MRONJ is treated conservatively with antibiotics, topical disinfectants, and sequestrectomy. In severe and recalcitrant cases, extensive surgery and microvascular reconstruction might be beneficial.[31]

Impaired mastication

- For adequate mastication, functional nerves, muscles, jaws, and dentition are required. In addition, sufficient saliva (quality and quantity) and a functional tongue are essential for bolus formation. In oncology patients, mastication may be impaired by sensory and/or motor neurologic modifications, muscle fibrosis, jaw resection, rampant dental caries and loss of denture retention, hyposalivation, and a resected/fibrotic tongue (Fig. 8). These changes are progressive and may further impair the nutrition of the survivor owing to dysphagia, trismus, taste alteration, hyposalivation, oral mucosal pain, and depression. The enhancement of mastication ability in oncologic patients is a clinical challenge demanding a multidisciplinary approach.

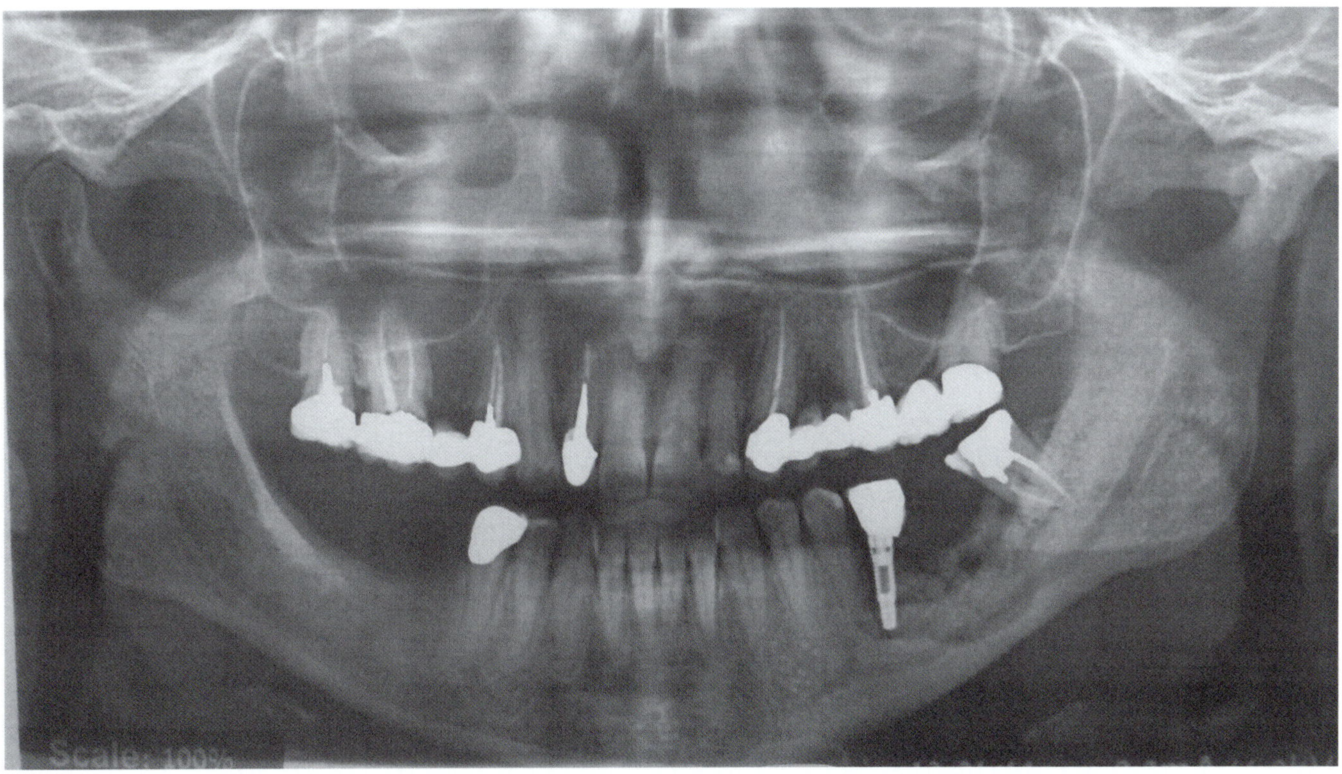

Fig. 7 Medication-related osteonecrosis of the jaw: radiologic presentation.

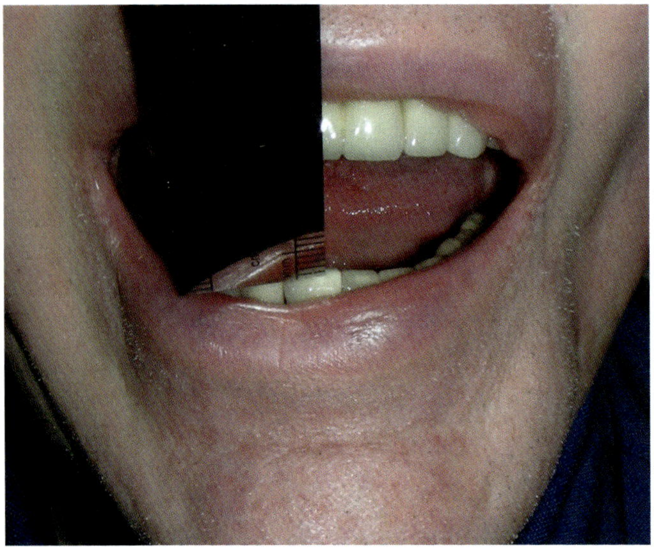

Fig. 8 Post-radiotherapy trismus (maximal mouth opening of 19 mm).

Swallowing dysfunction

- Dysphagia (swallowing dysfunction) is a common debilitating complication in head and neck cancer patients that may lead to aspiration pneumonia. Dysphagia and odynophagia (painful swallowing) are among the main obstacles of treatment intensification.[34]
- Up to two-thirds of patients present with dysphagia upon diagnosis of head and neck cancer. Approximately one-third of dysphagic patients develop aspiration pneumonia requiring treatment, with a high mortality rate (20%–65%).[35] Table 3 presents the common causes of dysphagia in cancer patients. Swallowing should be assessed before and after oncologic treatment, and early intervention by an experienced speech–language pathologist for safe swallowing strategies emphasizing avoiding aspiration is recommended (Table 4).

Speech disorder

- Disturbance of speech, voice, and resonance may impair the verbal communication of head and neck cancer survivors. Long-term postradiation cranial neuropathies (especially cranial nerves X and XII) may cause delayed speech or voice deterioration (eg, dysphonia and dysarthria, respectively).[36] New or worsening hoarseness or dysarthria may indicate a recurrence or a new malignancy and the patient should be examined accordingly. After ruling out malignancy, the patient should be evaluated by a speech–language pathologist, and behavioral voice–speech therapies and prosthetic rehabilitation should be considered. In patients after total laryngectomy, valved tracheoesophageal voice prosthesis may enhance speech intelligibility.[37] Prosthodontic obturators fabricated by an experienced maxillofacial prosthodontists may improve speech resonance in patients with palatal defects.

Restricted mouth opening in chronic graft-versus-host disease

- GVHD-related sclerodermatous disease of the tongue and perioral soft tissues impairs function of the muscles in that area, restricts range of motion of the tissues and mouth opening, and reduces vestibular depth.[38] The sclerodermatous changes slowly and irreversibly progress and dysfunction is noted, for example, difficulty eating or speaking (Fig. 9).[39] The loss of vestibular depth can prevent adequate denture retention.
- The differential diagnosis includes restricted movement owing to painful intraoral lesions or scarring from intraoral lesions. Treatment methods are similar to those for trismus (Table 5).

Table 3 Common causes of dysphagia in cancer patients

Timing		Category	Causative	Comments
Pretreatment		Tumor mass effect	Disruption/compression of the swallowing structures	Mass or infiltration
			Disruption/compression of the cranial nerves	V, VII, IX, X, XI, XII CN; mass or infiltration
			Pain	Very common
Posttreatment	Early	Radiotherapy related	Edema	
			Mucositis	Very common
	Late		Fibrosis	
			Salivary modifications	Thick, mucouslike saliva and hyposalivation; very common
			Functional modifications of sensory and motor neurons	For example, taste changes
		Surgery related	Resection	Very common
			Scarring	Very common
			Neurologic modifications	
		Other modalities	Mucositis	Chemotherapy related
			Stomatitis	Targeted therapy-related (eg, mTOR)
			Pain	Very common

Most are relevant to head and neck or lung cancer patients; chemotherapy-related mucositis and targeted therapy-related stomatitis, can also affect other cancer patients.

Abbreviations: CN, cranial nerve; mTOR, mammalian target of rapamycin.

Table 4 Modalities for the prevention and treatment of dysphagia

Purpose	Category	Method	Comments	
Prevention	Treatment planning	Planning of radiation field	Consider preexisting dysphagia	
	Lifestyle	Restriction of smoking during and after radiotherapy		
Treatment	Dietary modifications	Experienced dietician	Consultation and follow-up to ensure adequate and safe intake	
	Rehabilitative interventions	Esophageal dilation	For patients with stricture	
		Sialagogue	For example, pilocarpine	
		Management of dental caries	Prevention and early treatment	
	Compensatory maneuvers	Postures/exercises for improving swallowing function	*Role*	*Exercise*
		Mendelsohn maneuver	Prolongation of laryngeal excursion and cricopharyngeal opening during swallowing	Initiate swallowing and hold the larynx in an elevated position for 5 s
		Shaker exercises	Targeting upper esophageal sphincter-related dysphagia	Lie flat on back, lift head 10 cm, and look at toes (without lifting shoulders)
		Effortful swallow	Targeting reduced pharyngeal peristalsis with residue after swallowing	Swallowing hard, squeezing the tongue and walls of the throat together
		Chin tuck/chin to chest	Targeting the reduced bolus control, premature spillage into the larynx and decreased tongue base movement	Head rotation toward affected side: compensatory measure for unilateral pharyngeal paresis or unilateral vocal fold dysfunction or cricopharyngeal dysmotility
		Oral exercises	Targeting restricted oral range of motion	Tongue retraction, yawn etc.

Sensory disturbances

Dysgeusia

- Up to 85% of cancer patients report taste changes.[40]
- These taste disturbances may be caused by damage to the gustatory system, loss or distortion of olfactory function, systemic co-diagnosis or local oropharyngeal conditions.[41] Chemotherapy and RT may damage the taste buds directly or indirectly via the neurotoxic effects of chemotherapy or by changes in saliva quality caused by both chemotherapy and RT.

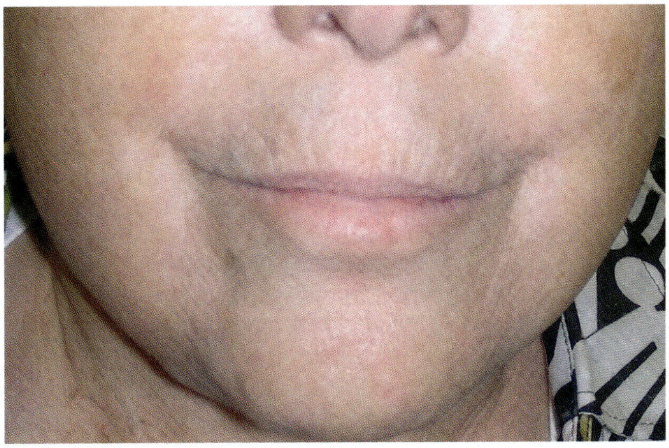

Fig. 9 Sclerodermatous graft-versus-host disease.

- Additionally, targeted therapy, such as tyrosine kinase inhibitors, have been reported to cause dysguesia[1,42]
- Dysguesia may be limited to certain types of taste. Altered taste or loss of taste may be experienced at rest, may limit oral intake, and has a marked impact on patient quality of life.
- Taste sensitivity may recover within several months, but some studies describe long-term taste change. About 20% of patients reported taste change at 6 years after HSCT.[43]

Neuropathy: tooth neuropathy and orofacial neuropathy

- Neuropathy was reported in patients treated with cytotoxics, such as vinca plant alkaloids, taxanes, bortezomib, and platinum derivatives.[44] Additionally, perioral neuropathy was found in patients treated with thalidomide, which is indicated in multiple myeloma and cGVHD. Dysesthesia was recently reported in association with targeted therapy, such as tyrosine kinase inhibitors[42]
- Oral neuropathic pain is typically described as burning, "pins and needles," numbness or tingling of the affected area. Usually no lesion is apparent at the site of the symptoms.
- Dental neurotoxicity is rare and was reported after cyclophosphamide use.[44] The pain was characterized as a severe, throbbing toothache, with no clinical or radiologic abnormalities. Palliative pulp extirpation relieved the pain, and the histologic evaluation of the pulp excluded inflammation or malignant cell infiltration.[44]

Table 5 Prevention and treatment of trismus in head and neck cancer patients and restricted mouth opening in cGVHD

Purpose	Category	Method	Comments
Prevention	Physiotherapy	Daily self-exercise of perioral/tongue muscles	Maintain the range of (vertical/horizontal) motion
	Basic oral care	Daily soft brushing and fluoride application	Maintain oral health
		Professional maintenance by dental hygienist	Every 3 mo
Treatment	Physiotherapy	Professional physiotherapy	Every 1–2 wk
		Forced opening of the jaws using the thumb and index finger	Daily self-exercise, repeated as prescribed is more important than professional physiotherapy
		Conical rubber plug	
		Stacking an increasing number of wooden tongue blades and placing them between the upper/lower incisors, 10 min, 3 times/d	
		Dynamic bite opener (Fig. 10)	
	Heat therapy	Specialized heat device	
		Placing a slightly moist warm towel on affected area, for 20 min, every 1–2 h	
		Warm intraoral saline rinse	
	Medication	Muscle relaxants (eg, benzodiazepines)	Avoid overdose and abuse
		Analgesics (eg, NSAIDs)	
		Pentoxifylline	
		Intralesional injection of corticosteroid	In cGVHD patients
		Halofuginone	Antifibrotic agent; In cGVHD patients
	Surgery	Relieving incisions in the corners of the mouth	For progressive restriction or when intraoral operation is needed
	Other	ECP	In cGVHD patients

Abbreviations: cGVHD, chronic graft-versus-host disease; ECP, extracorporeal photopheresis; NSAIDs, nonsteroidal anti-inflammatory drugs.

Data from Refs.[39,68–72]

Teeth and gingivae

Increased dental demineralization and caries (see dry mouth)

- The effects of cancer treatment, including reduced salivary flow, diet changes, and the low priority of oral hygiene, enable the oral flora to become more cariogenic.[45] These factors predispose the patient for tooth demineralization and dental caries. In cancer patients with extreme, irreversible hyposalivation, the development of dental caries is rapid, affecting tooth surfaces that are not usually affected in healthy individuals, and may result in tooth loss. Similarly, in patients diagnosed with HSCT and with oral cGVHD, salivary gland involvement may result in rampant caries and its sequalae.
- The prevalence of dental caries in cancer patients is 37.3%, 24%, and 21.4% for those treated with chemotherapy, RT, chemoradiotherapy, respectively.[46] After RT, this prevalence increase dramatically over time to 55% and 74% at 5 and 7 years after treatment, respectively.[45] In patients after HSCT, particularly those with oral cGVHD, dental caries was reported to increase during a 22-month median time period in at least 50% of the decay parameters tested.[47]
- Dental caries typically develops in fissures and proximal surfaces, and may be observed as discoloration of the dental crown. When hyposalivation is present, additional surfaces tend to be involved, such as the cervical surfaces, the roots, and to a lesser extent the incisal surfaces (Figs. 11 and 12). The early clinical presentation of demineralization is "white lesions" on the enamel. Later, the enamel becomes mottled with white-brownish stains that eventually chip off or break (Fig. 13). Often only a root will remain. Initially, the tooth may be sensitive to cold or sweet food, as decay progresses toward the pulp the patient may report pain. The sharp edges of carious teeth may irritate the oral mucosa, complicating the diagnosis of other mucosal conditions, such as chronic mucositis or oral cGVHD.[48]

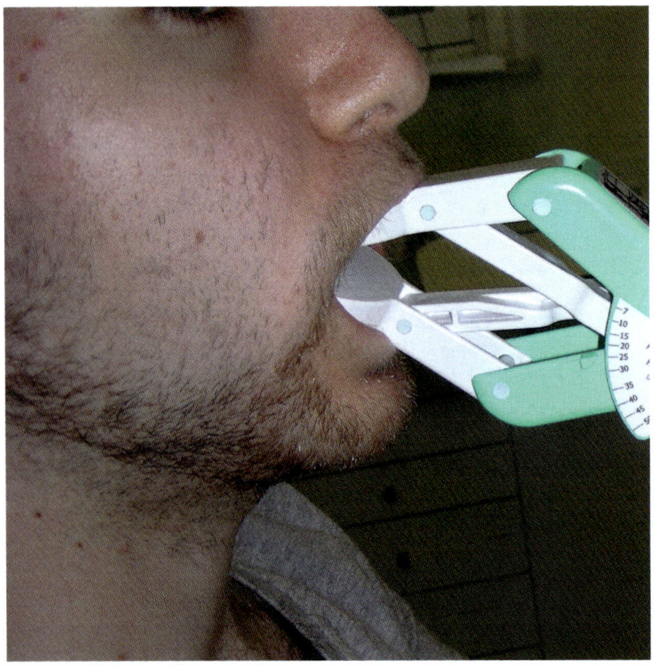

Fig. 10 Dynamic device to exercise mouth opening.

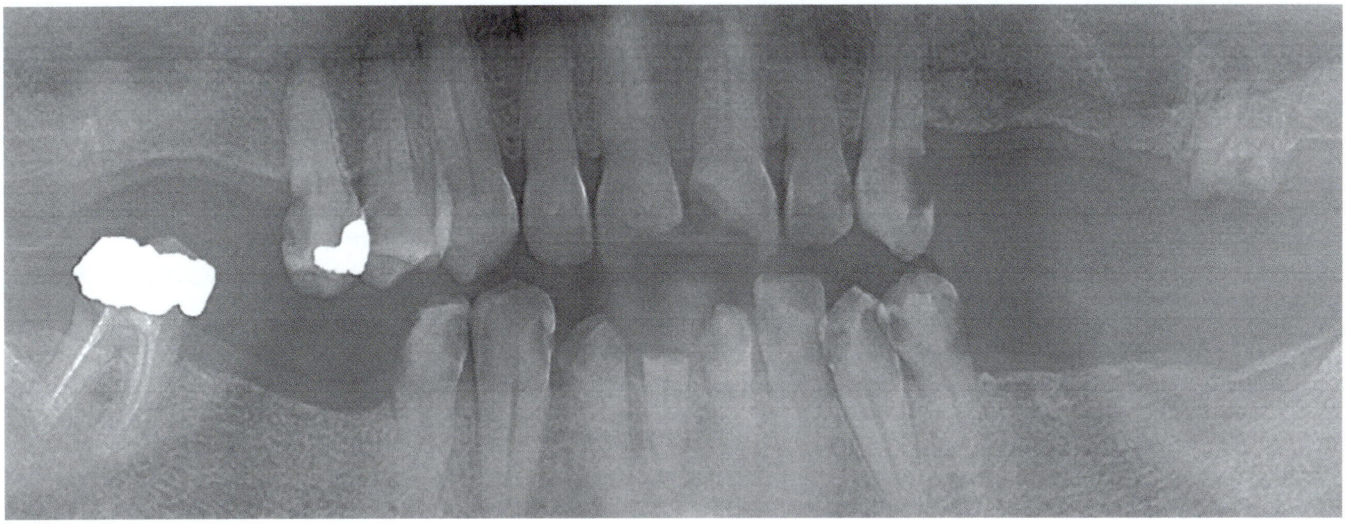

Fig. 11 Rampant caries after radiotherapy, panoramic radiographic view (sectioned).

- The main treatment objective is prevention. Before the initiation of cancer treatment, patients are advised have their teeth assessed and to remove nonrestorable teeth. They are also provided with instructions for oral hygiene and a healthy diet that minimizes caries risk. High-concentration fluoride preparations (varnish, toothpaste, gel) are applied or a prescription is provided, occasionally with customized trays. In patients with hyposalivation, such as those after RT or cGVHD, saliva stimulation using either gustatory–mechanical stimuli (chewing gum) or pharmacologic sialoguges, may slow down demineralization. Preparations based on calcium phosphate may retard the decay process by increasing remineralization. It has been suggested that preparations based on casein protein in combination with calcium and phosphate enhance remineralization and prevent dental decay.[49] In a 3-month follow-up study in head and neck cancer patients, subjects using casein protein in combination with calcium and phosphate with fluoride showed a trend toward lesser caries progression, whereas the controls using fluoride alone did not.[50] Frequent dental recalls are recommended to detect early signs of caries and initiate restorative treatment. In patients after RT or in patients with a history of bisphosphonates/denosumab, the restorative and endodontic treatment options should be maximized because extractions or implant placement increase the risk of ORN or MRONJ.

Pulp necrosis and obliteration (chronic graft-versus-host disease)

- cGVHD may manifest in the oral tissues as sclerodermatous changes. The characteristic progressive fibrosis of the soft oral tissues in scleroderma, may explain the generalized pulp calcifications observed in radiographs.[51]

Gingival enlargement

- Cyclosporine administered to prevent GVHD in patients undergoing HSCT may cause gingival enlargement. The differential diagnosis includes gingival enlargement induced by other medications or relapse of a hematologic malignancy.

Desquamative gingivitis (chronic graft-versus-host disease)

- Desquamative gingivitis is noted in several mucocutaneous diseases, including cGVHD. Desquamative gingivitis may be asymptomatic; however, some patients report

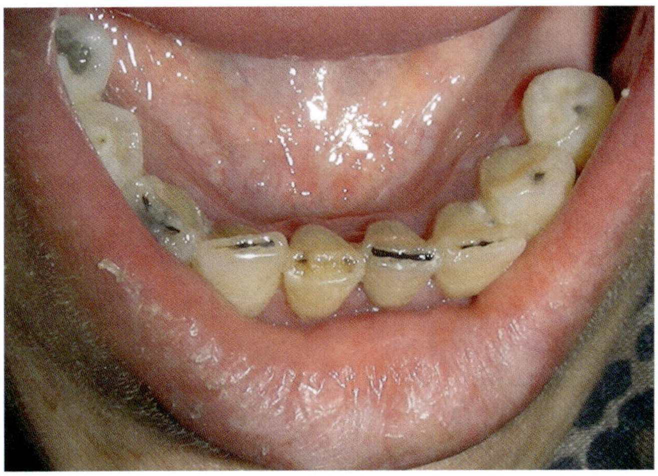

Fig. 12 Incisal edges caries in dry mouth.

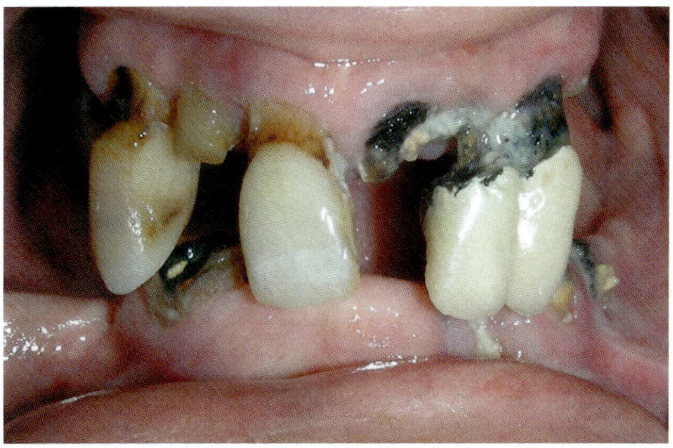

Fig. 13 Rampant caries 3 years after radiotherapy.

discomfort during brushing, resulting in increased dental plaque accumulation. The gingival desquamation may be accompanied by lichenoid changes on other mucosal surfaces (Fig. 14). The treatment is primarily with topical steroids.

Acute periodontal infections

- The myelosuppression induced by cytotoxic treatment increases infection risk. The periodontium may harbor pathogens that become the source of opportunistic infections, and preexisting periodontal disease may spread locally or systemically. The common bacteria implicated in periodontal infection in leukemic patients are *Staphylococcus epidermidis*, *S aureus*, and *Pseudomonas aeruginosa*.[52] However, the literature presents a broad range of opportunistic infections in the gingival or periodontal tissue, particularly in patients treated for hematologic malignancies. The consequences of an acute periodontal infection may be serious. In bone marrow transplantation patients, 35% of septicemias were caused by *S viridans* originating from the oral cavity.[53]

Bleeding

- Oral bleeding in cancer patients is an important complication requiring a prompt response to ensure hemodynamic stability.
- The main cause of this complication is thrombocytopenia induced by cytotoxic agents that develops a few days after treatment initiation. Platelets counts of less than $20{,}000 \times 10^6/L$ may lead to spontaneous bleeding. Another cause of bleeding in cancer patients is disseminated intravascular coagulation. In disseminated intravascular coagulation, the cancer or the cancer lysis products induce a procoagulation state, which uses up the circulating platelets, and therefore manifests as a bleeding tendency. Additionally, certain targeted therapies, such as bevacizumab (Avastin), are associated with increased risk of bleeding.

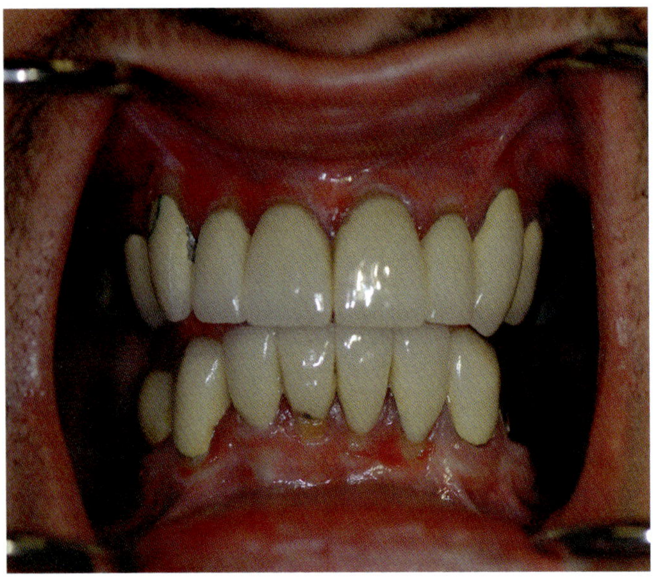

Fig. 14 Desquamative gingivitis in chronic graft-versus-host disease.

- Oral manifestations include submucosal bleeding in various sizes (hematoma, ecchymosis, petechia), or signs of fresh bleeding into the oral cavity (bloody-pinkish saliva, gingival oozing, fresh crusts on the lips, or active bleeding from traumatized soft tissues).
- The treatment for uncontrolled oral bleeding is mainly with local pressure and topical hemostatic agents. In severe cases, platelets or fresh frozen plasma may need to be transfused. Hydration and monitoring the red blood lineage counts is necessary to determine if a blood transfusion is needed. After hemostasis the patient should be instructed about avoiding local trauma and maintaining oral hygiene.

Infections: bacterial, viral, and fungal

- Oral infections are relatively common early and/or late complications of cancer treatment, potentially involving any oral tissue. Generally, the lower the white blood cell count, the higher risk of infection. This section focuses on acute infections of the oral mucosal surfaces.
- In cancer patients treated with chemotherapy, about 20% of the oral infections are of bacterial origin.[54] The main causative micropathogens are gram-negative bacilli (*Pseudomonas aeruginosa*, *Klebsiella pneumoniae*) and gram-positive cocci (*S aureus*, *S epidermidis*, and *S pyogenes*).[54,55] Cultures may show mixed infections. The clinical presentation is of a well-circumscribed ulceration covered with a central slightly raised whitish-yellowish pseudomembrane that may turn grayish over time. The lesions may be extremely painful.[54] Systemic antibiotics are the mainstay of treatment. Culture and sensitivity are beneficial to select second-line treatments. In HSCT patients, triple antibiotic–based protocols are commonly used.
- Fungal infections are common in cancer patients treated with chemotherapy or RT and estimated to affect 38% of the patients.[56] The most common oral fungal infection is candidiasis, which may manifest in several ways: pseudomembranous type (thrush), erythematous type, angular cheilitis, rhomboid glossitis, or hyperplastic type (Fig. 15). The most frequent sites are the dorsum of the

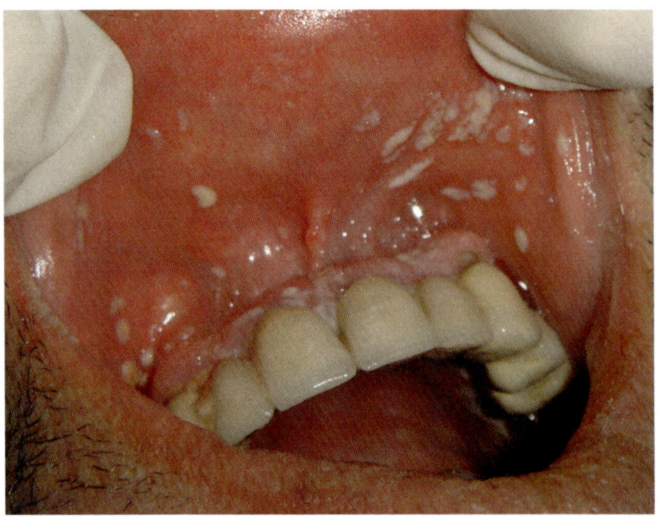

Fig. 15 Candidiasis, pseudomembranous type.

tongue, the palate, the commissures of the lips, and to a lesser extent the buccal and labial mucosa. The treatment varies from topical to systemic antifungals, depending on the extent of immunosuppression and presence of systemic signs of infection.

- Viral infections are common in patients treated with chemotherapy, particularly after myeloablative protocols. The oral lesions may appear as a local reactivation or may represent a manifestation of a systemic viral infection. The most common viral infection is herpes virus simplex (Figs. 16 and 17). Other oral herpetic infections (cytomegalovirus, varicella zoster virus, and Epstein–Barr virus) are rare. The prevalence of herpes simplex virus infection in patients treated with chemotherapy for hematologic malignancies was reported to be about 50%, from cultures of oral ulcerations. The prevalence of herpes simplex virus infection in patients treated with RT presenting with oral ulcers increased from none to 43% when adjunctive chemotherapy was added.[57] The treatment is mostly with systemic antivirals, such as acyclovir and valacyclovir.[58]

Malignancy

- A secondary oral cancer may be a complication of cancer treatment. Although the range of secondary oral cancers is broad, 2 malignancies tend to be more prevalent in patients after HSCT: posttransplant lymphoproliferative disorder (PTLD) and squamous cell carcinoma. Sarcoma tends to be associated with RT to the head and neck. Each of these malignancies has its own epidemiology, clinical features, histopathology, differential diagnosis, and treatment considerations. For the purpose of this article some key points are highlighted.
- PTLDs are a range of diseases from benign proliferations to malignant lymphomas[59] and predominantly occur early in the post-HSCT period. Oral PTLD is rare and has a variable presentation, including craterlike gingival defects, exophytic lesions, ulcerated swellings, gingival enlargement, and generalized erythematous to cyanotic gingiva.[60] Early treatment includes immune suppression reduction and rituximab. In Epstein–Barr virus–positive PTLD, antiviral therapy is recommended. More recent data suggest early use of rituximab. In aggressive forms of PTLD, chemotherapy may be needed.[59]
- Squamous cell carcinoma is one of the most frequent solid cancers after HSCT, and the most common oral second primary cancer.[61] The risk increases with time, reaching a more than 8-fold risk at 10 years after HSCT. Higher doses of total body radiation and longer exposure to azathioprine were suggested to be risk factors for second solid cancers after HSCT.[62] cGVHD and male gender increase the risk.[61,62] Oral squamous cell carcinomas after HSCT are frequently multifocal and recur locally suggesting aggressiveness (Fig. 18).[63] Vigilant follow-up and coordination of care are critical for the early detection of the cancer.

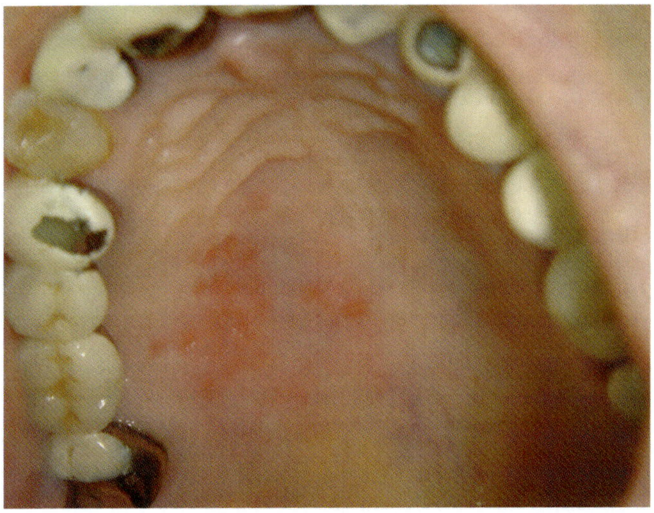

Fig. 16 Herpes simplex virus reactivation, hard palate.

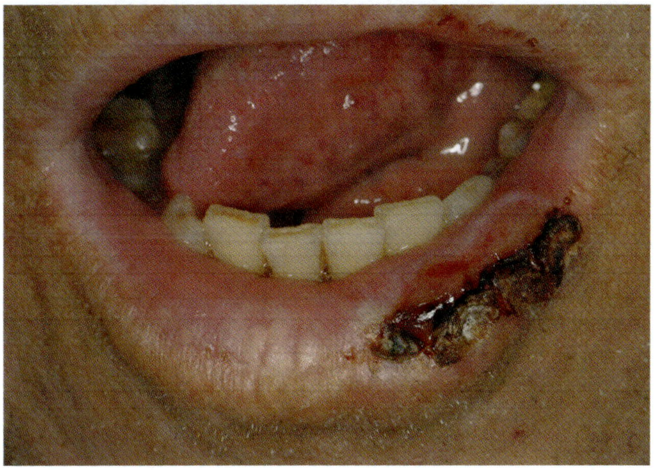

Fig. 17 Herpes simplex virus reactivation, lower lip.

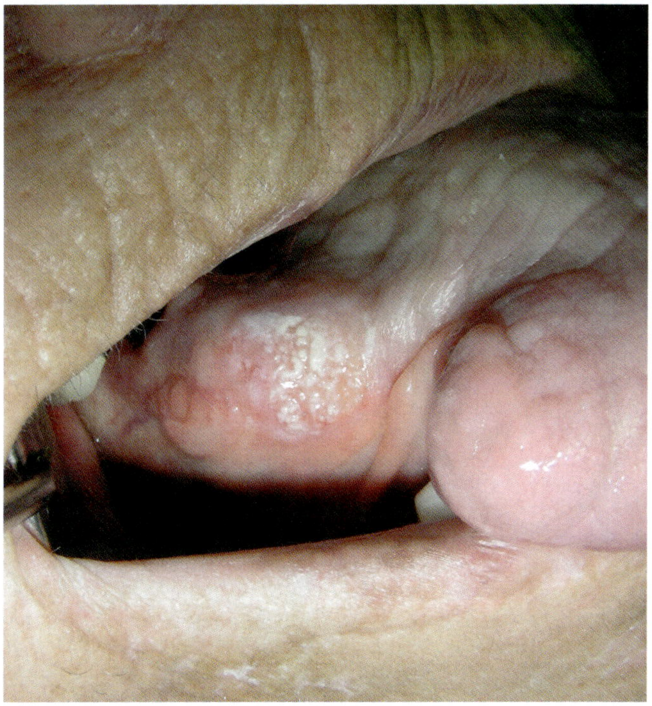

Fig. 18 Squamous cell carcinoma after hematopoietic stem cell transplantation.

- Postradiation sarcomas may develop locally 3 to 20 years after RT, rarely in the oral tissues.[64,65]

Developmental disturbances of teeth and craniofacial growth occur in pediatric patients.

- Cancer therapy delivered during the development of teeth and maxillofacial complex may result in dental abnormalities and growth disruptions. Enamel hypoplasia, hypodontia, microdontia, premature apical closure, root stunting, and lower root–crown ratio than in the general population have been reported. Minor changes such as enamel white spot or brown opacities and developmental grooves/pits may be an esthetic problem and increase the risk of caries. Some dental abnormalities may cause malocclusion.[66,67]

Summary

Oral complications of nonsurgical cancer therapy are variable and common, affecting numerous tissue types. These complications are often symptomatic, impairing oral function and quality of life. In neutropenic patients, oral complications have systemic implications. When curative treatment is unavailable, supportive and palliative management is essential for patient well-being.

References

1. Watters AL, Epstein JB, Agulnik M. Oral complications of targeted cancer therapies: a narrative literature review. Oral Oncol 2011; 47(6):441–8.
2. Vera-Llonch M, Oster G, Hagiwara M, et al. Oral mucositis in patients undergoing radiation treatment for head and neck carcinoma. Cancer 2006;106(2):329–36.
3. De Sanctis V, Bossi P, Sanguineti G, et al. Mucositis in head and neck cancer patients treated with radiotherapy and systemic therapies: literature review and consensus statements. Crit Rev Oncol Hematol 2016;100:147–66.
4. Sonis ST. Oral mucositis in head and neck cancer: risk, biology, and management. Am Soc Clin Oncol Educ book 2013:e236–40.
5. Elting LS, Cooksley C, Chambers M, et al. The burdens of cancer therapy. Clinical and economic outcomes of chemotherapy-induced mucositis. Cancer 2003;98(7):1531–9.
6. Lalla RV, Bowen J, Barasch A, et al. MASCC/ISOO clinical practice guidelines for the management of mucositis secondary to cancer therapy. Cancer 2014;120(10):1453–61.
7. Elad S, Zadik Y. Chronic oral mucositis after radiotherapy to the head and neck: a new insight. Support Care Cancer 2016;24(11): 4825–30.
8. Barrett AP. Neutropenic ulceration. A distinctive clinical entity. J Periodontol 1987;58(1):51–5.
9. Hasturk H, Tezcan I, Yel L, et al. A case of chronic severe neutropenia: oral findings and consequences of short-term granulocyte colony-stimulating factor treatment. Aust Dent J 1998;43(1):9–13.
10. Cheney-Peters D, Lund TC. Oral pyogenic granuloma after bone marrow transplant in the pediatric/adolescent population: report of 5 cases. J Pediatr Hematol Oncol 2016;38(7):570–3.
11. Kanda Y, Arai C, Chizuka A, et al. Pyogenic granuloma of the tongue early after allogeneic bone marrow transplantation for multiple myeloma. Leuk Lymphoma 2000;37(3–4):445–9.
12. Lee WJ, Lee JL, Chang SE, et al. Cutaneous adverse effects in patients treated with the multitargeted kinase inhibitors sorafenib and sunitinib. Br J Dermatol 2009;161(5):1045–51.
13. Martins F, de Oliveira MA, Wang Q, et al. A review of oral toxicity associated with mTOR inhibitor therapy in cancer patients. Oral Oncol 2013;49(4):293–8.
14. Peterson DE, O'Shaughnessy JA, Rugo HS, et al. Oral mucosal injury caused by mammalian target of rapamycin inhibitors: emerging perspectives on pathobiology and impact on clinical practice. Cancer Med 2016;5(8):1897–907.
15. Sonis S, Treister N, Chawla S, et al. Preliminary characterization of oral lesions associated with inhibitors of mammalian target of rapamycin in cancer patients. Cancer 2010;116(1):210–5.
16. Meleti M, Vescovi P, Mooi WJ, et al. Pigmented lesions of the oral mucosa and perioral tissues: a flow-chart for the diagnosis and some recommendations for the management. Oral Surg Oral Med Oral Pathol Oral Radiol Endod 2008;105(5): 606–16.
17. Wong M, Sade S, Gilbert M, et al. Oral melanosis after tyrosine kinase inhibition with Imatinib for chronic myelogenous leukemia: report of a case and review of the literature. Dermatol Online J 2011;17(5):4.
18. Resende RG, Teixeira RG, Vasconcelos Fde O, et al. Imatinib-associated hyperpigmentation of the palate in post-HSCT patient. J Craniomaxillofac Surg 2012;40(5):e140–3.
19. Jensen SB, Pedersen AM, Vissink A, et al. A systematic review of salivary gland hypofunction and xerostomia induced by cancer therapies: prevalence, severity and impact on quality of life. Support Care Cancer 2010;18(8):1039–60.
20. Wilberg P, Hjermstad MJ, Ottesen S, et al. Chemotherapy-associated oral sequelae in patients with cancers outside the head and neck region. J Pain Symptom Manage 2014;48(6): 1060–9.
21. Chaushu G, Itzkovitz-Chaushu S, Yefenof E, et al. A longitudinal follow-up of salivary secretion in bone marrow transplant patients. Oral Surg Oral Med Oral Pathol Oral Radiol Endod 1995;79(2): 164–9.
22. Buchali A, Feyer P, Groll J, et al. Immediate toxicity during fractionated total body irradiation as conditioning for bone marrow transplantation. Radiother Oncol 2000;54(2):157–62.
23. Jensen SB, Pedersen AM, Vissink A, et al. A systematic review of salivary gland hypofunction and xerostomia induced by cancer therapies: management strategies and economic impact. Support Care Cancer 2010;18(8):1061–79.
24. AAOM Clinical Practice Statement: subject: clinical management of cancer therapy-induced salivary gland hypofunction and xerostomia. Oral Surg Oral Med Oral Pathol Oral Radiol 2016;122(3): 310–2.
25. Keshet N, Abu-Tair J, Zaharia B, et al. Superficial oral mucoceles in cancer patient after radiation therapy: an overlooked yet imperative phenomenon. Oral Oncol 2016;52:e1–2.
26. De Felice F, Musio D, Tombolini V. Osteoradionecrosis and intensity modulated radiation therapy: an overview. Crit Rev Oncol Hematol 2016;107:39–43.
27. Peterson DE, Doerr W, Hovan A, et al. Osteoradionecrosis in cancer patients: the evidence base for treatment-dependent frequency, current management strategies, and future studies. Support Care Cancer 2010;18(8):1089–98.
28. Buglione M, Cavagnini R, Di Rosario F, et al. Oral toxicity management in head and neck cancer patients treated with chemotherapy and radiation: dental pathologies and osteoradionecrosis (Part 1) literature review and consensus statement. Crit Rev Oncol Hematol 2016;97:131–42.
29. Costa DA, Costa TP, Netto EC, et al. New perspectives on the conservative management of osteoradionecrosis of the mandible: a literature review. Head Neck 2016;38(11):1708–16.
30. Yarom N, Elad S, Madrid C, et al. Osteonecrosis of the jaws induced by drugs other than bisphosphonates - a call to update terminology in light of new data. Oral Oncol 2010;46(1):e1.
31. Ruggiero SL, Dodson TB, Fantasia J, et al. American Association of Oral and Maxillofacial Surgeons position paper on medication-related osteonecrosis of the jaw—2014 update. J Oral Maxillofac Surg 2014;72(10):1938–56.

32. Lazarovici TS, Yahalom R, Taicher S, et al. Bisphosphonate-related osteonecrosis of the jaws: a single-center study of 101 patients. J Oral Maxillofac Surg 2009;67(4):850–5.
33. Yarom N, Yahalom R, Shoshani Y, et al. Osteonecrosis of the jaw induced by orally administered bisphosphonates: incidence, clinical features, predisposing factors and treatment outcome. Osteoporos Int 2007;18(10):1363–70.
34. Robbins KT. Barriers to winning the battle with head-and-neck cancer. Int J Radiat Oncol Biol Phys 2002;53(1):4–5.
35. Russi EG, Corvo R, Merlotti A, et al. Swallowing dysfunction in head and neck cancer patients treated by radiotherapy: review and recommendations of the supportive task group of the Italian Association of Radiation Oncology. Cancer Treat Rev 2012;38(8):1033–49.
36. Jacobi I, van der Molen L, Huiskens H, et al. Voice and speech outcomes of chemoradiation for advanced head and neck cancer: a systematic review. Eur Arch Otorhinolaryngol 2010;267(10):1495–505.
37. Xi S. Effectiveness of voice rehabilitation on vocalisation in post-laryngectomy patients: a systematic review. Int J Evid Based Healthc 2010;8(4):256–8.
38. Zadik Y. Restricted mouth opening in chronic graft-versus-host disease. Oral Surg Oral Med Oral Pathol Oral Radiol 2016;121(2):201–2.
39. Elad SH, Horowitz R, Zadik Y. Supportive and palliative care in dentistry and oral medicine. In: Smith HS, Pilitsis JG, editors. The art and science of palliative medicine. Hong Kong (China): AME Publishing Company; 2014. p. 385–405.
40. Hovan AJ, Williams PM, Stevenson-Moore P, et al. A systematic review of dysgeusia induced by cancer therapies. Support Care Cancer 2010;18(8):1081–7.
41. Epstein JB, Smutzer G, Doty RL. Understanding the impact of taste changes in oncology care. Support Care Cancer 2016;24(4):1917–31.
42. Yuan A, Kurtz SL, Barysauskas CM, et al. Oral adverse events in cancer patients treated with VEGFR-directed multitargeted tyrosine kinase inhibitors. Oral Oncol 2015;51(11):1026–33.
43. Hull KM, Kerridge I, Schifter M. Long-term oral complications of allogeneic haematopoietic SCT. Bone Marrow Transplant 2012;47(2):265–70.
44. Zadik Y, Vainstein V, Heling I, et al. Cytotoxic chemotherapy-induced odontalgia: a differential diagnosis for dental pain. J Endod 2010;36(9):1588–92.
45. Deng J, Jackson L, Epstein JB, et al. Dental demineralization and caries in patients with head and neck cancer. Oral Oncol 2015;51(9):824–31.
46. Hong CH, Napenas JJ, Hodgson BD, et al. A systematic review of dental disease in patients undergoing cancer therapy. Support Care Cancer 2010;18(8):1007–21.
47. Castellarin P, Stevenson K, Biasotto M, et al. Extensive dental caries in patients with oral chronic graft-versus-host disease. Biol Blood Marrow Transplant 2012;18(10):1573–9.
48. Curtis JW Jr, Caughman GB. An apparent unusual relationship between rampant caries and the oral mucosal manifestations of chronic graft-versus-host disease. Oral Surg Oral Med Oral Pathol 1994;78(2):267–72.
49. Singh ML, Papas AS. Long-term clinical observation of dental caries in salivary hypofunction patients using a supersaturated calcium-phosphate remineralizing rinse. J Clin Dent 2009;20(3):87–92.
50. Sim CP, Wee J, Xu Y, et al. Anti-caries effect of CPP-ACP in irradiated nasopharyngeal carcinoma patients. Clin Oral Investig 2015;19(5):1005–11.
51. Gomes CB, Treister NS, Miller B, et al. Pulp obliteration in a patient with sclerodermatous chronic graft-versus-host disease. J Endod 2016;42(4):678–80.
52. Epstein JB, Stevenson-Moore P. Periodontal disease and periodontal management in patients with cancer. Oral Oncol 2001;37(8):613–9.
53. Heimdahl A, Nord CE. Colonization of the oropharynx with pathogenic microorganisms—a potential risk factor for infection in compromised patients. Chemioterapia : Int J Mediterr Soc Chemother 1985;4(2):186–91.
54. Dreizen S, Bodey GP, Valdivieso M. Chemotherapy-associated oral infections in adults with solid tumors. Oral Surg Oral Med Oral Pathol 1983;55(2):113–20.
55. Khan SA, Wingard JR. Infection and mucosal injury in cancer treatment. J Natl Cancer Inst Monographs 2001;(29):31–6.
56. Lalla RV, Latortue MC, Hong CH, et al. A systematic review of oral fungal infections in patients receiving cancer therapy. Support Care Cancer 2010;18(8):985–92.
57. Elad S, Zadik Y, Hewson I, et al. A systematic review of viral infections associated with oral involvement in cancer patients: a spotlight on Herpesviridea. Support Care Cancer 2010;18(8):993–1006.
58. Elad S, Ranna V, Ariyawardana A, et al. A systematic review of oral herpetic viral infections in cancer patients: commonly used outcome measures and interventions. Support Care Cancer 2016;25(2):687–700.
59. Singavi AK, Harrington AM, Fenske TS. Post-transplant lymphoproliferative disorders. Cancer Treat Res 2015;165:305–27.
60. Elad S, Meyerowitz C, Shapira MY, et al. Oral posttransplantation lymphoproliferative disorder: an uncommon site for an uncommon disorder. Oral Surg Oral Med Oral Pathol Oral Radiol Endod 2008;105(1):59–64.
61. Curtis RE, Rowlings PA, Deeg HJ, et al. Solid cancers after bone marrow transplantation. N Engl J Med 1997;336(13):897–904.
62. Curtis RE, Metayer C, Rizzo JD, et al. Impact of chronic GVHD therapy on the development of squamous-cell cancers after hematopoietic stem-cell transplantation: an international case-control study. Blood 2005;105(10):3802–11.
63. Mawardi H, Elad S, Correa ME, et al. Oral epithelial dysplasia and squamous cell carcinoma following allogeneic hematopoietic stem cell transplantation: clinical presentation and treatment outcomes. Bone Marrow Transplant 2011;46(6):884–91.
64. Bingol UA, Arslan H, Cinar C. Postradiation sarcoma from a free flap. J Craniofac Surg 2013;24(6):2160–2.
65. Bonetta A, Gelli MC, Zini G, et al. Postradiation sarcoma of head and neck: report of two cases. Tumori 1996;82(3):270–2.
66. Effinger KE, Migliorati CA, Hudson MM, et al. Oral and dental late effects in survivors of childhood cancer: a Children's Oncology Group report. Support Care Cancer 2014;22(7):2009–19.
67. van der Pas-van Voskuilen IG, Veerkamp JS, Raber-Durlacher JE, et al. Long-term adverse effects of hematopoietic stem cell transplantation on dental development in children. Support Care Cancer 2009;17(9):1169–75.
68. Bensadoun RJ, Riesenbeck D, Lockhart PB, et al. A systematic review of trismus induced by cancer therapies in head and neck cancer patients. Support Care Cancer 2010;18(8):1033–8.
69. Meier JK, Wolff D, Pavletic S, et al. Oral chronic graft-versus-host disease: report from the International Consensus Conference on clinical practice in cGVHD. Clin Oral Investig 2011;15(2):127–39.
70. Carpenter PA, Kitko CL, Elad S, et al. National Institutes of Health consensus development Project on Criteria for clinical Trials in chronic graft-versus-host disease: V. The 2014 ancillary therapy and supportive care Working group report. Biol Blood Marrow Transplant 2015;21(7):1167–87.
71. Rhodus NL. Cancer and oral care of the cancer patient. In: Little JW, Falace DA, Miller CS, et al, editors. Dental management of the medically compromised patient. 8th edition. St Louis (MO): Elsevier Mosby; 2013. p. 459–92.
72. Peterson DB, Jensen SB. Oral complications of nonsurgical cancer therapies: diagnosis and treatment. In: Glick M, editor. Burket's oral medicine. 12th edition. Shelton (CT): People's Medical Publishing House; 2015. p. 201–18.

Oral Manifestations of Hematologic Disease

Christina McCord, DDS, MSc, FRCD(C) [a,*], Lisa Johnson, DDS, MSc, FRCD(C) [b]

KEYWORDS

• Hematologic disease • Anemia • Leukopenia • Lymphoma • Leukemia • Thrombocytopenia • Bleeding disorders

KEY POINTS

- Iron deficiency and vitamin B_{12} deficiency should be considered in the differential diagnosis for patients presenting with atrophic glossitis.
- Susceptibility to oral infections, with clinical presentation of ulcers or gingivitis/periodontitis, may suggest underlying leukopenia, in particular neutropenia.
- Intraoral hematologic malignancies, in particular non-Hodgkin lymphomas (NHLs), can present with intrabony or soft tissue masses that may mimic other benign or malignant diseases.
- Langerhans cell histiocytosis (LCH) most commonly affects younger age groups and has characteristic radiographic and histologic features.
- Oral palatal petechiae may be a sign of underlying thrombocytopenia.

Introduction

Hematologic diseases with intraoral manifestations comprise a heterogeneous group of disorders. For the purposes of this chapter, a group of selected diseases and conditions are discussed, which are generally classifiable into four groups: white blood cell disorders, red blood cell disorders, histiocytic disorders, and bleeding disorders. Diagnosis of hematologic diseases can be challenging as many of these conditions share similar clinical and/or radiographic features. Careful history, clinical exam and ancillary testing, including radiography, blood investigations, and/or biopsy can aid in diagnosis. Provision of dental treatment in the context of unrecognized hematologic disease could result in life threatening bleeding or infection. Thus, a basic understanding of the oral complications of hematologic disease is an essential part of patient care.

White blood cell disorders

Lymphoma

Lymphomas include a diverse group of hematological malignancies, which can present as masses both within the lymphoid tissues and in extranodal locations. The World Health Organization classifies lymphomas based on their cells of origin (Table 1), including B cells, T cells, and natural killer (NK) cells. Hodgkin lymphomas are lymphomas of B-cell origin, which are classified separately from other B-cell and NK-cell/T-cell lymphomas (NHLs). Hodgkin lymphomas are exceptionally rare intraorally and, therefore, are not discussed further.

Non-Hodgkin lymphoma

NHL may have B-cell or T-cell/NK-cell origin, with B-cell lymphomas being more common. Immunodeficiency states and certain viruses, including Epstein-Barr virus, have been associated with increased risk and development of certain intraoral lymphomas.

Epidemiology

NHLs primary affect adults, with greater than 75% of cases diagnosed after the age of 55. The estimated incidence is more than 72,000 new cases per year.

Clinical presentation

- Nodal involvement consists of a slowly enlarging, nontender mass that gradually becomes affixed to adjacent tissues.
- Extranodal intraoral involvement
  - May manifest as a diffuse, nontender submucosal swelling, with or without surface ulceration (Fig. 1).
  - The palate is the most commonly affected intraoral site (Fig. 2).
  - Central lesions often are present as an ill-defined radiolucency (Fig. 3) and may involve the periodontal ligament space or the follicle of a developing tooth.
  - Pain and/or paresthesia may accompany lesions with bone involvement.

The authors have nothing to disclose.

[a] Division of Oral Pathology, Department of Pathology and Laboratory Medicine, Schulich School of Medicine and Dentistry, Western University, 1151 Richmond Street, HSA 418A, London, Ontario N6A 5C1, Canada

[b] Department of Oral and Maxillofacial Sciences, Faculty of Dentistry, Dalhousie University, 5981 University Avenue, Room 5124, PO Box 15000, Halifax, Nova Scotia B3H 4R2, Canada

* Corresponding author.

E-mail address: christina.mccord@schulich.uwo.ca

Atlas Oral Maxillofacial Surg Clin N Am 25 (2017) 149–162

http://dx.doi.org/10.1016/j.cxom.2017.04.007

Table 1 World Health Organization classification of lymphoid neoplasms

Category	Lymphoma subtypes
Precursor B-cell neoplasm	B-cell acute lymphoblastic leukemia/lymphoblastic lymphoma
Peripheral B-cell neoplasms	Chronic lymphocytic leukemia/lymphoma, B-cell prolymphocytic leukemia, lymphoplasmacytic lymphoma, splenic and marginal zone lymphoma, extranodal marginal zone lymphoma, mantle cell lymphoma, follicular lymphoma, marginal zone lymphoma, hairy cell leukemia, plasmacytoma/ plasma cell myeloma, diffuse large B-cell lymphoma, Burkitt lymphoma
Precursor T-cell neoplasms	T-cell acute lymphoblastic leukemia/lymphoblastic lymphoma
Peripheral T-cell and NK-cell neoplasms	T-cell prolymphocytic leukemia, large granular lymphocytic leukemia, mycosis fungoides, peripheral T-cell lymphoma not otherwise specified, anaplastic large cell lymphoma, angioimmunoblastic T-cell lymphoma, enteropathy-associated T-cell lymphoma, panniculitis-like T-cell lymphoma, hepatosplenic $\gamma\delta$T-cell lymphoma, adult T-cell leukemia/lymphoma, extranodal NK-cell/T-cell lymphoma, NK-cell lymphoma
Hodgkin lymphoma	Classic subtypes: nodular sclerosis, mixed cellularity, lymphocyte rich, lymphocyte depletion Lymphocyte predominant

Adapted from Kumar V, Abbas AK, Asster JC. Robbins and cotran pathologic basis of disease. 9th edition. Philadelphia: Elsevier, 2015.

Histopathology

Histopathology is variable depending on subtype. NHLs generally present as infiltrative sheets of lymphocyte-like cells showing varying degrees of differentiation with nodular, follicular, or diffuse growth patterns (Fig. 4). Diffuse large B-cell lymphoma is the most common intraoral subtype.

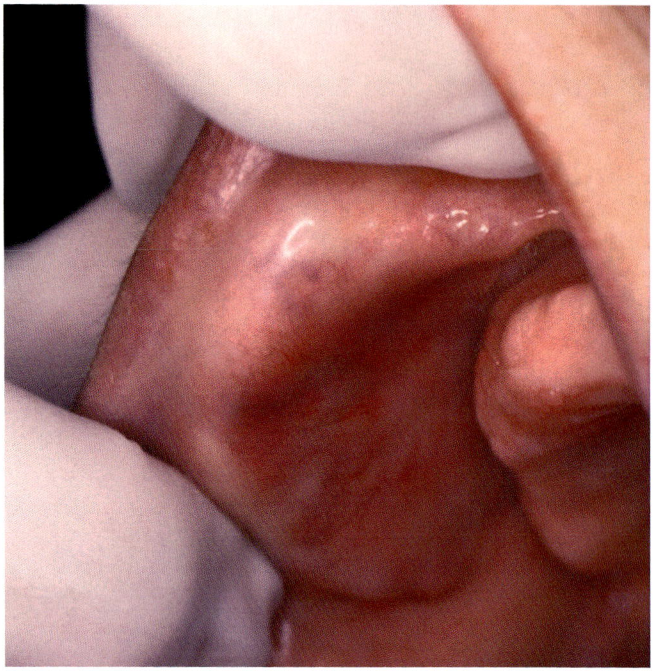

Fig. 1 Example of extranodal B-cell NHL presenting as a submucosal swelling of the labial and buccal mucosa.

Immunohistochemistry and cytogenetics are needed for definitive subtyping.

Differential diagnosis

- Nodal or extranodal involvement must be differentiated from reactive, benign, malignant, or metastatic processes.
- Radiographically, intraoral lymphomas may mimic periapical inflammatory disease, periodontal disease, osteomyelitis, or other malignancies.

Treatment

- Treatment is highly variable depending on subtype, ranging from no treatment with close follow-up to radiation and chemotherapy.

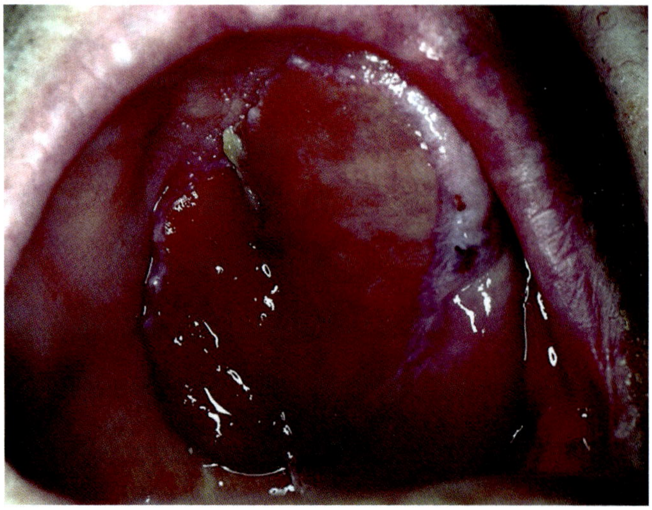

Fig. 2 Extranodal B-cell NHL in an older man presenting as a palatal swelling.

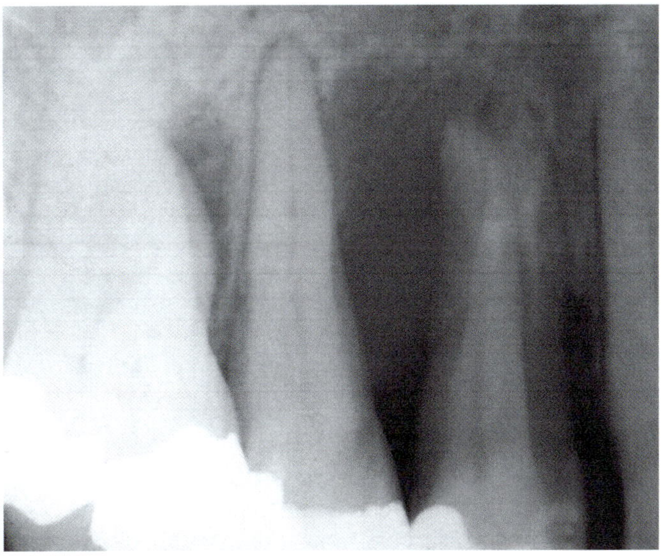

Fig. 3 Example of the radiographic features of extranodal B-cell NHL showing an ill-defined, infiltrative radiolucency affecting the right posterior maxilla. Concomitant widening of periodontal ligament space is also present.

T-cell lymphoma

Oral involvement of T-cell/NK-cell lymphomas is uncommon. Mycosis fungoides, for example, is a cutaneous lymphoma of T-cell origin more common in men, which can demonstrate oral involvement, usually in the later stages of disease. It is a slowly progressive, incurable disease, with normal life expectancy for patients in which the disease remains limited. Extranodal NK-cell/T-cell lymphoma is another uncommon hematologic malignancy that presents clinically with extensive destruction of the palate and nasal regions in the midline (midfacial destructive disease). It is known to have strong associations with Epstein-Barr virus. This condition occurs in adults and has a male predominance.

Multiple myeloma

Multiple myeloma (MM) is a multifocal disease of monoclonal neoplastic plasma cells, which proliferate in the bone marrow and produce abnormal immunoglobulins. MM is characterized by lytic bone lesions, myelophthisic anemia, and immune dysfunction. Solitary plasmacytoma is an uncommon, unifocal presentation of plasma cell malignancy. Localized extrabony presentations are termed extramedullary plasmacytoma.

Epidemiology

MM is an uncommon cancer with an estimated incidence of 6.5 cases per 100,000 per year. MM is a disease of older adults with most cases diagnosed after age 65. Men are predominantly affected, and the incidence of disease is greater in individuals of African descent.

Clinical presentation

The clinical signs and symptoms of MM are related to the proliferation of plasma cells, production of immunoglobulins, and suppression of normal immunity; the salient signs and symptoms are summarized in Table 2. Figs. 5 and 6 depict the radiographic features of MM.

Histopathology

Microscopically, MM shows sheets of variably differentiated cells with plasmacytic features (Fig. 7), showing immunohistochemical evidence of plasma cell differentiation (CD138 and CD38) and monoclonality for kappa or lambda light chains. Amyloid deposition may also be seen.

Differential diagnosis

- Clinically MM can mimic other conditions that can cause myelophthisic anemia, including other types of malignancy, granulomatous conditions, myelofibrosis, and lipid storage disorders.
- Radiographic disease may mimic metastatic cancer or osteomyelitis.
- Intraorally, MM may mimic periapical inflammatory disease, gingivitis, or periodontitis.
- LCH may also show punched-out, well-defined radiolucencies but typically affects a younger age group.

Treatment

In general, treatment involves a combination of immunomodulators, corticosteroids, and proteasome inhibitors.

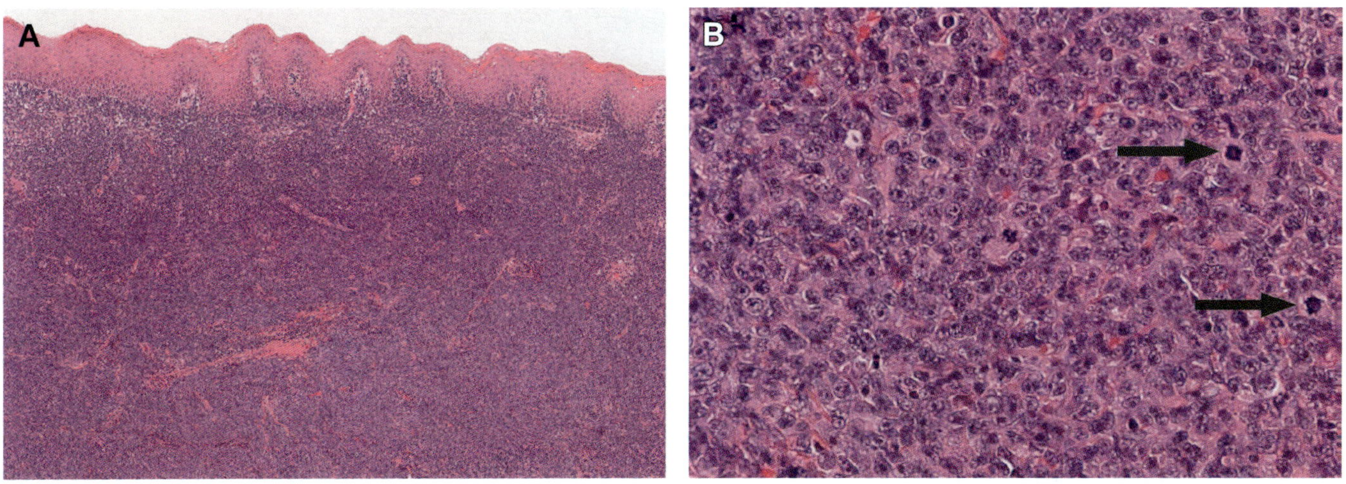

Fig. 4 Microscopic features of diffuse large B-cell lymphoma. (*A*) Shows a diffuse lymphocytic infiltrate, which has effaced the normal tissue architecture (hematoxylin-eosin, original magnification ×5). (*B*) Shows a high-power image depicting an irregular lymphocytic infiltrate with abundant mitotic figures (hematoxylin-eosin, original magnification ×40 [*arrows*]).

Table 2 Clinical features of multiple myeloma

Signs and symptoms	Oral manifestations
Lytic bone lesions causing bone pain	Multiple, well-defined punched-out radiolucent lesions of the jaws
Normocytic normochromic anemia causing weakness, fatigue, pallor	Amyloid deposits presenting as nodular masses ± ulceration
Thrombocytopenia	Gingival hemorrhage or petechiae due to thrombocytopenia
Infections due to leukopenia and hypogammaglobulinemia	Signs and symptoms related to anemia and leukopenia
Hypercalcemia	
Renal disease	Pain
Peripheral neuropathy and headache due to central nervous system involvement	Paresthesia
Serum or urinary M protein	
Bence-Jones proteinuria	

Hematopoietic stem cell transplantation may be used in eligible patients less than 65 years of age. Palliative radiation and bisphosphonates may be used to treat bone pain and prevent fracture. Solitary plasmacytomas are most commonly treated with radiation therapy.

Leukemia

Leukemias are a group of hematopoietic malignancies derived from hematopoietic stem cells. Leukemias can have either lymphoid or myeloid origin, and their clinical course is generally classified as acute or chronic. The four main types of leukemia are acute myelogenous leukemia (AML), chronic myelogenous leukemia (CML), acute lymphoblastic leukemia (ALL), and chronic lymphoblastic leukemia (CLL).

Epidemiology

The overall incidence of leukemias in the United States is 13.5 per 100,000 population. Different types of leukemia have different incidence rates within the population (Table 3).

Clinical presentation

Clinical signs and symptoms related to leukemia are generally the result of malignant infiltration of the bone marrow, resulting in a pancytopenia called myelophthisic anemia. Some leukemias may be asymptomatic and diagnosis is made with routine blood investigations.

General signs and symptoms

- Pallor, weakness, and fatigue as a result of anemia
- Fever and infections due to neutropenia
- Ecchymosis, epistaxis, spontaneous gingival bleeding, and petechial hemorrhages due to thrombocytopenia
- Leukemia cutis, myeloid sarcoma
- Organomegaly, lymphadenopathy

Oral signs and symptoms

- Neutropenic ulcers, spontaneous gingival bleeding, and petechial hemorrhages of palate
- Gingival enlargement (in myelomonocytic types) or myeloid sarcoma (Figs. 8 and 9)
- Opportunistic infections, for example, *Candida albicans*
- Paraneoplastic pemphigus can occur with CLL

Histopathology

Microscopically, leukemia shows effacement and destruction of normal tissues by malignant infiltrates with immature myeloid or lymphoid features, as determined by immunohistochemial staining.

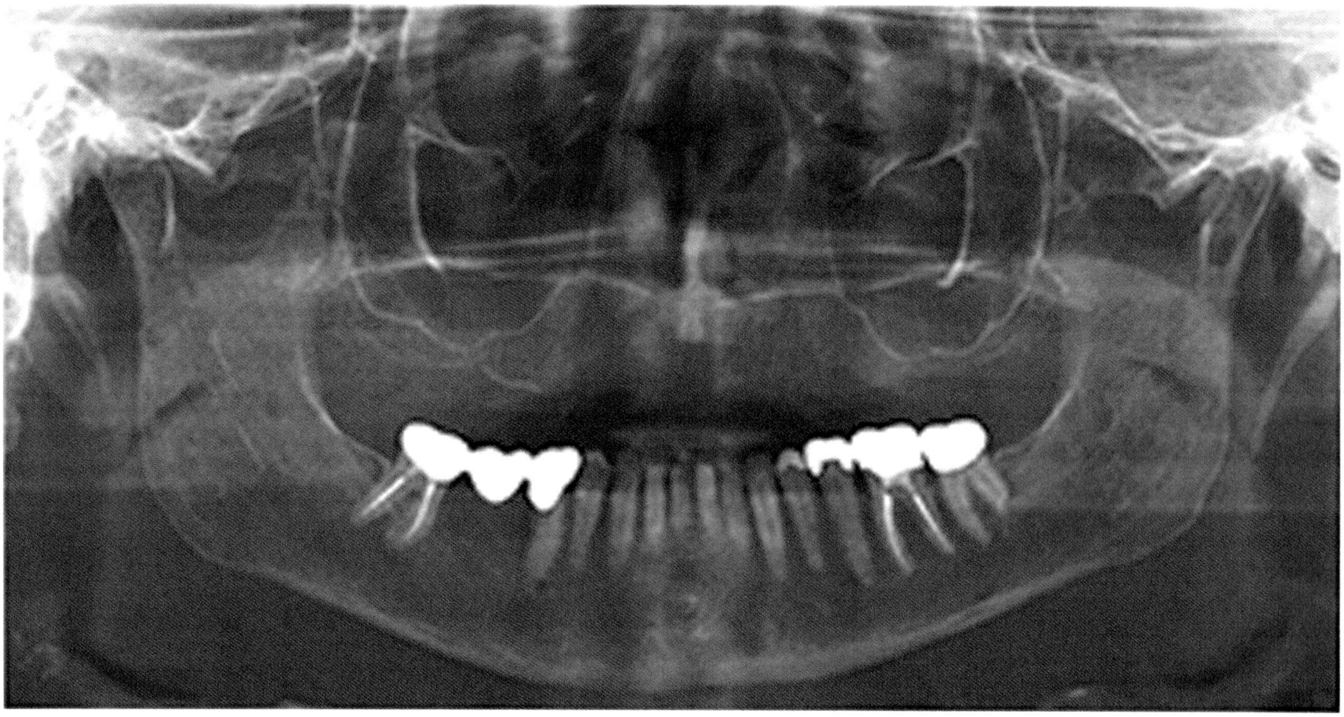

Fig. 5 Panoramic radiograph of MM showing multiple, well-defined, punched-out radiolucencies affecting the mandible. (*Courtesy of* Dr K.C. Chan, New York, NY.)

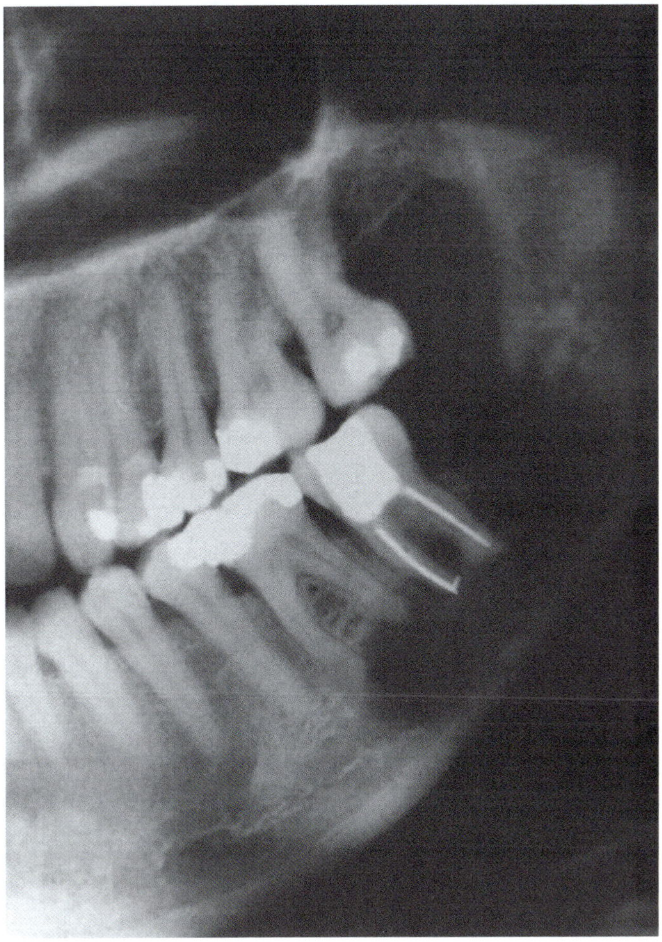

Fig. 6 Radiographic example of MM showing an ill-defined, infiltrative radiolucency affecting the left posterior mandible. (*Courtesy of* the Oral Pathology Archives, Western University, London, Ontario.)

Table 3 Leukemia: incidence and prognosis

Type	Incidence	Prognosis
AML	Incidence rises with age Peak incidence >60 13,000 new cases annually	AML with genetic aberrations (favorable to poor) AML with myelodysplasia -like features (poor) AML, therapy related (very poor) AML, not otherwise specified (intermediate)
CML	Adults, but can affect children and adolescents Peak incidence 5th–6th decades 4500 new cases annually	Sustained remission in >90% of patients with *BCR-ABL* inhibitors Stem cell transplants curative in 75% of younger patients
ALL	B-cell ALL manifests in childhood, most common cancer of childhood 2500 new cases annually Peak incidence at age 3 y	With treatment, complete remission in 95% and 75%–85% cured 35%–50% of adults achieve complete cure
CLL	Older adults, 60 median age at diagnosis 15,000 new cases annually 2:1 male predominance	Median survival is 4–6 y Many patients survive >10 y Large cell transformation associated with poor prognosis

Differential diagnosis

- Clinically and radiographically, leukemia may mimic periapical inflammatory disease.
- Oral manifestations of pancytopenia due to leukemia are indistinguishable from other causes of pancytopenia, such as adverse drug reactions, immune conditions, and viral infections.
- Other causes of gingival enlargement, such as drug-induced or inflammatory hyperplastic gingivitis can also mimic leukemia clinically.

Treatment

Treatment of leukemia is centered on chemotherapy; however, the choice of chemotherapeutic agent differs depending on

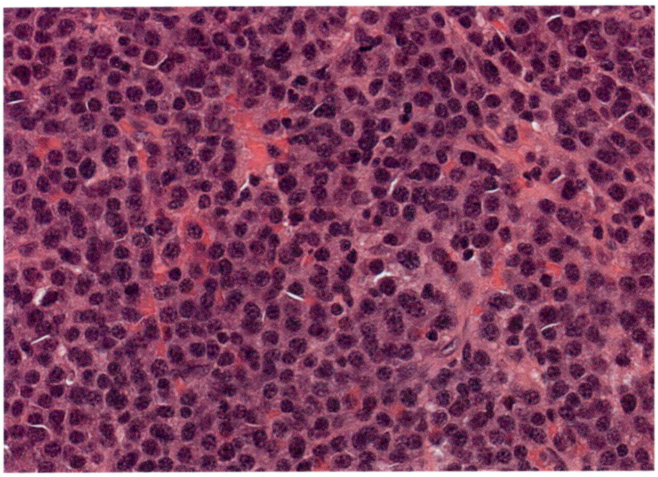

Fig. 7 Microscopic features of plasma cell myeloma. Diffuse sheet of atypical cells with plasmacytic features (hematoxylin-eosin, original magnification ×40).

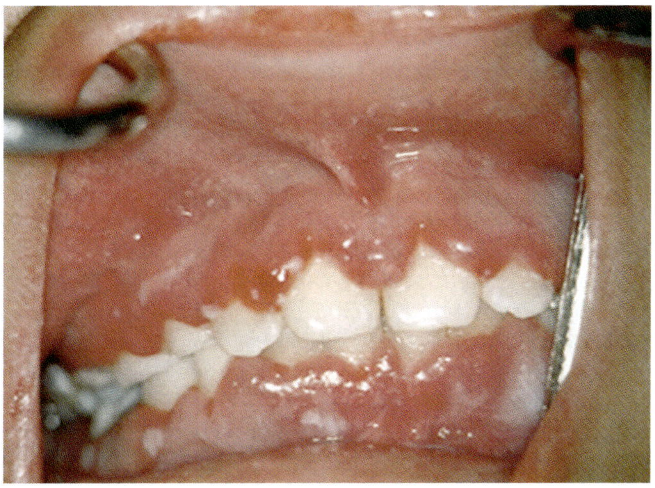

Fig. 8 Leukemic gingivitis in a patient with AML. (*From* Sapp JP, Eversole LR, Wysocki GP. Contemporary oral and maxillofacial pathology. 2nd edition. St Louis (MO): Mosby; 2004; with permission.)

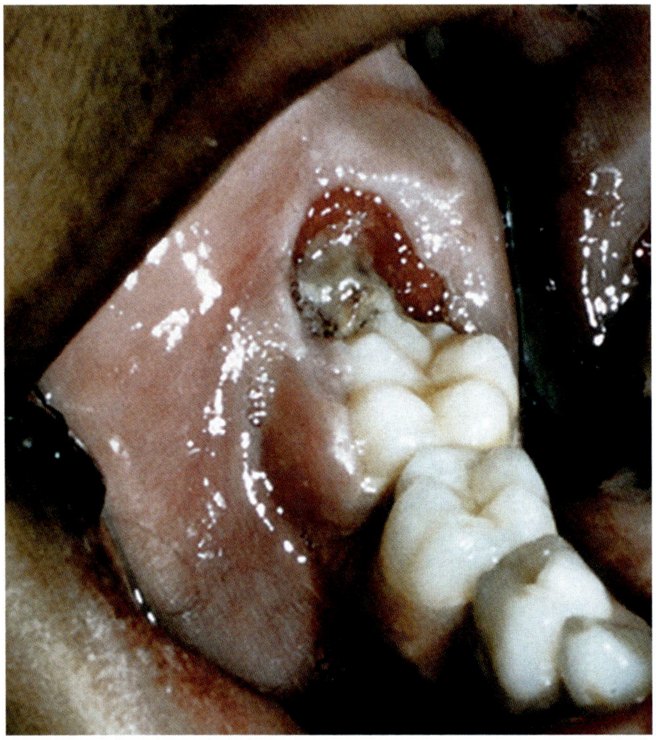

Fig. 9 An ulcerated masslike proliferation in a patient with leukemia (myeloid/granulocytic sarcoma). (*From* Sapp JP, Eversole LR, Wysocki GP. Contemporary oral and maxillofacial pathology. 2nd edition. St Louis (MO): Mosby; 2004; with permission.)

Table 4 Causes of neutropenia

Etiology	Underlying disease state
Inadequate or ineffective neutrophil production	Aplastic anemia Myelodysplastic syndromes and hematological malignancies Marrow space occupying diseases, for example, Gaucher disease, osteopetrosis Nutritional deficiencies, including vitamin B_{12} and folate Congenital conditions, for example, Severe congenital neutropenia, Kostmann syndrome Drug toxicity, for example, chemotherapeutics
Accelerated destruction of circulating neutrophils	Microbial infections, for example, hepatitis A, hepatitis B, rubella, varicella, HIV, tuberculosis Drug exposure, for example, antibiotics, diuretics Autoimmune disease, for example, systemic lupus erythematosus Idiopathic

the type of leukemia. Cytogenetic and molecular information guide treatment choice in some forms of leukemia, particularly in CML. Stem cell transplantation is also a consideration in some cases of ALL, CML (high-risk forms), and CLL. Many asymptomatic cases of CLL are not treated. Detailed discussion of specific chemotherapeutic regimens is beyond the scope of this text. Prognostic information is summarized in Table 3.

Dental considerations

- Evaluation and treatment of dental disease before the initiation of chemotherapy
- Maintenance of good oral hygiene while undergoing chemotherapy
- Invasive dental procedures may require prophylactic antibiotics and/or platelet replacements

Neutropenia

Neutropenia is a clinical condition defined as a decrease in circulating neutrophils ($<1500/mm^3$) within the blood. It may be caused by a variety of clinical conditions that result in a decrease in overall neutrophil production or an increase in neutrophil destruction (Table 4). Agranulocytosis is a deficiency of granulocytic cells, which is commonly drug related and shares clinical features with neutropenia. Cyclic neutropenia is a specific form of neutropenia characterized by cycling neutrophil counts, with patients tending to become asymptomatic after childhood.

Epidemiology

Neutropenia may present in any age group, with cases due to congenital causes presenting in infancy and acquired neutropenia presenting in adulthood. Certain ethnic groups have increased prevalence of low neutrophil counts, which are clinically insignificant, termed benign ethnic neutropenia.

Clinical presentation

- Neutropenia may be associated with increased susceptibility to bacterial infections, most commonly affecting the oral cavity, ear, and perirectal areas.
- Neutropenic ulcers preferentially affect the gingiva.
- Loss of attachment and periodontal destruction may be seen, with reported premature exfoliation of deciduous teeth.

Differential diagnosis

- Cyclic neutropenia if presenting in a child
- Other causes of chronic oral ulceration, such as mucocutaneous conditions
- Necrotizing ulcerative gingivitis

Treatment

Systemic antibiotics are given to address bacterial infections. Granulocyte colony-stimulating factor may be required to promote neutrophil production. Hematopoietic stem cell transplantation may be considered in severe cases.

Red blood cell disorders

Abnormalities in red blood cells results in a decrease in the oxygen carrying capacity of the blood, thus giving rise to anemia. In general, patients with anemias present with classic signs and symptoms, including shortness of breath, pallor, fatigue, and a compensatory increase in heart rate. Anemias are subcategorized based on the red blood cell defect, which gives rise to pathognomonic changes in red blood cell morphology.

Iron deficiency anemia

A state in which iron stores in the blood are depleted, resulting in malfunctioning of the hemoglobin molecule and its ability to bind and carry oxygen. Iron deficiency anemia is characterized by hypochromic, microcytic anemia, low serum iron and ferritin, and low transferrin saturation.

Causes of iron deficiency anemia

- Inadequate dietary intake or increased iron demand (eg, pregnancy)
- Reduced gastrointestinal absorption (eg, after gastric bypass surgery, *Helicobacter pylori* infection, or celiac disease)
- Blood loss (eg, gastrointestinal bleeding due to occult malignancy, menorrhagia, or chronic disease)

Epidemiology

Population studies estimate that iron deficiency is present in 9% to 11% of women of childbearing age, with 2% to 5% showing anemia. Less than 1% of men are thought to be affected.

Clinical presentation

- Shortness of breath, pallor, fatigue, and increased heart rate
- Koilonychia (nails become thin and concave) (Fig. 10)
- Alopecia (hair loss)
- Atrophy of the mucosa of the tongue (Fig. 11) or gastrointestinal tract
- Predisposition to candidiasis, in particular angular cheilitis (see Fig. 11)
- Aphthous-like ulcers (Fig. 12)
- Esophageal webs resulting in dysphagia

Differential diagnosis

- Intraoral atrophy seen due to iron deficiency anemia can resemble erythematous candidiasis and B vitamin deficiency, including vitamin B_2, vitamin B_3, vitamin B_6, and vitamin B_{12}.
- Endocrine disturbances, such as hypothyroidism, may show clinical overlap with some of the features of iron deficiency anemia.

Treatment

Oral or parenteral iron supplementation, with iron stores and blood abnormalities typically returning to normal after 1 month to 2 months of treatment. Close follow-up is recommended if iron deficiency anemia is accompanied by esophageal webs and atrophic glossitis, a condition termed, Plummer-Vinson syndrome. Patients with this condition are at increased risk for upper aerodigestive tract malignancies.

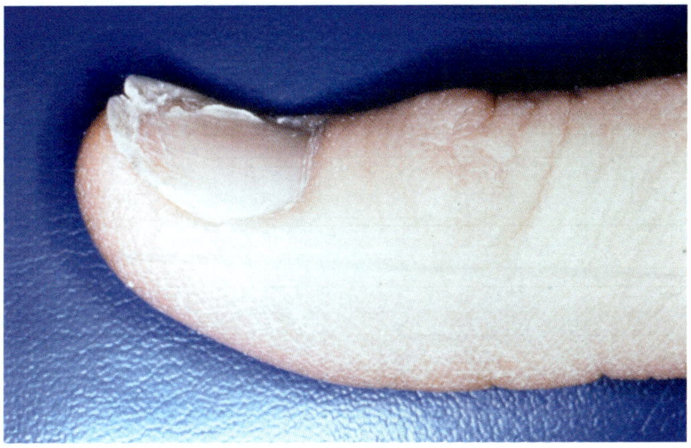

Fig. 10 Koilonychia in a case of severe iron deficiency anemia. (*Courtesy of* the Oral Pathology Archives, Western University, London, Ontario.)

Pernicious anemia

Pernicious anemia is the most common form of vitamin B_{12} (cobalamin) deficiency. It is caused by autoimmune gastritis, which results in failure of intrinsic factor production in the gut leading to vitamin B_{12} malabsorption. Vitamin B_{12} deficiency resulting directly from malabsorption is distinct from intrinsic factor deficiency and is often the result of restrictive diets and gastric bypass surgery.

In all instances of vitamin B_{12} deficiency, the resulting underproduction of red blood cells leads to abnormal enlargement of the red blood cells and their precursors, giving rise to megaloblastic anemia. A deficiency in folic acid gives rise to a comparable state.

Epidemiology

Pernicious anemia primary affects individuals 40 years to 70 years of age. Increased prevalence is noted in certain ethnic groups, including northern Europeans, African Americans, and Hispanics.

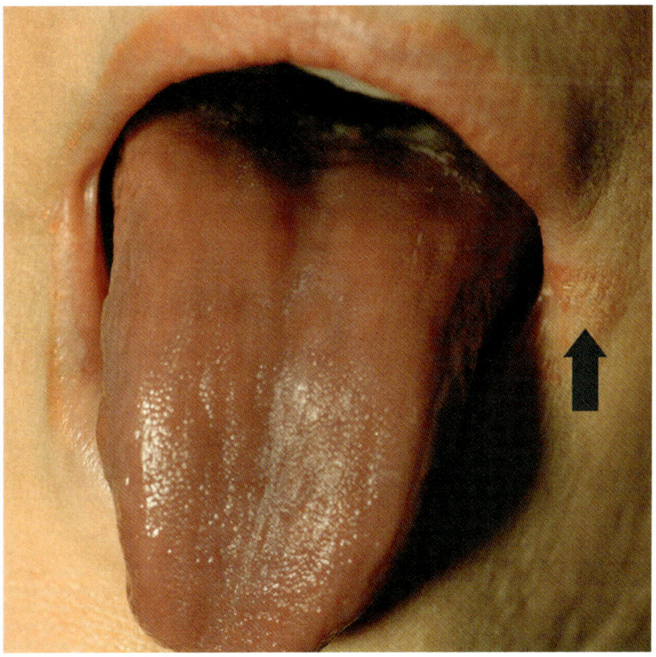

Fig. 11 Atrophic glossitis due to iron deficiency anemia. Patient also has concomitant angular cheilitis (*arrow*).

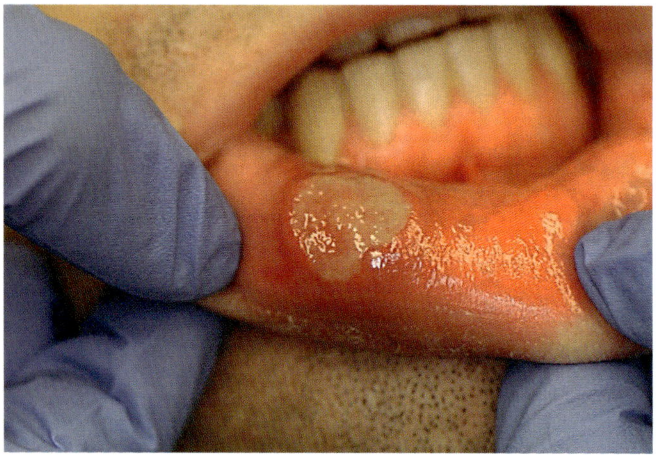

Fig. 12 Aphthous like ulcer in 20-year-old male patient with iron deficiency anemia.

Clinical presentation

- Insidious onset of classic anemia symptoms, including shortness of breath, pallor, fatigue, and increased heart rate
- Intraoral burning with erythema and atrophy of the oral mucosa, most commonly affecting the tongue (Fig. 13)
- Neurologic changes, including paresthesia, tingling, or numbness of the extremities
- Memory loss, irritability, depression, and dementia

Treatment

Pernicious anemia is treated with intramuscular vitamin B_{12} injections or high-dose oral cobalamin supplementation. Patients with long-standing pernicious anemia are at increased risk of gastric carcinoma, cardiovascular disease, neuromuscular and neuropsychiatric disorders.

Sickle cell anemia

Sickle cell anemia is an inheritable form of hemolytic anemia, associated with a point mutation in the β-globin gene resulting in an abnormal hemoglobin S chain. The hemoglobin S chain is prone to aggregation and polymerization, leading to deformation and eventual lysis of the red blood cell. This form of hemolytic anemia has a wide range of clinical presentations, with patients heterozygous for the disease (sickle cell trait) having milder presentations than those that are homozygous for the condition (sickle cell disease).

Epidemiology

An increased prevalence of sickle cell anemia is noted in African, Mediterranean, and Asian populations due to its protective affect against malaria. Sickle cell disease is thought to affect up to 100,000 Americans.

Clinical presentation

- Pain, ischemia, and infarction due to sickle cell crisis, most commonly affecting long bones, lungs, liver, brain, and spleen
- Increased susceptibility to infection and cerebrovascular accident

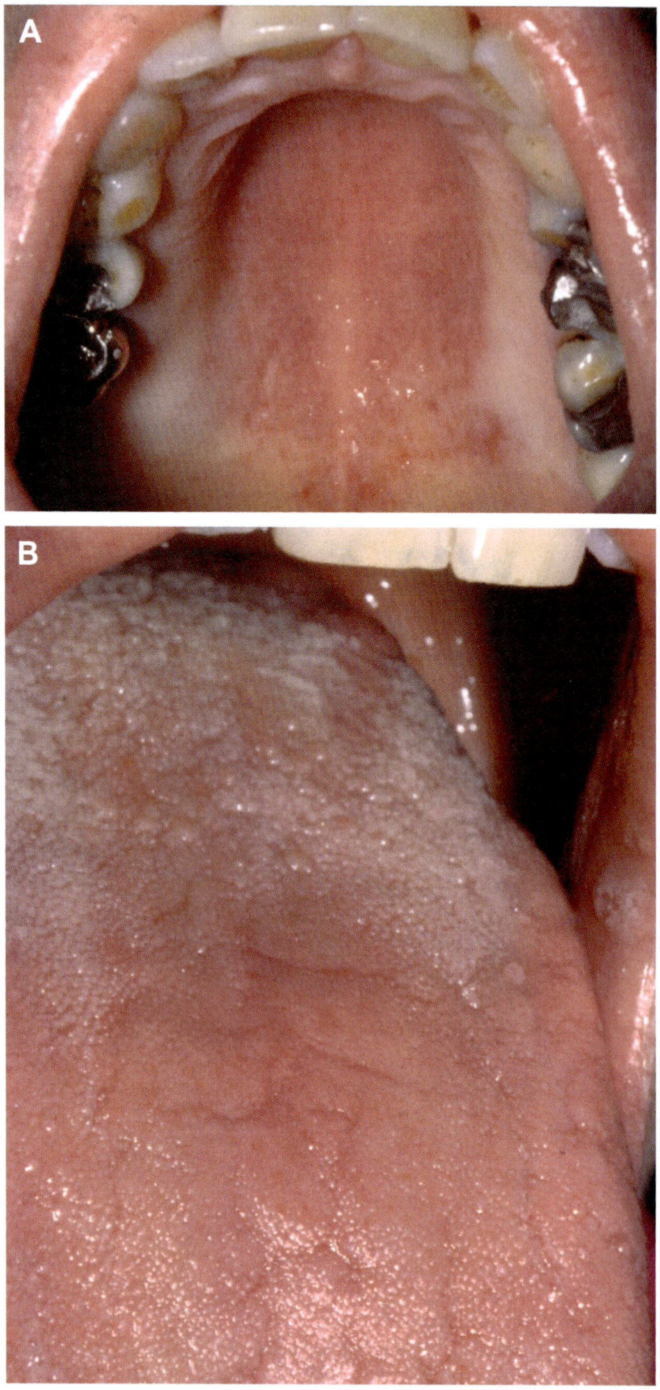

Fig. 13 Erythematous candidiasis (*A*) and atrophic glossitis (*B*) due to pernicious anemia. (*Courtesy of* Dr John Lovas, Halifax, Nova Scotia.)

- Non-specific intraoral changes such as reduced trabecular bone pattern in the mandible (Fig. 14), hair-on-end appearance on skull radiographs, and increased prevalence of osteomyelitis

Differential diagnosis

- Radiographically, sickle cell disease may mimic other conditions association with generalized rarefaction of bone, such as osteoporosis, osteomyelitis, and thalassemia.

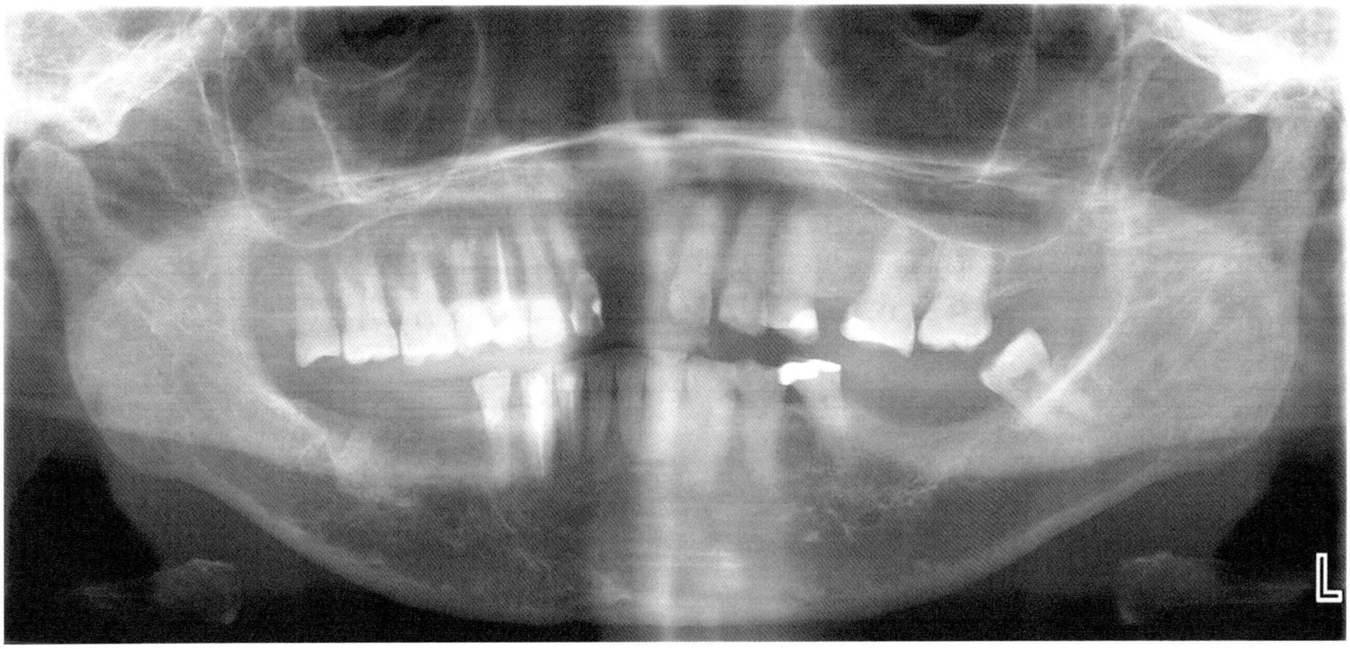

Fig. 14 Reduced trabecular bone pattern caused by sickle cell anemia in a 52-year-old African American woman. (*Courtesy of* Niloufar Amintavakoli, DDS, MSc, Diplomate of ABOMR, FRCD (C), Clinical Assistant Professor, Department of Oral and Maxillofacial Pathology, Radiology & Medicine, New York University College of Dentistry, New York, NY.)

Treatment

Sickle cell disease is treated supportively and with hydroxyurea to increase fetal hemoglobin. Hematopoietic stem cell transplantation is curative but is generally reserved for severe cases. Prophylactic antibiotics may be indicated for major surgical procedures.

Thalassemia

Thalassemia is an inherited condition associated with a mutation in the α-hemoglobin or β-hemoglobin genes, resulting in a reduction in the synthesis of 1 or more of the α-chain or β-chain(s). This condition results in inadequate hemoglobin production. Accumulation of excess globin chains lead to abnormal erythrocytes that rapidly undergo cell lysis, leading to hypochromic, microcytic anemia. This condition is subcategorized into β-thalassemia, when 1 or more of the 2 β-globin genes are affected, and α-thalassemia, when 1 or more of the 4 α-globin genes are mutated.

Epidemiology

Increased prevalence rates of thalassemia are reported in individuals of Mediterranean, African, Indian, and Southeast Asian descent due to its protective effect against malaria.

Clinical presentation

β-Thalassemia

- Patients with 1 defective β-hemoglobin chain are considered to have thalassemia minor and have no significant clinical presentation.
- Patients with 2 defective genes have thalassemia major and present with severe microcytic, hypochromic anemia.
- May show bone marrow hyperplasia, with enlargement of the jaws, reduced trabeculation (Fig. 15), and hair-on-end appearance on skull radiographs.
- If untreated, typically results in death in the first year of life, due to infection or cardiovascular complications.

α-Thalassemia

- When 1 of the 2 α-genes are mutated, no disease is present.
- When 2 genes are mutated (α-thalassemia trait), a patient has mild anemia of no clinical significance.
- When 3 genes are mutated (hemoglobin H disease), a patient suffers from hemolytic anemia and splenomegaly.
- Mutation of all 4 genes results in hydrops fetalis and death within the first few hours of life.

Differential diagnosis

- Thalassemia may mimic other conditions association with generalized bone rarefaction, such as osteoporosis, osteomyelitis, and sickle cell anemia.

Treatment

Frequent blood transfusions with concurrent iron chelating agent (eg, deferoxamine) to prevent hemochromatosis. Hematopoietic bone marrow transplant in eligible individuals is curative.

Histiocytic disorders: Langerhans cell histiocytosis

LCH is a group of conditions characterized by the proliferation of immature dendritic cells called Langerhans cell histiocytes, with variable biologic behavior.

Epidemiology

LCH is a rare disease, primarily affecting children, with equal gender predilection. Oral and maxillofacial cases are predominantly seen in patients less than 40 years of age, with 50% of cases presenting as unifocal single system disease.

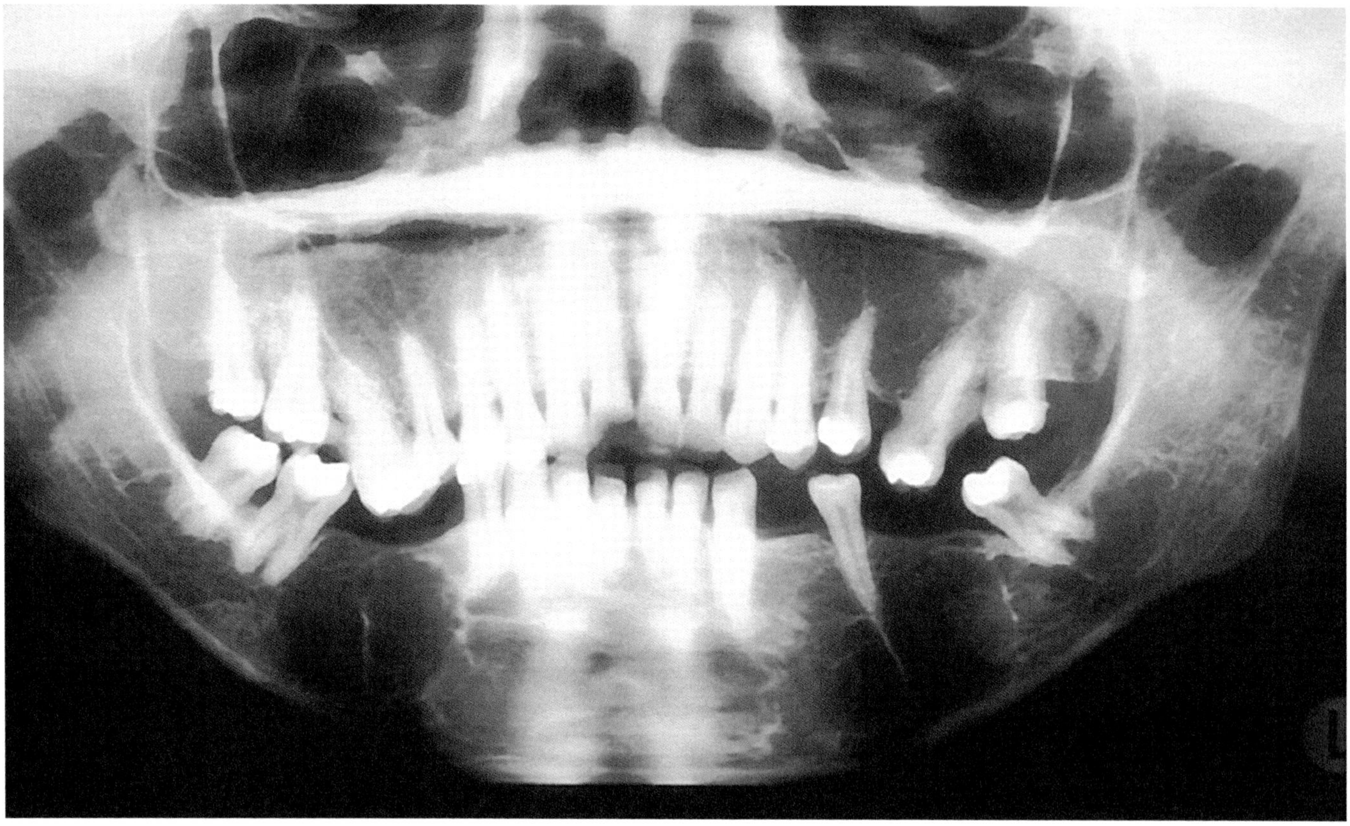

Fig. 15 Enlargement of the marrow spaces affecting the mandible and maxilla in a patient with thalassemia. (*From* Sapp JP, Eversole LR, Wysocki GP. Contemporary oral and maxillofacial pathology. 2nd edition. St Louis (MO): Mosby; 2004; with permission.)

Clinical presentation

Currently, the preferred classification of LCH, proposed by the Histiocyte Society, is based on the extent and localization of disease (Table 5).

Table 5 Clinical classification of Langerhans cell histiocytosis

Disease category	Clinical features
Single-system unifocal disease	Unifocal bone, skin, or lymph node Older children and adults Good prognosis
Single-system multifocal disease (several lesions in a single organ system)	Multifocal bone or multiple lymph nodes Young children Intermediate prognosis
Multifocal, multisystem disease (low risk)	Involvement of 2 or more organs, with or without organ dysfunction, no involvement of high risk organs Excellent prognosis
Multifocal, multisystem disease (high risk)	Involvement of at least 1 or more high-risk organs: lungs, liver, spleen, hematopoietic system Young children and infants Poor prognosis

Clinical features of oral and maxillofacial lesions

- Most commonly presents as single or multiple bone lesions with no systemic or visceral involvement
- Posterior mandible > maxilla > soft tissue lesions
- Bone pain, soft tissue mass, gingivitis, mucosal ulceration, and loosening of teeth may be present (Fig. 16)
- Well defined and noncorticated radiographic appearance often showing a scooped-out appearance (Fig. 17)
- Periosteal new born formation and root resorption can be seen

Histopathology

Microscopically, LCH shows a proliferation of pale-staining histiocyte-like cells with nuclear grooves or folds (Fig. 18). These cells are situated in a background of mixed inflammatory cells invariably containing eosinophils, lymphocytes, plasma cells, and multinucleated giant cells. Langerhans cell histiocytes are positive for CD1a and or langerin (CD207) by immunohistochemistry and show Birbeck granules on electron microscopy.

Differential diagnosis

- Periodontal disease
- Periapical inflammatory disease
- Malignancy, primary or metastatic

Treatment

Solitary lesions are treated by curettage and/or low-dose radiation. Chemotherapy or intralesional steroid injections may also be used. Oral and maxillofacial LCH in the absence of visceral involvement has a good prognosis, but recurrence of

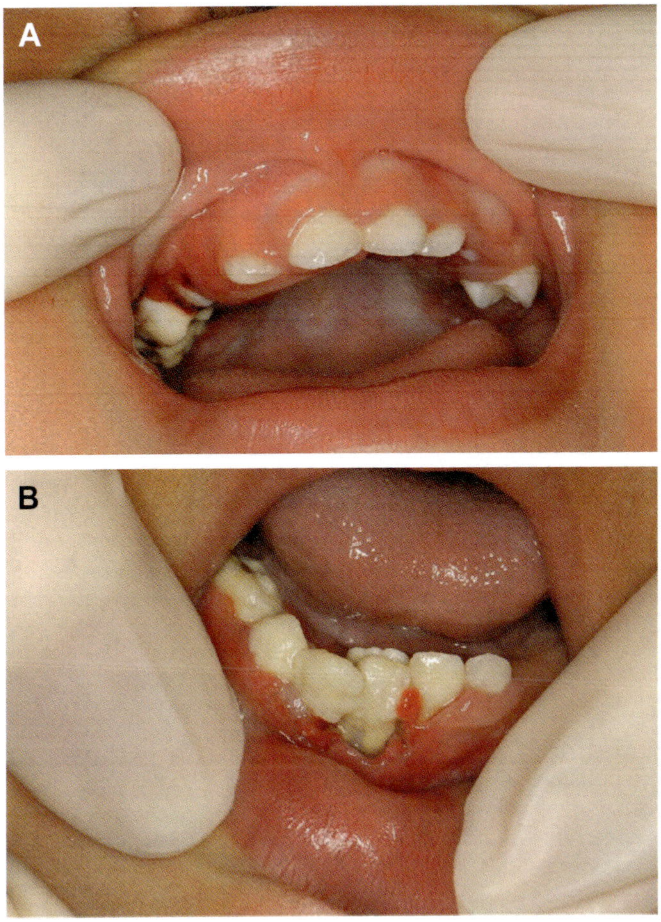

Fig. 16 LCH affecting the bone and soft tissues of the maxilla (*A*) and mandible (*B*) in a young male patient. The patient was known to have skin but not visceral involvement.

disease has been reported, particularly in patients with multifocal bone disease. In patients with multisystem disease, treatment involves multidrug chemotherapy and is associated with a poorer prognosis.

Bleeding disorders

Thrombocytopenia

Thrombocytopenia is a reduced platelet count as a result of decreased platelet production, survival or sequestration of platelets in the spleen. Potential causes for decreased platelet count are listed in Table 6.

Clinical presentation

- Oral manifestations may be the presenting sign of disease and include petechial hemorrhages (Fig. 19), spontaneous gingival hemorrhage, and bleeding from minor trauma.

Differential diagnosis

- Palatal petechiae are not specific to thrombotic disorders and can occur in coagulation disorders, trauma, viral infections, amyloidosis, vitamin C deficiency, and systemic lupus erythematosus.
- Condition, such as aplastic anemia, malignancy, and HIV, can also cause thrombocytopenia and may have similar intraoral manifestations.

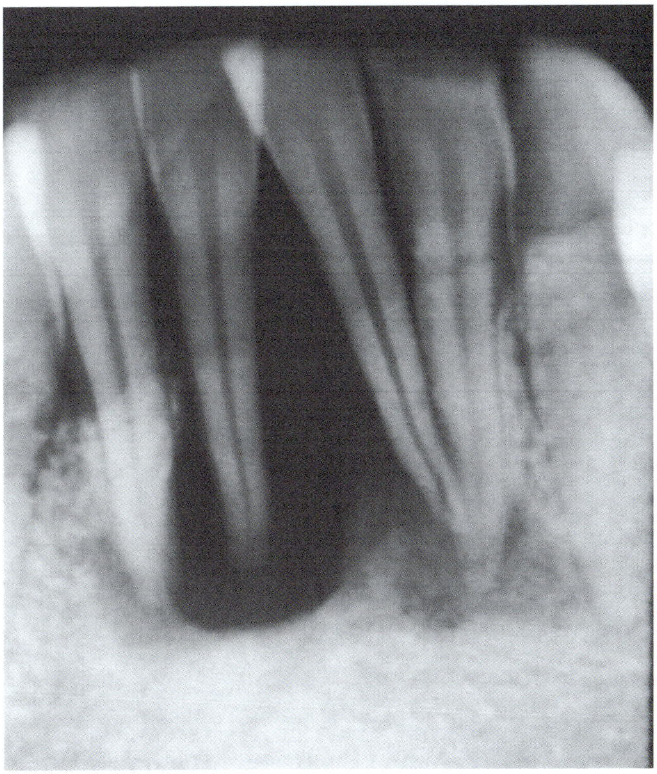

Fig. 17 Radiographic features of LCH in a 26-year-old female patient. The radiograph shows a scooped-out radiolucency, giving the appearance of teeth standing in space.

Treatment

Treatment depends on the severity of disease as well as the underlying cause. Platelet transfusions, corticosteroids or intravenous immune globulin may be required. Drug-associated cases require immediate discontinuation of offending drug.

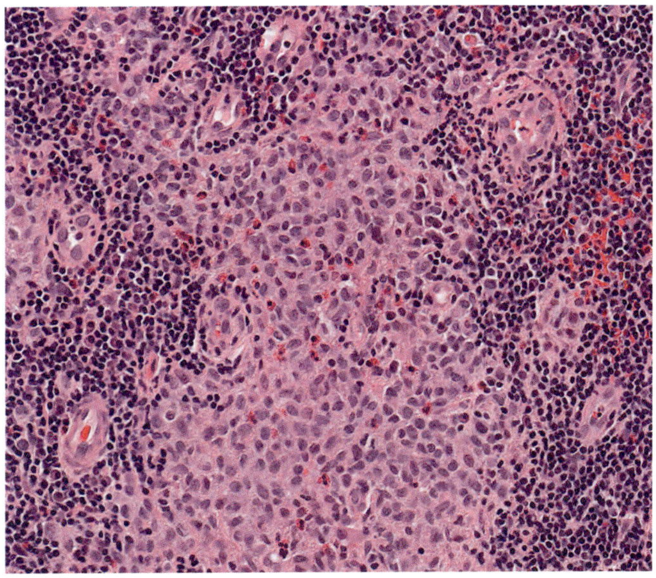

Fig. 18 Microscopic appearance of LCH. Pale staining cells with irregular nuclear contours (Langerhans cells) are admixed with eosinophils and other inflammatory cells (hematoxylin-eosin, original magnification ×20).

Table 6 Causes of thrombocytopenia

Etiology	Underlying disease state
Decreased platelet production	Bone marrow suppression (eg, leukemia, aplastic anemia) Drugs, alcohol, HIV, myelodysplastic syndrome
Decreased platelet survival	Immunologic (primary and secondary ITP, drug associated, HIV-associated) Nonimmunologic (DIC, injury due to mechanical heart valves)
Platelet sequestration	Liver disease, tumors, Gaucher disease

Abbreviations: DIC, disseminated intravascular coagulation; ITP, idiopathic thrombocytopenic purpura.

Hereditary hemorrhagic telangiectasia (Osler-Weber-Rendu disease)

Hereditary hemorrhagic telangiectasia (HHT) is an inherited condition resulting in structural anomalies of blood vessels. Two subtypes of HHT have been identified. HHT type 1 presents primarily with arteriovenous abnormalities (AVMs) affecting the lungs and brain, whereas HHT type 2 presents primarily with hepatic involvement. The clinical hallmark of HHT is telangiectatic lesions affecting mucous membranes of the gastrointestinal tract, including the mouth, nasal cavity and eyes.

Epidemiology

HHT has an incidence of 1:5000 to 18,000 with geographic variance. HHT type 1 is caused by mutation in *ENG* (endoglin), whereas HHT type 2 is caused by mutation of *ACVRL1* (activin receptor–like kinase 1). An HHT juvenile polyposis overlap syndrome has been identified in patients with *MADH4* mutation.

Clinical presentation

- Epistaxis, arteriovenous malformations (AVMs) of lung, brain, or liver.

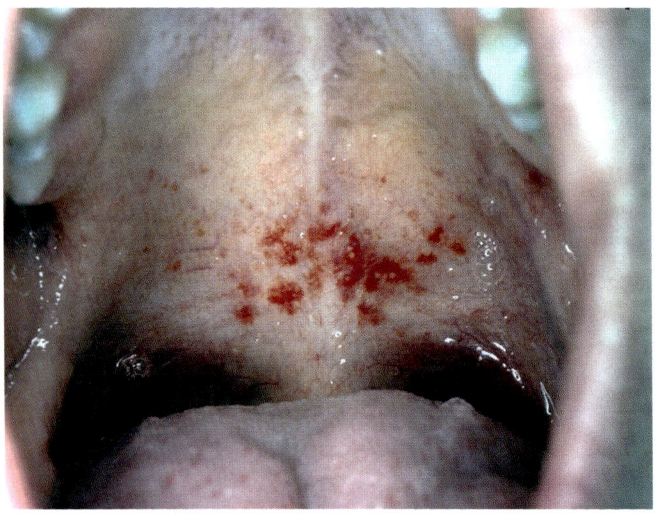

Fig. 19 Palatal petechial hemorrhages.

- Small 1-mm to -2-mm vascular lesions, which blanch with pressure, called telangiectasias, affecting the skin and mucous membranes. The vermilion, tongue, and buccal mucosa are common sites of involvement (Fig. 20).

Differential diagnosis

- Other causes of recurrent epistaxis, such as bleeding diatheses and neoplasms.
- Limited cutaneous systemic sclerosis (calcinosis cutis, Raynaud phenomenon, esophageal dysfunction, sclerodactyly and telangiectasia, or CREST syndrome) ataxia-telangiectasia, or chronic liver disease may also present with telangiectasias.

Treatment

Cutaneous and gastrointestinal lesions may be treated by laser ablation. Embolization or surgical treatment may be required for large pulmonary AVMs or cerebral arteriovenous shunts. Blood transfusion and iron therapy may be needed following dental extraction and antibiotic prophylaxis may be indicated in patients with pulmonary AVMs to prevent brain abscess.

Hemophilia

Hemophilia is an inherited bleeding disorder associated with a quantitative defect in a particular clotting factor. Hemophilia A is caused by deficiency of factor VIII and hemophilia B is caused by deficiency of factor IX.

Epidemiology

Hemophilia A is an X-linked disorder affecting 1 in 5000 boys and men. Up to 30% of cases represent spontaneous mutations. Hemophilia B is also X-linked, but less common, affecting 1 in 30,000 boys and men.

Clinical presentation

- The clinical hallmark is prolonged bleeding due to a delay in clotting
- Clinical manifestations depend on the severity of the disease:
  - Mild disease (6%–50% of normal clotting factor)
  - Moderately severe disease (2%–5% of normal clotting factor)
  - Severe disease (<1% of normal clotting factor)
- Uncontrolled or delayed bleeding after surgical procedures, extractions, or periodontal procedures
- Easy bruising and spontaneous hemorrhage in areas susceptible to trauma
- Bleeding into joints (hemarthrosis) causing deformity and disability

Differential diagnosis

- Bleeding is a complication of many inherited and acquired disorders. von Willebrand disease, and other factor deficiencies may present with similar clinical features.

Treatment

- Clotting factor replacement depends on the severity of the disease and the intervention planned.
- Antifibrinolytics are often given prior to and after surgery.

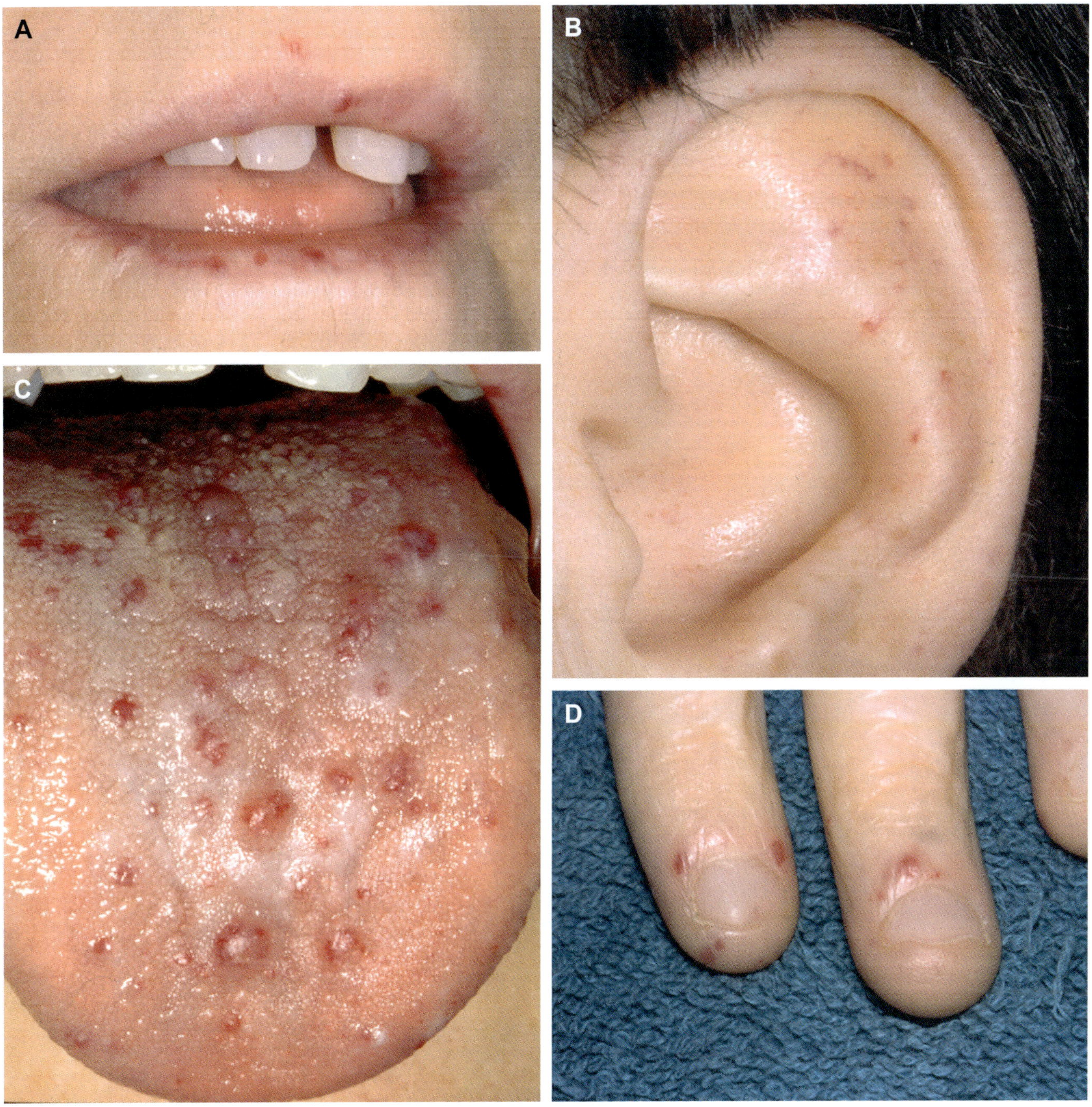

Fig. 20 Multiple superficial, small, dilated blood vessels (telangiectasias) affecting the lips (*A*), skin of the ear (*B*), dorsal tongue (*C*), and finger tips (*D*) in a patient with HHT. (*Courtesy of* Dr John Lovas, Halifax, Nova Scotia.)

Further readings

Abla O, Egeler RM, Weitzman S. Langerhans cell histiocytosis: current concepts and treatments. Cancer Treat Rev 2010;36(4):354–9.

Arber DA, Orazi A, Hasserjian R, et al. The 2016 revision to the World Health Organization classification of myeloid neoplasms and acute leukemia. Blood 2016;127(20):2391–405.

Cardoso RC, Gerngross PJ, Hofstede TM, et al. The multiple oral presentations of multiple myeloma. Support Care Cancer 2014;22(1):259–67.

Dagenais M, Pharoah MJ, Sikorski PA. The radiographic characteristics of histiocytosis X. A study of 29 cases that involve the jaws. Oral Surg Oral Med Oral Pathol 1992;74(2):230–6.

Faughnan ME, Palda VA, Garcia-Tsao G, et al. International guidelines for the diagnosis and management of hereditary haemorrhagic telangiectasia. J Med Genet 2011;48(2):73–87.

Hazza'a AM, Al-Jamal G. Radiographic features of the jaws and teeth in thalassaemia major. Dentomaxillofac Radiol 2006;35(4):283–8.

Heiland M, Weber M, Schmelzle R. Life-threatening bleeding after dental extraction in a hemophilia A patient with inhibitors to factor VIII: a case report. J Oral Maxillofac Surg 2003;61(11):1350–3.

Hicks J, Flaitz CM. Langerhans cell histiocytosis: current insights in a molecular age with emphasis on clinical oral and maxillofacial pathology practice. Oral Surg Oral Med Oral Pathol Oral Radiol Endod 2005;100(2 Suppl):S42–66.

Hou GL, Huang JS, Tsai CC. Analysis of oral manifestations of leukemia: a retrospective study. Oral Dis 1997;3(1):31–8.

Kelleher M, Bishop K, Briggs P. Oral complications associated with sickle cell anemia: a review and case report. Oral Surg Oral Med Oral Pathol Oral Radiol Endod 1996;82(2):225–8.

Kolokotronis A, Konstantinou N, Christakis I, et al. Localized B-cell non-Hodgkin's lymphoma of oral cavity and maxillofacial region: a clinical study. Oral Surg Oral Med Oral Pathol Oral Radiol Endod 2005;99(3):303–10.

Kumar R, Carcao M. Inherited abnormalities of coagulation: hemophilia, von Willebrand disease, and beyond. Pediatr Clin North Am 2013;60(6):1419–41.

Kumar V, Abbas AK, Asster JC. Robbins and cotran pathologic basis of disease. 9th edition. Phildadelphia: Elsevier; 2015.

Little JW, Falace DA, Miller CS, et al. Little and Falace's dental management of the medically compromised patient. 8th edition. St Louis (MO): Elsevier; 2013.

Looker AC, Dallman PR, Carroll MD, et al. Prevalence of iron deficiency in the United States. JAMA 1997;277(12):973–6.

Modell B, Darlison M. Global epidemiology of haemoglobin disorders and derived service indicators. Bull World Health Organ 2008;86(6): 480–7.

Neville BW, Damm D, Allen CM, et al. Oral and maxillofacial pathology. 4th edition. St Louis (MO): Elsevier; 2016.

Rees DC, Williams TN, Gladwin MT. Sickle-cell disease. Lancet 2010; 376(9757):2018–31.

Siegel RL, Miller KD, Jemal A. Cancer statistics, 2016. CA Cancer J Clin 2016;66(1):7–30.

Swerdlow SH, Campo E, Harris NL, et al. WHO classification of tumours of hematopoietic and lymphoid tissues. 4th edition. Lyon (France): International Agency for Research on Cancer (IARC); 2008.

Swerdlow SH, Campo E, Pileri SA, et al. The 2016 revision of the World Health Organization classification of lymphoid neoplasms. Blood 2016;127(20):2375–90.

te Veldhuis EC, te Veldhuis AH, van Dijk FS, et al. Rendu-Osler-Weber disease: update of medical and dental considerations. Oral Surg Oral Med Oral Pathol Oral Radiol Endod 2008;105(2):e38–41.

Yamamoto JF, Goodman MT. Patterns of leukemia incidence in the United States by subtype and demographic characteristics, 1997-2002. Cancer Causes Control 2008;19(4):379–90.

Zapater E, Bagan JV, Carbonell F, et al. Malignant lymphoma of the head and neck. Oral Dis 2010;16(2):119–28.

Zimmermann C, Meurer MI, Grando LJ, et al. Dental treatment in patients with leukemia. J Oncol 2015;2015:571739.

Oral Manifestations of Viral Infections

Mahnaz Fatahzadeh, DMD, MSD

KEYWORDS

• Herpes simplex • Varicella zoster • Human papilloma • Coxsackie • Viral infection

KEY POINTS

- A plethora of symptomatic or asymptomatic viral conditions may affect the oral cavity.
- Clinical presentation of viral infections range from no change to epithelial ulcerations, benign soft tissue growths and malignancy.
- Definitive diagnosis of oral ulcerations caused by varicella, Coxsackie and herpes simplex viruses relies on history, physical exam and diagnostic tests.
- Educating Patients about the contagious nature of viral conditions is essential for preventing spread of infections.

Introduction

Viruses cause a plethora of symptomatic or asymptomatic infections in the oral cavity, with clinical manifestations ranging from no change to epithelial ulcerations, benign soft tissue growths, and malignancy. The host's intact innate and adaptive immunity is often adequate for viral recognition and mounting a protective response. Those with a defective immune system, however, often experience more severe sequelae.

Ulcerative manifestations of various viral infections are often difficult to discern from each other and from clinically similar conditions of different etiology. This article reviews presentation, diagnosis, and the management approach for major viral conditions of oral cavity such as herpes simplex virus type 1 (HSV1), varicella zoster virus (VZV), coxsackie viruses, and human papilloma virus (HPV).

Herpes simplex type

Description

The herpesviridae group of viruses includes more than 80 herpesviruses; for 8 viruses, people are the natural host. All human herpes viruses (HHVs) have a double-stranded DNA core within a protein capsid, enclosed by a tegument and an envelope, and are capable of causing life-long latency. Herpes simplex virus (HSV) has 2 serotypes, HSV1 and HSV2, which are partially homologous in their DNA core but have different antigenic properties.

Although HSV1 and HSV2 primarily infect orofacial and genital regions, respectively, sexual practices could result in cross-over infections. Herpes simplex viruses are highly transmissible through contact with oral or genital secretions of individuals with active lesions as well as asymptomatic shedding. Spread of infection to other mucocutaneous sites occurs through autoinoculation.

Epidemiology

HSV-1 prevalence varies depending on age, race, geographic location, and socioeconomic status. In the underdeveloped countries, HSV-1seroconversions is not only higher but also occurs at a younger age.

Primary oral herpes

Primary herpetic gingivostomatitis (PHGS) develops when a nonimmune individual is exposed to HSV-1 for the first time.

Clinical presentation and differential diagnosis

Most cases affect children 1 to 5 years of age and are often subclinical. Symptomatic patients present with lymphadenopathy, fever, sore throat, and vesiculo-ulcerative lesions affecting the oral and perioral regions (Fig. 1). Both movable and nonmovable oral mucosa may be affected, and acute onset of generalized gingival inflammation and pain is a classic feature (Figs. 2 and 3).

Differential diagnosis includes herpangina, erythema multiforme, allergic stomatitis, acute necrotizing ulcerative gingivitis, and acute eruptions of vesiculobullous diseases.

Management

The condition is self-limiting in healthy individuals. When oral pain and dysphagia pose risk of dehydration and poor nutritional intake, palliation and off-label antiviral therapy with acyclovir or valacyclovir may be indicated.

Antipyetics such as acetaminophen may be used to treat fever, and anesthetic rinses may be used for palliation. Hydration and a bland, soft diet should also be encouraged. Patients should be educated about the contagious nature of the virus and potential for spread of infection to others or autoinoculation to other body sites.

Disclosure: None.

Department of Diagnostic Sciences, Rutgers School of Dental Medicine, Room D-855, 110 Bergen Street, Newark, NJ 07103, USA
E-mail address: fatahza@sdm.rutgers.edu

Atlas Oral Maxillofacial Surg Clin N Am 25 (2017) 163-170
1061-3315/17/
http://dx.doi.org/10.1016/j.cxom.2017.04.008

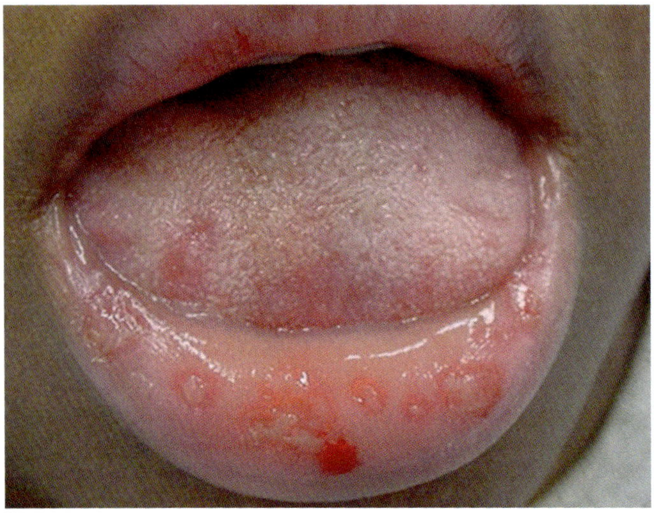

Fig. 1 Primary herpetic gingivostomatitis affecting the lower lip.

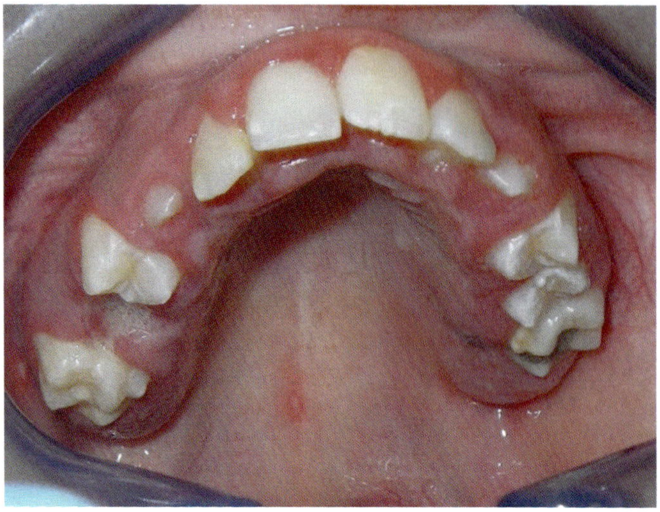

Fig. 3 Gingival erythema and edema in primary herpetic gingivostomatitis.

Secondary oral herpes

HSV 1 establishes life-long latency in trigeminal ganglion. Internal and external triggers such as stress, fatigue, fever, menstruation, immunosuppression, and exposure to heat, cold, or sunlight could cause viral reactivation. Viral reactivation may occur in up to 40% of individuals testing positive for HSV1 antibodies and lead to asymptomatic viral shedding (recurrence) or clinical disease (recrudescence).

Clinical presentation

Recrudescence may affect mucocutaneous junction of the lips (Figs. 4 and 5) or keratinized intraoral tissues (Figs. 6 and 7). Unlike PHGS, there are no systemic symptoms with recrudescence. However, onset of HSL is often preceded by a local prodrome of tingling, burning, or itching. Recrudescent intraoral herpes (RIH) is less common than herpes simplex labialis (HSL), and in the immunocompetent host, it affects keratinized tissues such as gingiva and palate.

Differential diagnosis

Differential diagnosis for RIH includes herpes zoster, herpetiform aphthous ulcers, and traumatic ulcers. Vesicular onset and localization to nonmovable mucosa often help differentiate RIH from recurrent aphthous ulcerations. Diagnosis of both primary and secondary HSV1 infections relies on history and clinical presentation. However, Tzanck smear, viral culture, tissue biopsy, serology, or polymerase chain reaction (PCR) may prove beneficial in atypical cases.

Management

In the immunocompetent host, HSL heals within 7 to 14 days without scarring. Frequent or disfiguring recurrences of HSL and severe or chronic HSV outbreaks in the immunosuppressed host may require antiviral therapy. US Food and Drug Administration (FDA)-approved medications for HSL include topical deconasol and penciclovir, as well as systemic valacyclovir. Maximal therapeutic efficacy requires early recognition of signs and symptoms of an outbreak and initiation of antiviral therapy during the prodrome.

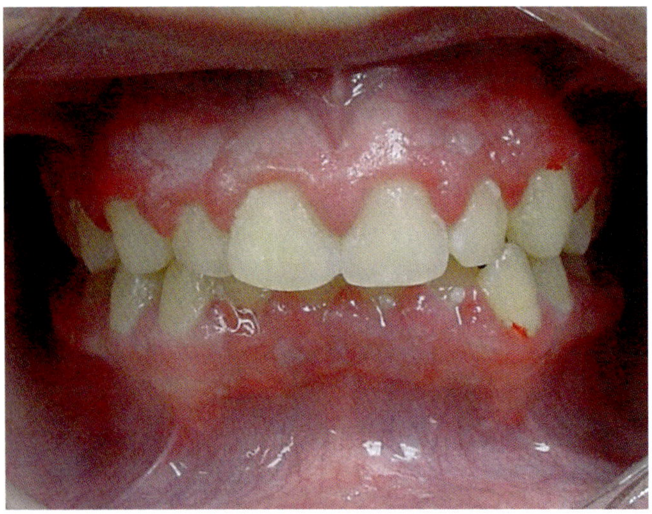

Fig. 2 Gingival erythema and focal ulcerations in primary herpetic gingivostomatitis.

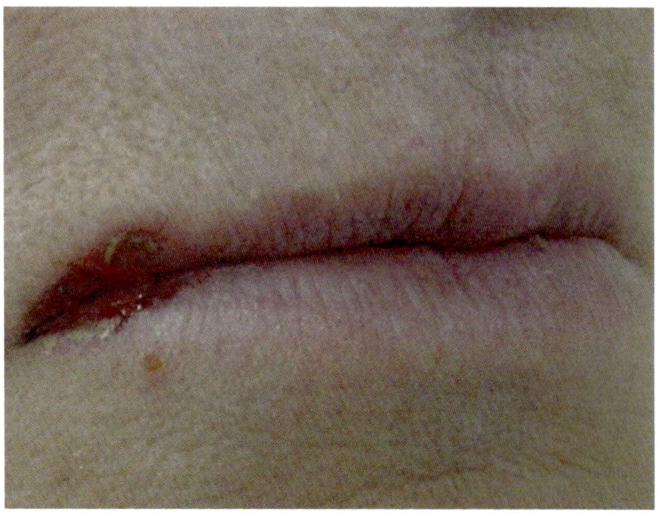

Fig. 4 Herpes simplex labialis affecting right labial commissures.

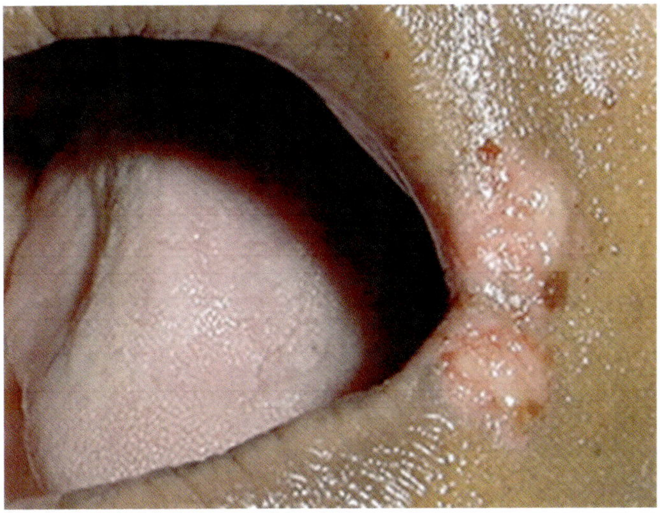

Fig. 5 Herpes simplex labialis affecting left labial commissures.

Varicella-zoster virus

Varicella zoster (chicken pox)

Description

Varicella zoster virus (VZV) is one of human herpes group of viruses capable of developing primary and secondary disease. Primary exposure to VZV in a nonimmunized person results in an acute disease known as chicken pox. The main route of viral transmission is through respiratory tracts or conjunctiva.

Clinical presentation and management

A prodrome may precede development of a generalized, pruritic skin rash, which spread centripetally. Fever and malaise may also be present. Lesions progress through macular to papular, vesicular, pustular, and crusted stages. Although mouth and oropharynx may be affected, intraoral lesions are minimally symptomatic.

In healthy individuals, recovery is uneventful and leads to life-long immunity. Condition is highly contagious and measures to prevent transmission to other should be considered.

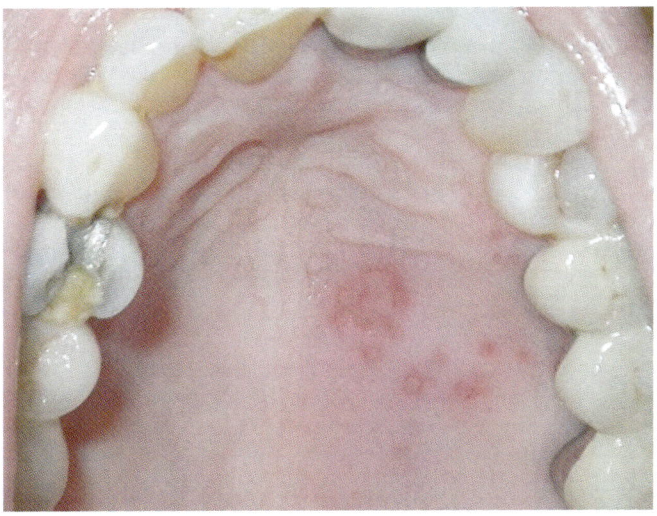

Fig. 6 Recurrent intraoral herpes on left palatal mucosa.

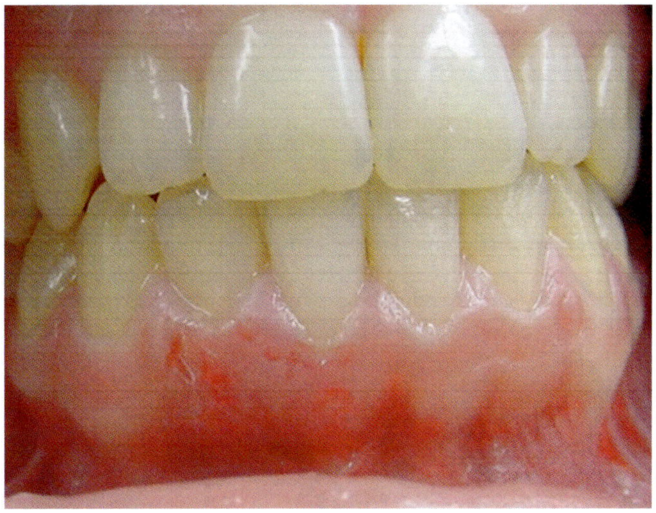

Fig. 7 Recurrent intraoral herpes on lower right attached gingiva.

Herpes zoster (shingles)

Description

Reactivation of VZV dormant in a sensory nerve ganglion results in herpes zoster (HZ) or shingles in a sensory dermatome (Fig. 8). Reactivation occurs in 5 out of 1000 individuals testing seropositive for VZV. Cytotoxic drugs, immunosuppression, internal malignancies, and aging are among the risk factors for viral reactivation.

Clinical presentation

Herpes zoster presents with a prodrome of mild fever, malaise and pain, burning, itching, or paresthesia in the affected area. This is followed by regional lymphadenopathy and unilateral vesicular rash in dermatome of a sensory nerve. Involvement of bilateral or multiple dermatomes is uncommon and should raise concerns about immunosuppression.

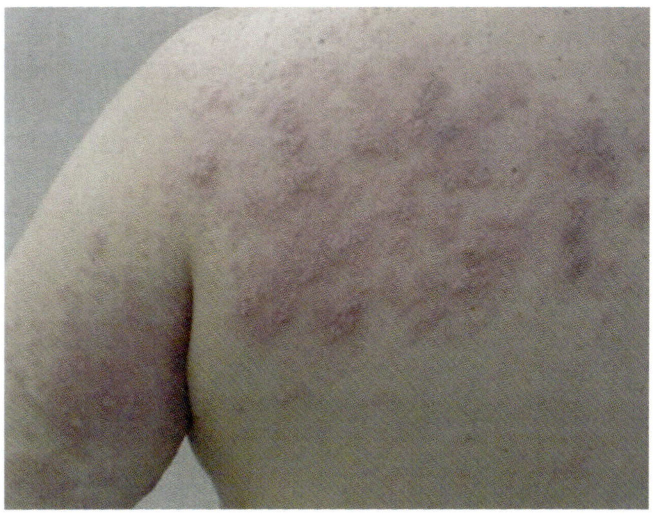

Fig. 8 Vesicular eruptions of herpes zoster in upper arm and back dermatome.

Up to 15% of HZ cases may involve mucocutaneous distribution of trigeminal nerve with predilection for ophthalmic division. The latter may lead to serious ocular complications such as corneal ulceration and blindness necessitating urgent medical attention. Involvement of maxillary division of CN5 leads to ipsilateral vesicular eruptions in midface and mucous membranes of nose, nasopharynx, palate and tonsils (Fig. 9).

HZ affecting the mandibular nerve leads to ipsilateral lesions involving side of the head, ear, lower lip, and corresponding oral mucosa. Lesions may only affect oral mucosa and spare cutaneous dermatome. Potential oral complications of HZ include exfoliation of teeth, root esorption, and osteonecrosis.

Postherpetic neuralgia (PHN), characterized by severe, refractory pain following resolution of lesions, is a serious complication of HZ. It is most common in the ophthalmic division of trigeminal nerve, and individuals older than 50 are particularly at risk.

Reactivation of latent VZV in the geniculate ganglion causes Ramsey Hunt syndrome characterized by cranial nerve 7 and sometimes cranial nerve 8 dysfunction. Affected patients may experience a vesicular rash affecting the ear and pharynx, together with ipsilateral facial paralysis, earache, taste changes, vertigo, tinnitus, and hearing loss.

Differential diagnosis

Oral HZ may be mistaken for RIH. However, the former generally has more severe prodrome, distinctly unilateral outbreaks, ipsilateral cutaneous rash, and potential complications such as postherpetic neuralgia. Both HSV and HZV have positive Tzanck smears and require additional laboratory testing for differentiation. In immunocompetent individuals, prodromal pain and itching, unilateral vesicular eruptions, and dermatomal rash help exclude herpangina and aphthous ulceration.

Weakness, hypoesthesia, or severe pain in the sensory distribution of a given nerve in the absence of classic zoster rash is known as Zoster sine herpete. In the oral region, the latter may mimic odontogenic pain, and its exclusion is critical in order to avoid unnecessary dental interventions such as endodontics or extractions. Zoster sine herpete affecting head and neck region may also be confused with trigeminal neuralgia.

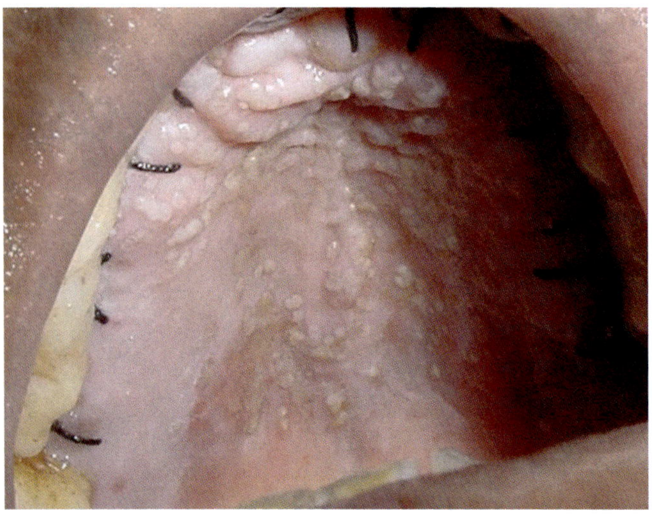

Fig. 9 Vesicular eruptions of herpes zoster on left palatal mucosa.

Vesicular eruptions of HZ resemble vesiculobollous diseases such as pemphigus and pemphigoid. Involvement of geniculate ganglion may mimic sign and symptoms resembling Bell palsy.

Diagnosis and management

Diagnosis of HZ often relies on history and clinical findings. However, laboratory investigations such as viral culture, PCR, or serologic testing and epidemiologic linkage may be used for confirmation.

Management of HZ depends on the age, immune status, symptoms, and clinical presentation. Depending on severity, topical anesthetics, analgesics, anticonvulsants, tricylic antidepressants, or their combinations may be used to manage pain and pruritis. When indicated, timely intervention with high-dose antivirals with or without corticosteroids helps control symptoms and reduces the likelihood of PHN in susceptible patients.

Coxsackievirus infections

Description

Coxsackieviruses belong to the genus Enterovirus and contain a single strand of RNA with no envelope. Primary mode of transmission is through fecal-oral route and respiratory droplets and patients are most contagious in the first few days of illness. Coxsackieviruses are divided into 2 groups, each with multiple serotypes. Group A coxsackieviruses have a predilection for mucocutaneous tissues and cause herpangina or hand-foot-mouth disease (HFMD). In contrast, group B coxsackieviruses often infect visceral organs.

Epidemiology

Global distribution of coxsackievirus infections is broad, with predominance in tropical regions. In the United States, many enteroviral infections are associated with coxsackieviruses. The incidence of coxsackievirus infections is higher in infants and children younger than 10 years of age with a 2:1 male predilection.

Clinical presentation

Most coxsackievirus infections are subclinical or manifest with a nonspecific rash or febrile illnesses. Complications are more likely in neonates and the immunocompromised.

Herpangina

Herpangina primarily affects young children, causing fever, malaise, and symptomatic oral lesions. The latter occur in clusters and progress through macular, popular, and vesicular stages before diffuse erythema and punctate erosions develop in posterior oral cavity (Fig. 10).

Lesions affect the soft palate, uvula, posterior pharygeal wall, and tonsils, causing sore throat, odynophagia, dysphagia, and occasionally throat exudates. Headache, vomiting, and abdominal pain may also be present.

Herpangina symptoms may overlap with those of streptococcal pharyngitis and tonsilitis. The latter may be excluded by a throat culture. Pharyngitis of streptococcal origin does not present with vesicular lesions seen in herpangina.

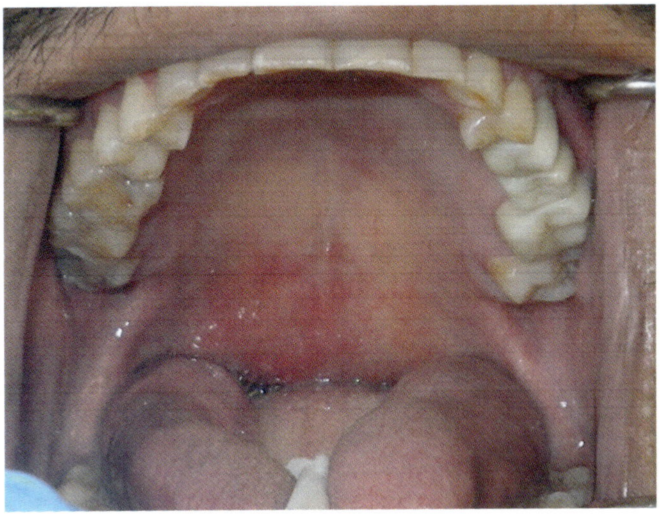

Fig. 10 vesicular eruptions of herpangina in posterior oral cavity.

Hand-foot-mouth disease
HFMD primarily affects children and is highly transmissible. Patients experience low-grade fever and vesicular sores that coalesce to form symptomatic oral erosions (Figs. 11 and 12). Typical locations include tongue, palate, and buccal mucosa.

Nearly $^3/_4$ of patients will also experience nonpruritic cuanteous papules and vesicles on dorsal and lateral aspects of hands and feet (Fig. 13). Coxsackievirus A16 is the predominant serotype in most cases. Severe outbreaks of HFMD often involve coxsackievirus A6.

Diagnosis

Differential diagnosis includes PHGS and HZ, both of which have multinucleated giant cells on Tzanck smear. Lesions of HFM show inter/intracellular edema and intracytoplasmic viral particles on microscopic examination.

Systemic symptoms of HFM are minimal compared with PHGS and VZV. Cutaneous lesions of HFMD differ from centripetal rash seen in VZV. Definitive diagnosis relies on identification of coxsackievirus virus by PCR or isolation in cell culture. Patients develop neutralizing antibodies upon exposure to coxsackieviruses and a fourfold rise in titer between exposure, and recovery from the illness supports the diagnosis.

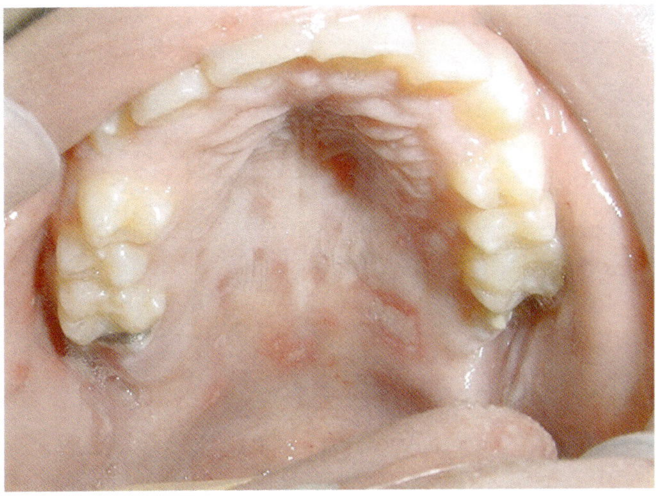

Fig. 11 Coalesced erosions of hand foot mouth disease on palatal mucosa.

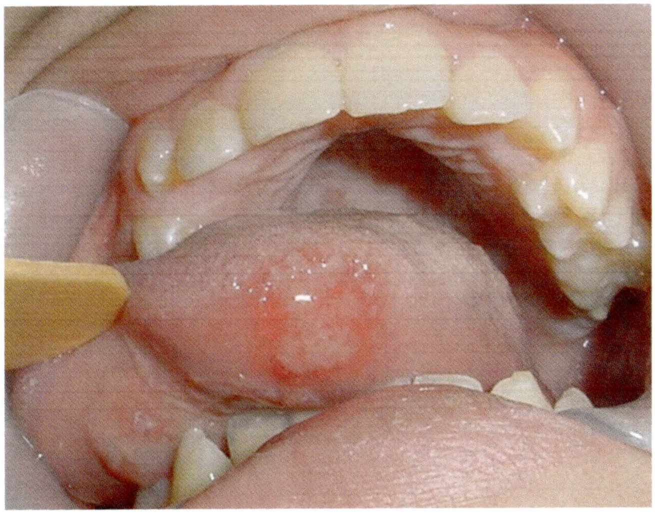

Fig. 12 Coalesced erosions of hand-foot-mouth disease on left tongue.

Management

No vaccine or specific antibiotic for coxsackievirus infections is available. Both HFMD and herpangina are generally self-limiting with good prognosis, and treatment is primarily supportive.

Antipyetics such as acetaminophen may be used to treat fever, and anesthetic rinses may be used to alleviate oral discomfort. Hydration and bland, soft diet should also be encouraged. Educating patients about hand washing, not sharing of utensils, and minimizing contact with those affected are key to preventing transmission.

Human papillomavirus

Description

A group of DNA viruses with predilection for mucocutaneous tissues. Human papilloma virus (HPV) is most frequently

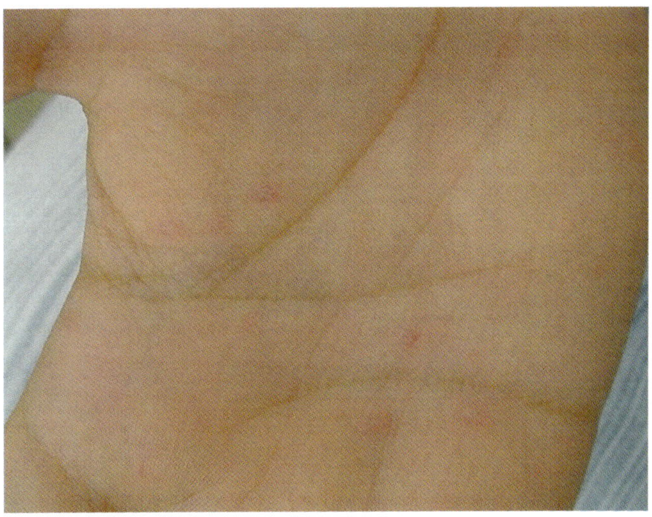

Fig. 13 Papular lesions of hand foot mouth disease affecting palm.

transmitted through intimate vaginal, anal, or oral contact, and it is widely distributed throughout the world. Multiple sexual exposures and immunocompromised status increase likelihood of HPV infection. There are over 120 types of HPV, of which 40 types infect mucosal epithelium. Most HPVs are classified as low risk for malignant epithelial transformation. Thirteen strains are considered high risk for mucocutaneous malignancy.

Natural history

HPV infections are asymptomatic, and in immunocompetent individuals frequently cleared within 2 years. Therefore, HPV infections do not require treatment.

Human immunodeficiency virus (HIV)-positive individuals not only have more frequent oral HPV infections but also are more likely to have persistent infection of basal epithelium and to be infected with multiple strains. Current heavy smoking also increases the risk of oral HPV infection.

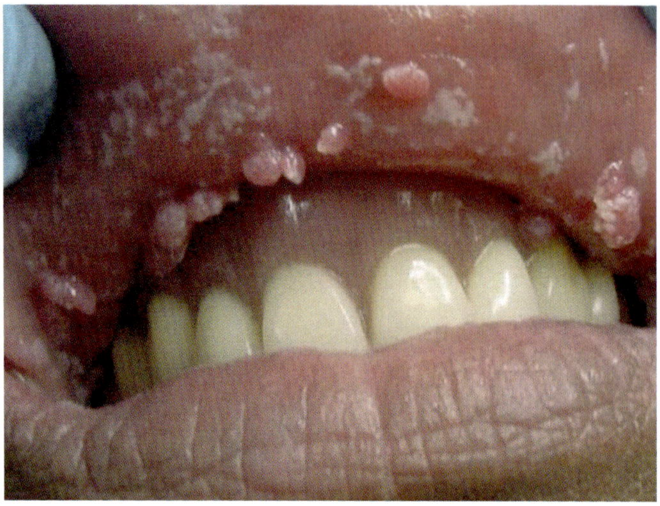

Fig. 15 Multiple squamous papillomas affecting upper labial mucosa.

Clinical presentation

Clinical manifestations of HPV include mucocutaneous warts (oral, anal, genital), respiratory papillomatosis, mucocutaneous epithelial dysplasia and a variety of epithelial cancers (cervical, vaginal, vulvar, penile, anal and oropharyngeal). Oral manifestations of HPV infection include

1. Respiratory papillomatosis resulting from maternal transmission of low-risk HPV to the newborn during vaginal birth and development of papillomas in the nasal passages, mouth, and lung
2. Oral warts resulting from focal epithelial proliferations caused by persistent low-risk HPV infection of oral epithelium—further subdivided into
   a. Squamous papilloma, the most common epithelial growths in the oral cavity, caused by HPV 6 and 11; Squamous papillomas are small, exophytic, and pedunculated with a papillary surface texture and can be found anywhere in the oral cavity (Figs. 14 and 15)
   b. Verruca vulgaris or common wart, presenting as a solitary or multiple broad-based lesions with cauliflower surface texture; common locations are lips, palate and gingiva; most often associated with HPV 2 and 4 (Figs. 16–19)
   c. Condyloma acuminatum or genital warts, which may develop in the oral cavity in association with oro-genital sex with a partner having genital lesions; lesions are larger, sessile, and clustered with predilection for non-keratinized oral mucosa such as soft palate, lingual frenum, and labial mucosa; associated with HPV 6, and 11 (Figs. 20 and 21).
   d. Focal epithelial hyperplasia or Heck disease, presenting with multiple small, smooth-surfaced papules affecting labial and buccal mucosa; condition is associated with HPV13 and 32 and typically regresses without treatment (Figs. 22 and 23)

Diagnosis

Microscopic evaluation of oral warts reveals HPV-infected keratinocytes with koilocytic changes (nuclear enlargement, nuclear membrane irregularity and hyperchromasia). Depending on type of wart, varying degree of acanthosis, parakeratosis, and verrucous epithelial proliferation may be

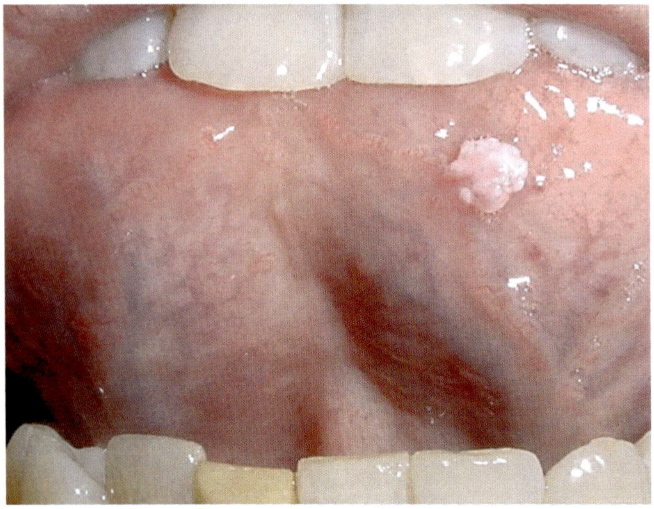

Fig. 14 Solitary squamous papilloma on ventral tongue.

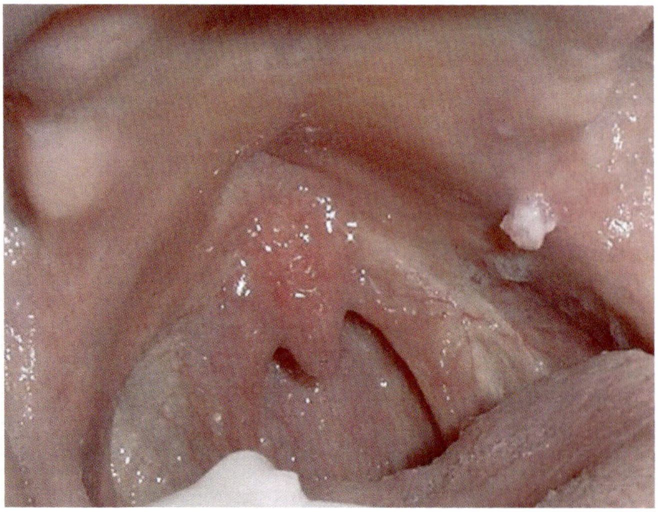

Fig. 16 Verruca vulgaris as a papillary growth on palate.

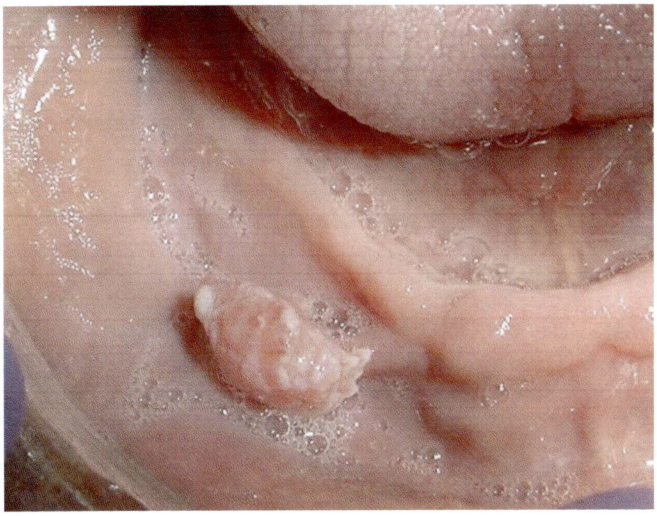

Fig. 17 Verruca vulgaris as a papillary growth on right buccal vestibule.

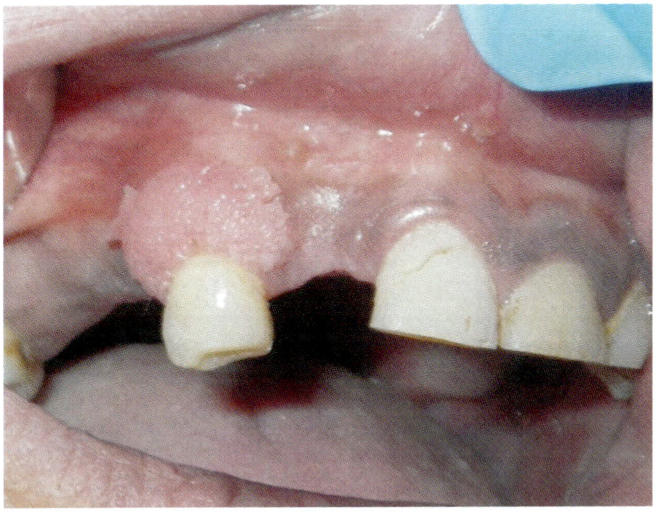

Fig. 18 Verruca vulgaris as a papillary growth on tooth #6 buccal gingiva.

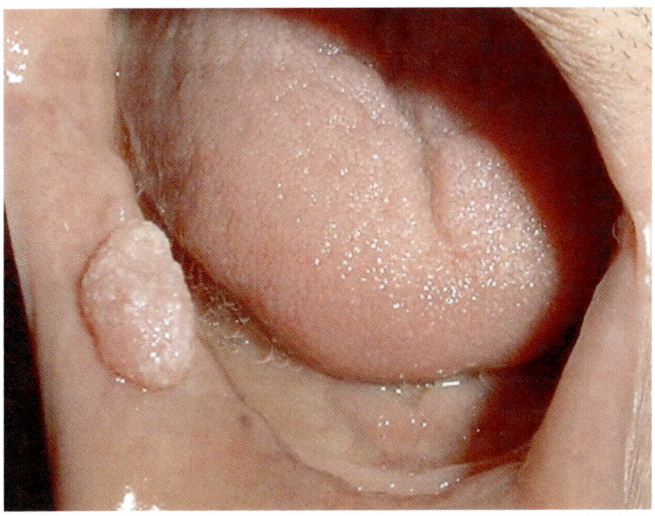

Fig. 19 Verruca vulgaris as a papillary growth on lower labial mucosa.

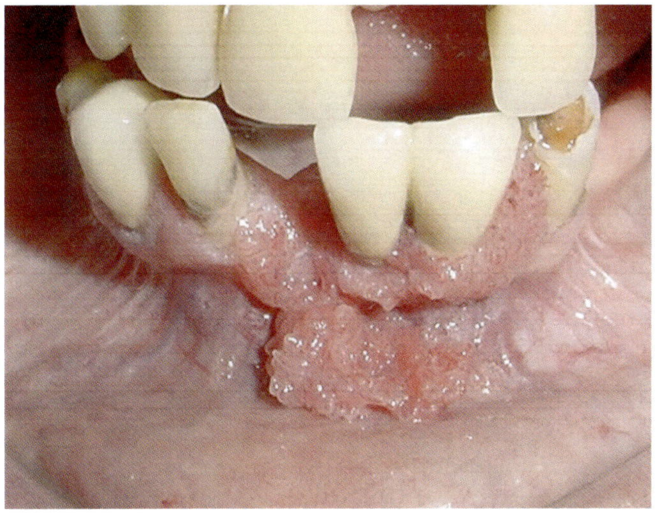

Fig. 20 Condyloma acuminatum on lower labial vestibule and attached gingiva.

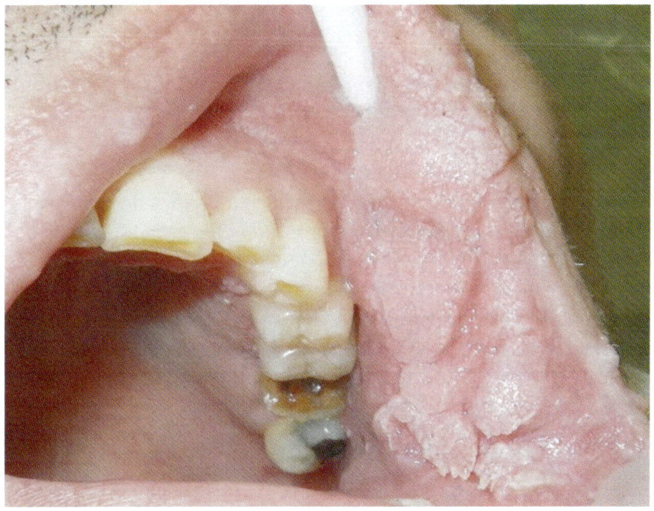

Fig. 21 Condyloma acuminatum on left anterior buccal mucosa.

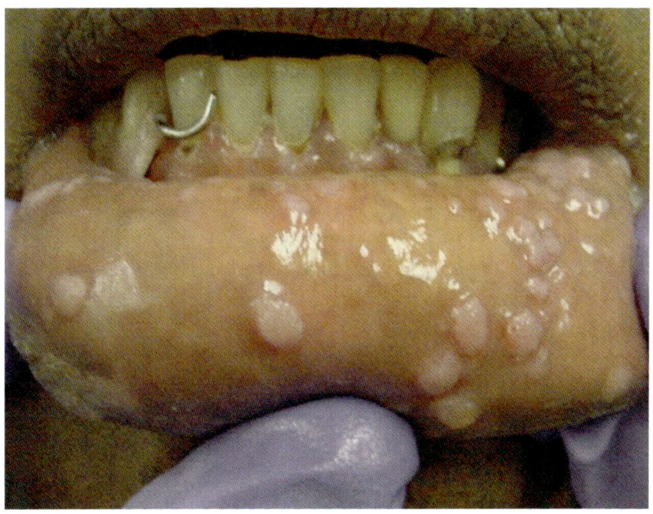

Fig. 22 Multiple papules of focal epithelial hyperplasia on lower labial mucosa.

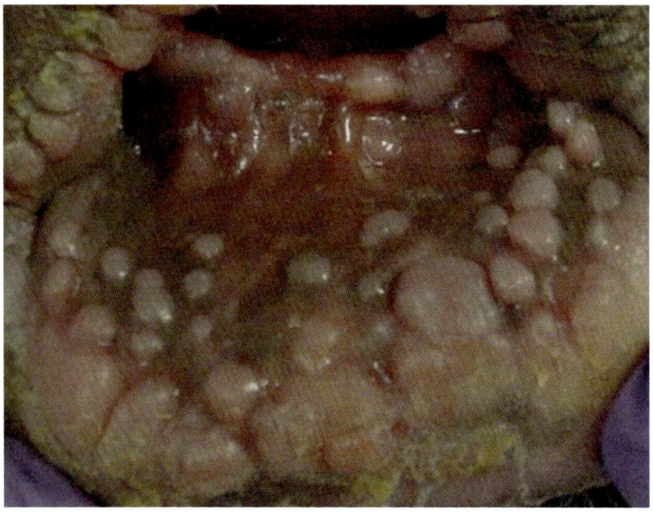

Fig. 23 Multiple papules of focal epithelial hyperplasia on lower labial mucosa.

present. Virally infected cells with condensed, hyperchromatic nuclei known as mitosoid bodies are frequently found on microscopoic examination of focal epithelial hyperplasia.

Management

Oral warts may be treated by surgical excision, laser ablation or cryotherapy with liquid nitrogen. There are no approved medical therapy for oral warts. However, frequent and refractory lesions in the immunocompromised may improve with topical application of imiquimod 5% cream, cidofovir gel, podofilox solution, or intralesional injection of interferon alpha. Identifying the source of infection (eg, patient's digital warts or partner's genital warts) may help prevent reinfection.

Oropharyngeal cancer

Persistence of high-risk HPV 16 in the posterior oral cavity increases the risk of oropharyngeal cancers affecting the base of tongue, posterior throat, and tonsillar structures. HPV16-associated cancer in these anatomic sites is the fastest growing subset of oropharyngeal cancers and frequently affects white men 35 to 55 years of age who do not smoke or drink.

The rise in the incidence of oropharyngeal cancers among those without traditional risk factors has been tied to lifestyle changes such as having multiple sex partners or engaging in oral sex. Clinical signs and symptoms of HPV positive oropharyngeal cancers include persistent sore throat or hoarseness, a neck mass, bloody sputum on coughing, and lingual paresthesia or ear pain. At times, there are no symptoms. HPV carcinogenesis may involve viral-coded proteins that inactivate tumor-suppressor genes p53 and retinoblastoma gene products and promote uncontrolled cell proliferation.

Diagnosis

Any warty growth in the posterior oral cavity should be biopsied and microscopically examined for dysplastic changes. Fine need aspiration of a neck swelling may also be diagnostic. HPV status of oropharyngeal lesions is frequently determined by testing for presence of HPV DNA or staining for P16, a surrogate marker for HPV infection.

Management

HPV-associated oral malignancies are treated with surgery, chemotherapy, and/or radiation. They not only have a better prognosis than oropharyngeal cancers caused by traditional risk factors but also lower likelihood of recurrence or second primaries.

Knowing the HPV status of oropharyngeal cancers may help stratify treatment planning for affected patients. There are no approved tests for HPV infection of the throat or oral cavity, because testing positive at a given time does not indicate persistence.

Dental providers should perform a focused review of systems and inquire about the clinical signs and symptoms of oropharyngeal cancer as part of initial or recall dental visits. Risk factors associated with oral HPV infection and oropharyngeal cancer should also be discussed with patients. HPV vaccines directed at HPV strains causing genital warts and cervical cancer may prove beneficial in protection against oropharyngeal cancer.

Further readings

Cohen JI. Herpes zoster. N Engl J Med 2013;369(18):1766–7.

Fatahzadeh M, Schwartz RA. Human herpes simplex virus infections: epidemiology, pathogenesis, symptomatology, diagnosis, and management. J Am Acad Dermatol 2007;57:737–63.

Fatahzadeh M, Schwartz RA. Herpes simplex labialis. J Cli Exp Dermatol 2007;32:625–30.

Gordon S. Viral infections of the mouth. In: James WD. e medicine. 2016. Available at: http://emedicine.medscape.com/article/1079920-overview. Accessed November 5, 2016.

Janniger C. Herpes zoster. In: Elston D, et.al. e medicine. 2016. Available at: http://emedicine.medscape.com/article/1132465-overview. Accessed November 5, 2016.

Muller ML. Coxsackie viruses. In: Bronze MS, et.al. e medicine. 2016. Available at: http://emedicine.medscape.com/article/215241-overview. Accessed November 5, 2016.

Slots J. Oral viral infections of adults. Periodontol 2000 2009;49:60–86.

Varicella. Centers for Disease Control and Prevention epidemiology and prevention of vaccine-preventable diseases. 13th edition. 2015. p. 353–76. Available at: http://www.cdc.gov/vaccines/pubs/pinkbook/index.html. Accessed November 5, 2016.

Weiss A, Dym H. Oral lesions caused by human papillomavirus. In: Clinical advisor. 2011. Available at: www.clinicaladvisor.com. Accessed November 5, 2016.

Oral Manifestations of Immunologically Mediated Diseases

Lisa Johnson, DDS, MSc, FRCD(C) [a,*], Kristina Perschbacher, DDS, MSc, FRCD(C) [b], Iona Leong, BDS, MSc, FRCD(C) [c], Grace Bradley, DDS, MSc, FRCD(C) [d]

KEYWORDS

• Oral • Mucosa • Swelling • Ulcer • Erythema • Stomatitis • Inflammation

KEY POINTS

- Oral mucosal swelling, ulceration or red-white lesions may be caused by an aberrant immune response.
- Clinical history is important to identify any trigger for the aberrant immune response; removal of the trigger will lead to resolution of the mucosal lesion.
- Clinical investigations may be needed to determine if the oral lesions are associated with extraoral lesions, which may indicate an underlying systemic disease.
- Incisional biopsy is useful for diagnosis of some conditions, whereas other conditions are diagnosed by clinical history and appearance.
- Symptomatic treatment may be provided if no known trigger or causative factor can be found.

Introduction

Immune-mediated conditions represent a spectrum of diseases characterized by an individual's immune system mounting an aberrant attack leading to tissue damage. In this article, we address immune-mediated conditions in which an inappropriate inflammatory reaction results in oral mucosal diseases that range from swelling to ulceration to red/white lesions. The inciting factor for the immune reaction is often difficult or impossible to identify. We highlight the clinical history and appearance of each condition and describe the role of laboratory tests and biopsy in diagnosis. The management of these conditions varies and may include removal of any demonstrable trigger, topical steroid, and other immunosuppressive agents. Conditions that present with self-limited oral lesions only require supportive care. In those conditions where oral lesions are associated with extraoral lesions, timely investigations are important to detect and treat systemic manifestations of disease.

The authors have nothing to disclose.

[a] Department of Oral and Maxillofacial Sciences, Faculty of Dentistry, Dalhousie University, 5981 University Avenue, Room 5124, PO Box 15000, Halifax, Nova Scotia B3H 4R2, Canada

[b] Oral Pathology and Oral Medicine, Faculty of Dentistry, University of Toronto, 124 Edward Street Room 308, Toronto, Ontario M5G 1G6, Canada

[c] Oral Pathology and Oral Medicine, Faculty of Dentistry, University of Toronto, 124 Edward Street Room 311, Toronto, Ontario M5G 1G6, Canada

[d] Oral Pathology and Oral Medicine, Faculty of Dentistry, University of Toronto, 124 Edward Street Room 315C, Toronto, Ontario M5G 1G6, Canada

* Corresponding author.

E-mail address: lisa.johnson@dal.ca

Swellings

Orofacial granulomatosis

Description

- Characterized by persistent swelling of one or both lips and/or intraoral swelling; biopsy shows inflammation with noncaseating granulomas.
- The etiology and pathogenesis are not fully understood; there may be multiple pathogenetic pathways leading to a common set of clinical manifestations.
- Patients who are known to have Crohn's disease or sarcoidosis may rarely develop orofacial swelling with clinical and histologic features nearly identical to orofacial granulomatosis (OFG); it is a matter of debate whether such patients should be classified as having OFG.
- OFG presenting in childhood is associated with an increased probability of Crohn's disease, although the signs and symptoms of Crohn's disease may only appear after an interval of several years.
- A minority of OFG have been shown to be associated with allergy to food, food preservatives and flavoring agents and oral hygiene products; both type I (immediate, IgE-mediated) hypersensitivity and type IV (delayed, cell-mediated) hypersensitivity have been shown to be associated with OFG.
- The remainder of OFG cases are idiopathic with no associated gastrointestinal tract abnormality and no identifiable allergen.

Prevalence

- OFG is an uncommon condition, but the exact prevalence has not been determined.
- Median age at onset is between 15 and 30 years of age in the majority of case series.

Atlas Oral Maxillofacial Surg Clin N Am 25 (2017) 171-185
1061-3315/17/
http://dx.doi.org/10.1016/j.cxom.2017.04.009

- Males and females are almost equally affected.
- Firm swelling of one or both lips is seen in more than 90% of cases; upper and lower lips are equally likely to be affected (Fig. 1A); the swelling varies in severity and may be symmetric or affect one side more than the other (Fig. 2A).
- Lip swelling may be associated with perioral erythema, angular cheilitis, and vertical fissures of the lip.
- The swelling is usually painless, although severe swelling with scaling and fissuring of the mucosa may cause discomfort.
- Lip swelling accompanied by fissured tongue and facial paralysis is known as Melkersson–Rosenthal syndrome.
- Intraoral lesions include diffuse or segmental swelling of the attached gingiva (see Fig. 1B), cobblestone appearance of the buccal mucosa, linear ulceration and swelling of the buccal vestibule (see Fig. 2B), and swelling of the anterior floor of mouth over Wharton's ducts.
- Clinical and laboratory investigations are required to determine if there is an underlying systemic disease (Table 1) or a local cause (Table 2).
- Patients with Crohn's disease who have orofacial lesions along with intestinal lesions ("oral Crohn's disease") may present clinically similar to OFG patients, but are more likely to have involvement of the mandibular buccal sulcus (Fig. 3A,B); it has also been shown that patients with OFG who have ulcers and swelling of the buccal sulcus are more likely to have concurrent Crohn's disease upon investigation than OFG patients with predominantly lip swelling.

Histopathology

- Edema in the lamina propria, chronic inflammatory infiltrate with nonnecrotizing granulomas consisting of epithelioid macrophages, and lymphocytes, often with multinucleated giant cells.
- Nonnecrotizing granulomas may be absent in the biopsy because of sampling problems or fluctuations in the disease process; a repeat biopsy of deeper tissues may be helpful to demonstrate the granulomatous inflammation.
- Special stains are negative for the presence of acid-fast bacilli and fungal organisms.
- No detectable foreign bodies by conventional or polarized light examination.

Diagnosis

- Based on clinical presentation and biopsy findings.
- Clinically, the lip swelling of OFG can be distinguished from that of angioedema because the latter condition has a rapid onset and resolves after 24 to 72 hours.
- Biopsy to demonstrate nonnecrotizing granulomas is useful to support the diagnosis of OFG.
- Clinical and laboratory investigations are required to determine if there is an underlying systemic disease or an allergy (see Tables 1 and 2).

Treatment

- Investigate for an underlying systemic disease (eg, Crohn's disease); the orofacial lesions should resolve upon treatment of the systemic disease.
- Treatment of odontogenic infections may lead to resolution of OFG.
- Perform cutaneous patch tests and urticarial tests if allergy is suspected; avoid exposure to allergens, for example, by instituting an elimination diet for patients who are found to have an associated allergy.
- Intralesional injections of triamcinolone acetonide are effective in the majority of patients in reducing lip and oral mucosal swelling; the injections are given every 2 to 4 weeks, typically for 4 to 6 months.
- Topical corticosteroids or calcineurin inhibitors (tacrolimus, pimecrolimus) may be used as an adjunct to intralesional injections of corticosteroid.
- Immunosuppressants such as azathioprine, or tumor necrosis factor-α inhibitors such as infliximab may be used in severe cases.
- Pediatric patients (age < 16 years) with OFG but no gastrointestinal disease should be monitored for signs and symptoms of Crohn's disease, because a number of

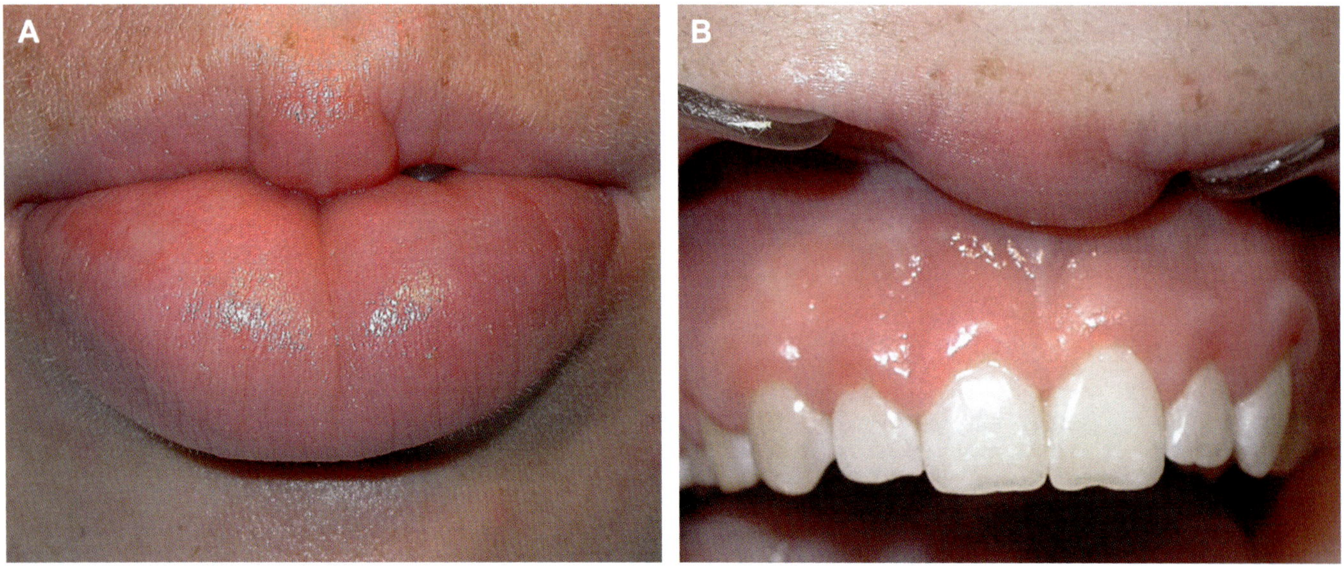

Fig. 1 (*A*) Diffuse, firm swelling of the lower lip and less extensive swelling of the upper lip in a 22 year-old female. The patient had a surgical reduction of the lower lip 7 years earlier but the swelling has slowly recurred. Biopsy showed nonnecrotizing granulomatous inflammation, consistent with a diagnosis of orofacial granulomatosis. (*B*) Same patient as *A*, showing diffuse swelling and erythema of the maxillary labial gingiva. Similar changes were noted in the mandibular anterior gingiva.

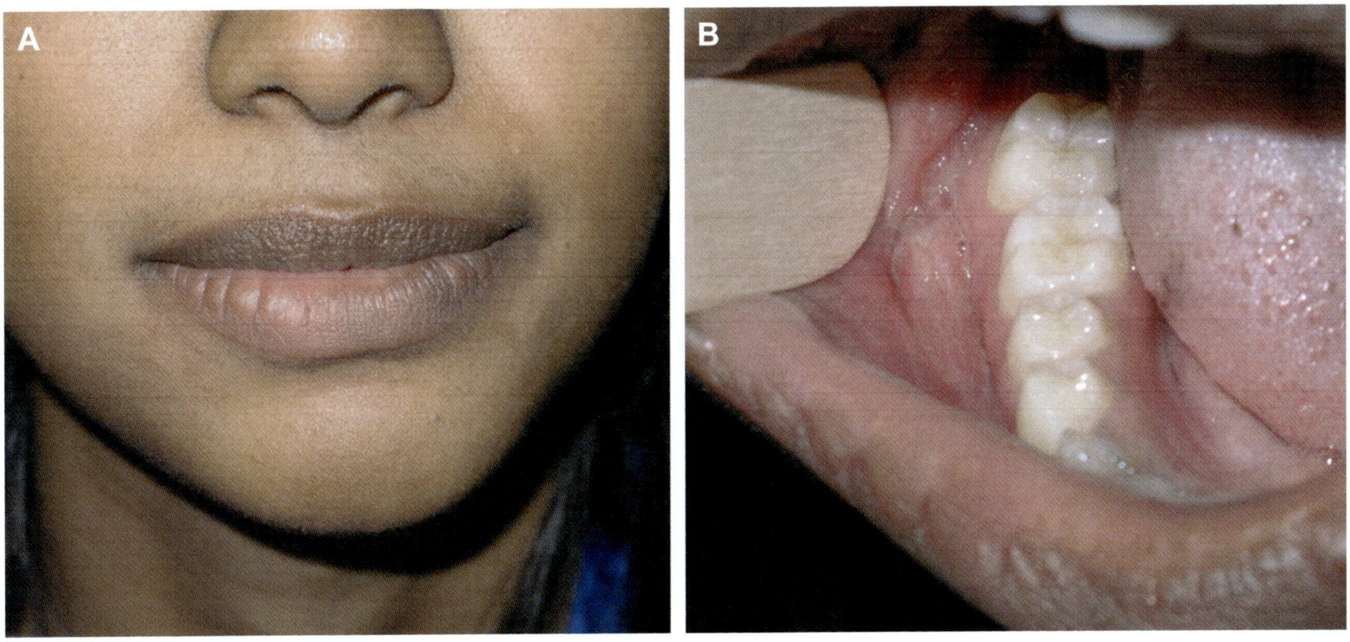

Fig. 2 (*A*) A 14-year-old healthy female with painless swelling of the right lower lip of several months' duration. The patient reported no gastrointestinal problems. (*B*) Same patient as *A*, showing a painless, deep fissured ulcer surrounded by raised linear folds of tissue in the right mandibular buccal vestibule. Biopsy demonstrated nonnecrotizing granulomatous inflammation, consistent with a diagnosis of orofacial granulomatosis.

studies have suggested that childhood onset of OFG is predictive of the development of Crohn's disease.
- Surgical reduction of lip enlargement has been used to improve facial appearance, but there is a risk of recurrence.[1–8]

Ulcers

Recurrent aphthous stomatitis

Description

- Painful, self-limited, recurrent oral ulcers.
- Unknown cause, but a variety of triggers have been reported, including stress, hormonal effects, food allergy, trauma, and smoking cessation.
- May also be triggered by use of systemic medications, including nonsteroidal antiinflammatory drugs, beta-blockers, and nicorandil.
- Decrease in mucosal barrier, antigenic stimulation, and T-cell–mediated immunologic reaction have been implicated in the pathogenesis.
- Three clinical forms: minor, major, and herpetiform.
- Predominantly on nonkeratinized mucosa.

Prevalence

- Common, affecting 20% of the population.
- Usually presents in childhood or adolescence.
- Eighty percent of affected individuals present with minor aphthous ulcers.

Clinical presentation

- All forms of aphthous ulcers are painful and characterized by a whitish-grey pseudomembrane and an erythematous halo.
- Minor aphthous ulcers (Fig. 4A, B).
  - Round ulcers, less than 1 cm in diameter.
  - Develop on nonkeratinized tissues; rare on dorsum of tongue, hard palate, and gingiva.
  - Predilection for the buccal and labial mucosa, followed by ventral tongue, soft palate, and floor of mouth.
  - Typically 1 to 5 are present at any given time.
  - Heal in 1 to 2 weeks with no scarring.
- Major aphthous ulcers (Fig. 5A, B).

Table 1 : Investigations of patients with orofacial granulomatosis to rule out systemic disease

Clinical presentation	Diagnostic tests	Diagnosis
• Gastrointestinal problems, such as bloating, cramps, and diarrhea; perianal symptoms in children • Laboratory findings of low hemoglobin, serum iron, vitamin B_{12}, folate • Elevated levels of inflammatory markers – erythrocyte sedimentation rate, C-reactive protein	• Endoscopy and biopsy	Crohn's disease
• Respiratory problems such as dyspnea • Salivary and lacrimal gland dysfunction • Elevated levels of inflammatory markers – erythrocyte sedimentation rate, C-reactive protein • Serum angiotensin-converting enzyme level	• Chest radiography to look for hilar lymphadenopathy • Bronchoscopy and biopsy	Sarcoidosis

Table 2 Investigations of patients with orofacial granulomatosis to rule out local causes

Clinical presentation	Diagnostic tests	Diagnosis
• Predominantly gingival involvement	• Vitality test, periodontal examination, and radiographs of teeth in the vicinity of orofacial swelling	Chronic dental infection
• Gingival swelling • History of scaling and polishing of teeth	• Identification of foreign material in gingival biopsy	Foreign body gingivitis
• History of atopy — asthma, eczema, allergic rhinitis • Association between exposure to suspected allergen and development/exacerbation of orofacial swelling	• Skin patch test against foods, food preservatives, and additives (eg, benzoates, monosodium glutamate, cinnamaldehyde), dental materials • Elevated serum IgE levels • Response to elimination diet	Allergy

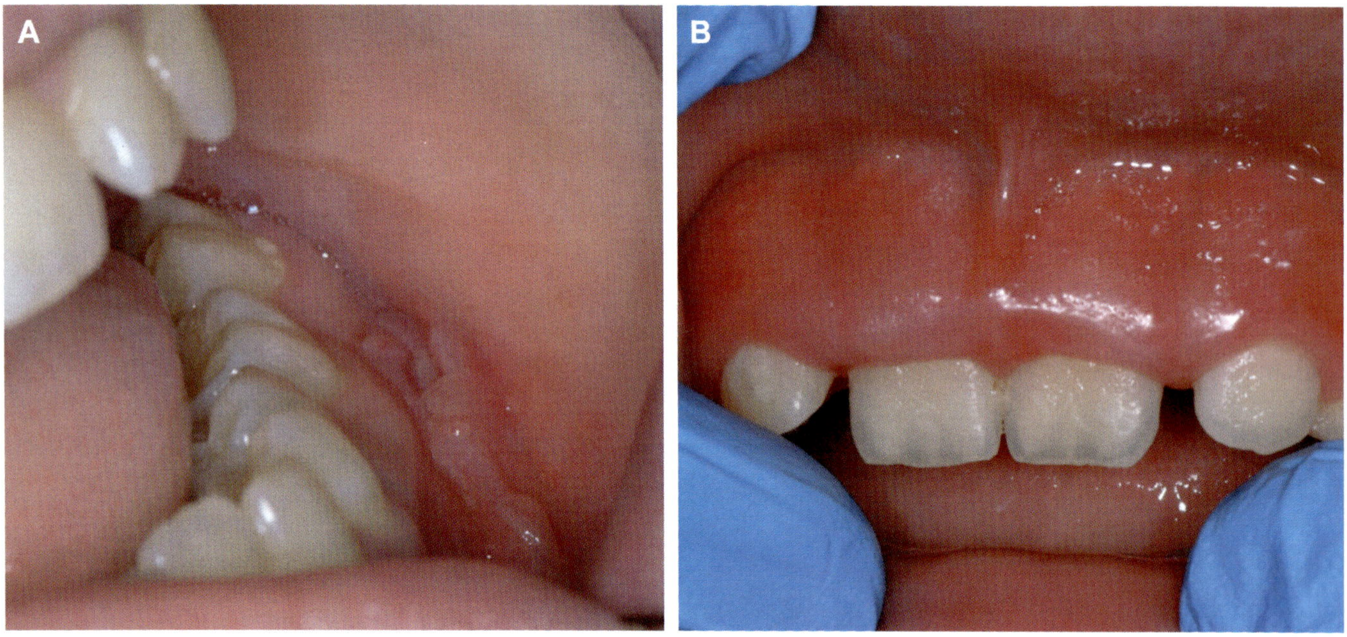

Fig. 3 (*A*) Elongated ulcer surrounded by thickened mucosa in the left mandibular buccal vestibule in a patient with Crohn's disease. Note the similarity to Fig. 2*B*. (*B*) Diffuse swelling of the maxillary labial gingiva in a patient with Crohn's disease.

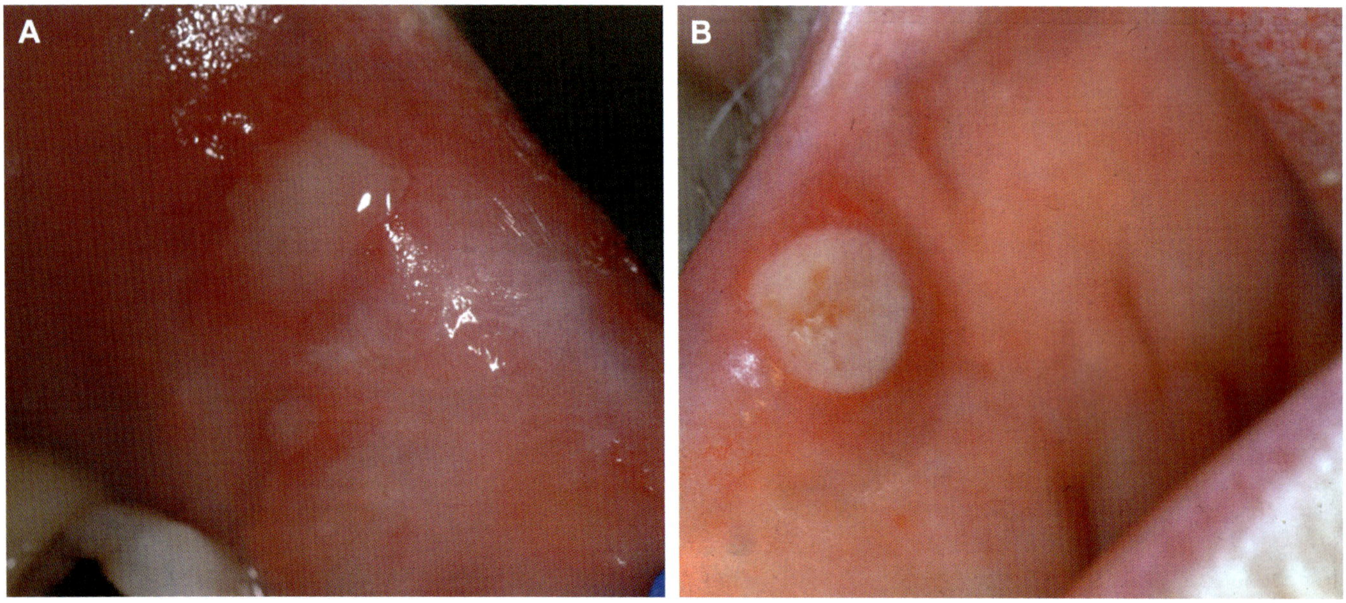

Fig. 4 (*A*) Minor aphthous ulcers. A 40-year-old female with 2 aphthous ulcers of the labial mucosa. The patient has a history of recurrent oral ulcers since childhood. (*B*) Aphthous ulcer on the labial mucosa with the characteristic appearance of a round ulcer covered by a whitish-grey pseudomembrane and surrounded by an erythematous halo.

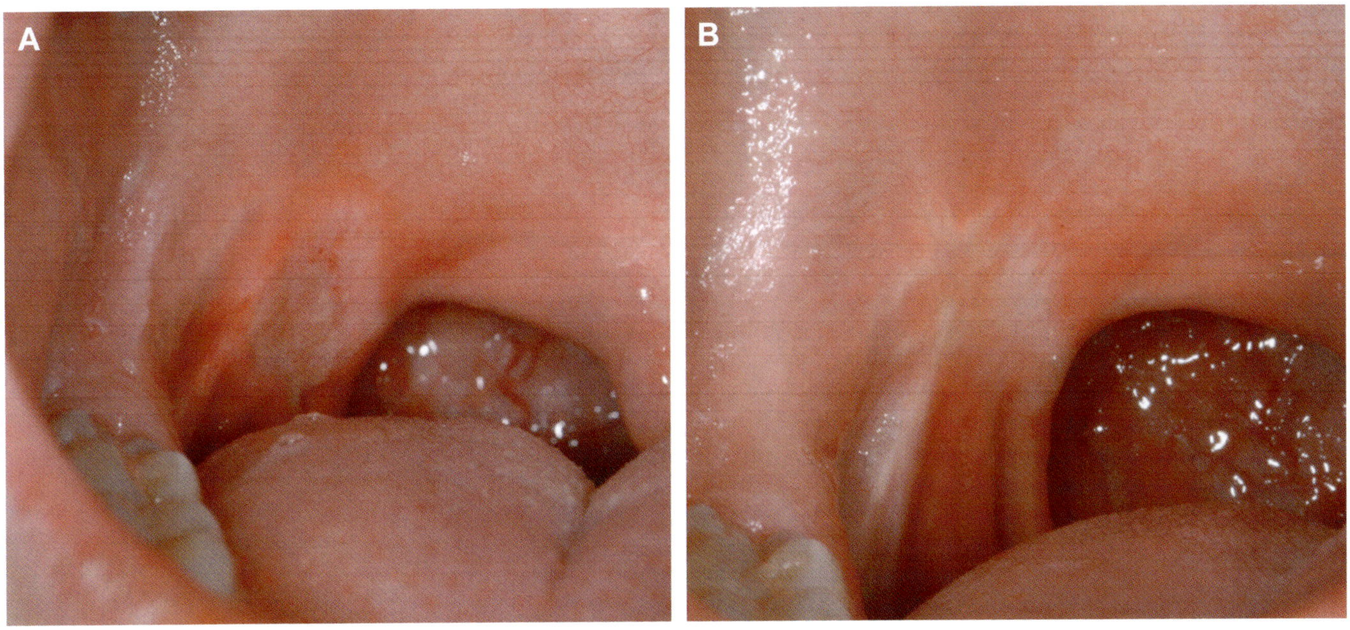

Fig. 5 (*A*) Major aphthous ulcer. Adolescent male presented with an ulcer of the right soft palate of 4 weeks' duration. He has a history of minor aphthous ulcers. (*B*) Same patient as *A*, 1 month later. The ulcer has healed, leaving a whitish scar.

  - Larger, deeper, and more irregular ulcers with a preference for tonsillar pillars, soft palate, and labial mucosa.
  - Diameter of 1 to 3 cm.
  - There may be 1 to 10 ulcers may be present at a time.
  - May extend from nonkeratinized to keratinized tissues.
  - Heal in 2 to 6 weeks, often with scarring.
- Herpetiform (Fig. 6A, B).
  - Least common form, representing only 5% of recurrent aphthous stomatitis cases.
  - Demonstrates a female predilection and may present in adulthood.
  - Numerous pinhead-sized ulcers, 1 to 3 mm in diameter, that coalesce to form larger ulcers, giving a resemblance to herpetic stomatitis.
  - Despite the name, infection with herpes virus has not been convincingly demonstrated.
  - Up to 100 ulcers may develop at 1 time, predominantly affecting nonkeratinized mucosa, but may affect keratinized mucosa as well.
  - Heal in 1 to 2 weeks, but frequent recurrences are typical.

Histopathology

- Nonspecific ulceration consisting of loss of surface epithelium with a mixed inflammatory infiltrate composed of neutrophils, lymphocytes, and histiocytes in the underlying connective tissue.
- The mucosa at the margins of the ulcer shows an inflammatory infiltrate of lymphocytes and histiocytes in the connective tissue and migration of inflammatory cells into the epithelium.

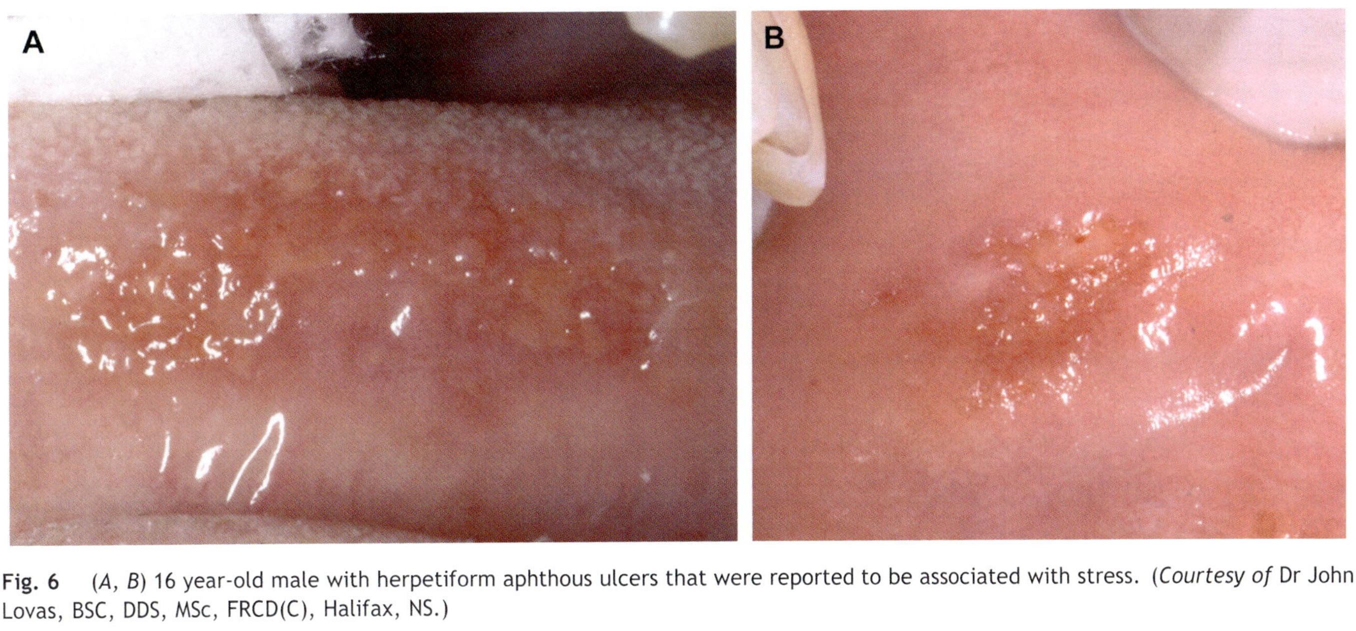

Fig. 6 (*A, B*) 16 year-old male with herpetiform aphthous ulcers that were reported to be associated with stress. (*Courtesy of* Dr John Lovas, BSC, DDS, MSc, FRCD(C), Halifax, NS.)

Diagnosis

- Based on history of self-limited, recurrent ulcers, characteristic clinical appearance and exclusion of underlying systemic disease (see below).
- Biopsy is not required except in rare occasions when a major aphthous ulcer has to be distinguished from malignant disease such as squamous cell carcinoma or lymphoma.
- Aphthous-like ulcers occur as part of several systemic diseases (Fig. 7A–D, Table 3); control of the systemic disease usually leads to improvement of the oral ulcers.
- A medical history should be taken to determine if the oral ulcers are associated with gastrointestinal problems including diarrhea, bloating, and signs of malabsorption, fever, lymphadenopathy, weight loss, skin lesions, ulcers on other mucosal surfaces, ocular inflammation, and joint pain.
- Laboratory investigation including complete blood count, red blood cell folate, serum iron, and vitamin B_{12} should be considered in case of onset of ulcers after adolescence or unusual number, frequency or location of ulcers.

Treatment

- A variety of treatments have been proposed, but none has been consistently effective in preventing recurrence or promoting healing of ulcers.
- Elimination of suspected triggers, for example, certain fruits, nuts, flavoring agents, and preservatives.
- Substitution of suspected medications with other medications, if possible.

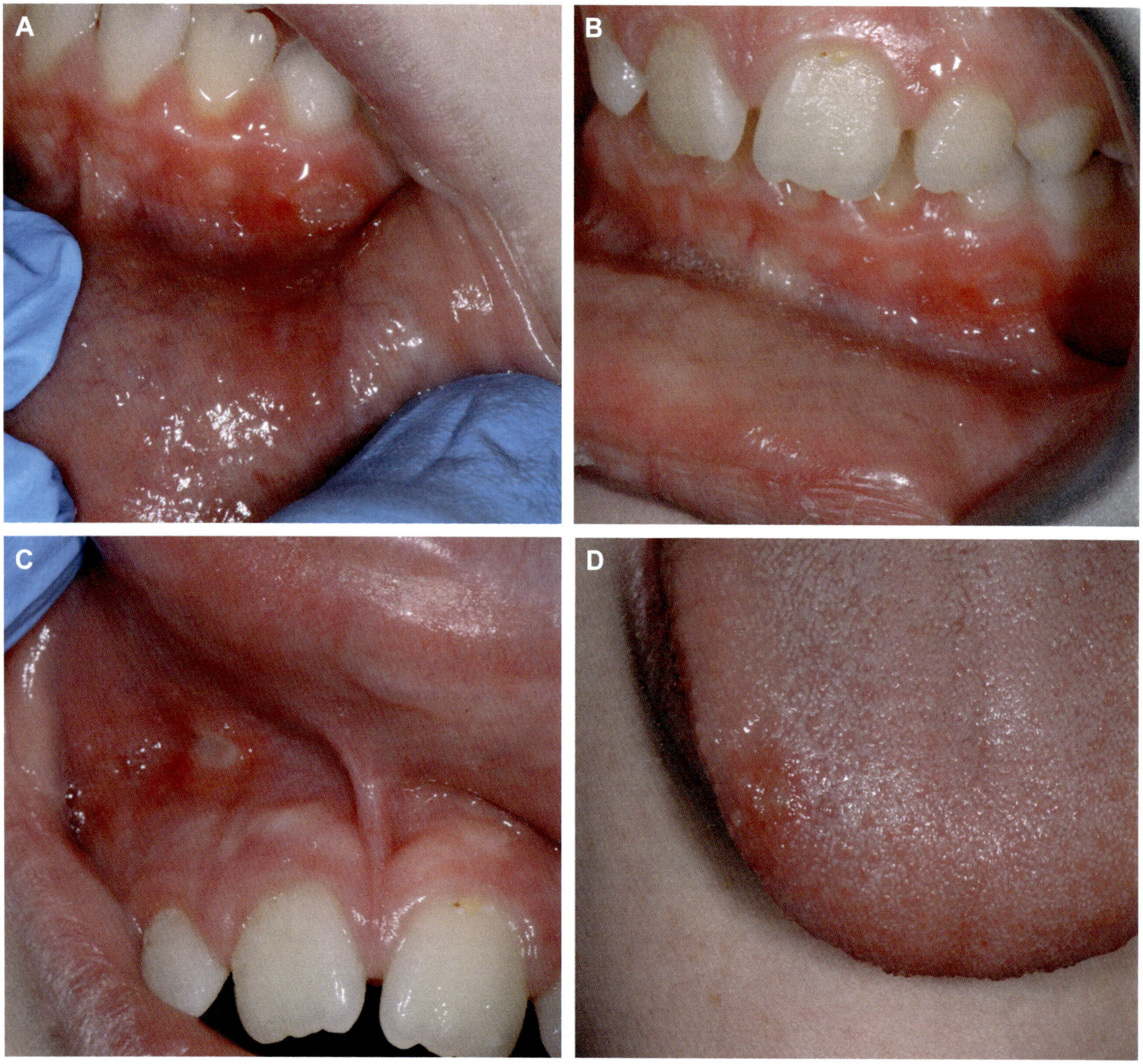

Fig. 7 (*A–D*) A 9-year-old male with ulcers of the maxillary and mandibular vestibules and lateral tongue. The patient has a history of ulcers starting at age 5 and experiences 1 to 2 outbreaks per month during which time he takes prednisolone. Diagnosis of periodic fever, aphthae, pharyngitis, adenitis (PFAPA) was made by a pediatric rheumatologist.

Table 3 Systemic disorders that are associated with aphthouslike oral ulcers

Systemic disorder	Clinical findings besides oral ulcers	Laboratory tests
Behçet syndrome	Genital ulcers, uveitis, skin lesions, joint lesions, central nervous system manifestations (see next section)	
Celiac disease (gluten sensitive enteropathy)	Gluten intolerance; bloating, diarrhea, weight loss, dental defects	Small intestine biopsy; antibodies to gliadin and tissue transglutaminase
Cyclic neutropenia	Presents in childhood with cyclical occurrence of fever and infections; usually improves in second decade	Complete blood count and correlation with development of ulcers
Nutritional deficiencies (iron, folate, vitamin B_{12})	Fatigue, weakness, pallor; atrophic glossitis, angular cheilitis	Serum iron, vitamin B_{12}, red blood cell folate
Immunocompromised conditions, eg, HIV infection	Candidiasis, hairy leukoplakia; Kaposi sarcoma, lymphoma	Complete blood count with immunodeficiency panel; HIV testing
Inflammatory bowel disease (ulcerative colitis and Crohn's disease)	Diarrhea, abdominal pain, weight loss	Endoscopy, biopsy
Mucosal and genital ulcers with inflamed cartilage	More common in the 4th–5th decades of life with oral and genital lesions with relapsing polychronditis	
Periodic fever, aphthae, pharyngitis, adenitis	Presents in young children and occurs in 3–5 wk intervals with fever, sore throat and cervical lymphadenopathy in the absence of upper respiratory tract infection	
Sweet syndrome (acute febrile neutrophilic dermatoses)	Sudden onset of fever, red papules and plaques on skin, mucosal ulcers, arthralgia/arthritis	
Reactive arthritis	Urethritis, arthritis, conjunctivitis; strong male predilection	

Abbreviation: HIV, human immunodeficiency virus.

- Laser therapy can provide pain relief and reduce healing time.
- Tetracycline rinse (contents of 250 mg capsule dissolved in 1 tbsp of water); doxycycline and minocycline gel or rinse are also effective.
- Chlorhexidine rinses 0.12%.
- Topical glucocorticosteroids, particularly 0.1% triamcinolone acetonide in orabase.
- Zylactin (over the counter) provides a covering film for symptomatic relief.
- Systemic glucocorticoids and other immune modulators may be considered in major aphthous stomatitis.[9–11]

Behçet disease

Description

- Behçets disease (BD) is a multisystem inflammatory disease of unknown etiology, currently considered to be a systemic vasculitis.
- Characterized by recurrent episodes of active disease and remissions, with different durations, most often manifesting as a triad of oral ulcers, genital ulcers, and ocular inflammation.

Prevalence

- BD is rare; the majority of cases are associated with HLA-B51 genotype, occurring more commonly in countries along the "silk route": Turkey, Japan, and the eastern Mediterranean countries.
- Usual age at onset is between the second and fourth decades.
- Males are more often diagnosed with BD than females and may have a worse clinical course.

Clinical presentation

- Oral ulcerations are similar in appearance to aphthous ulcers (both minor and major), with recurrent multifocal presentation, often lasting 1 to 4 weeks and healing without scarring.
  - Oral ulceration is seen in nearly all patients with BD and it is also the most frequent presenting symptom (see Fig. 8A–D).
- Genital lesions are similar to oral lesions and are present in approximately 75% of cases.
- Eye lesions are serious and may lead to severe vision loss and blindness.
  - Most commonly include posterior uveitis, conjunctivitis, conjunctival aphthosis, and scleritis.
- Typical skin lesions consist of erythematous papules, vesicles, or acnelike eruptions, as well as erythema nodosum.
- Arthritis, thrombophlebitis, gastrointestinal disease, and central nervous system involvement may be seen.

Histopathology

- Nonspecific ulceration of the epithelium.
- Most frequent pattern seen for skin lesions is leukocytoclastic vasculitis, consisting of infiltration of neutrophils and fibrinoid necrosis of the walls of small blood vessels, and extravasation of red blood cells.

Diagnosis

- Diagnosis of BD is difficult because it is based on clinical manifestations, which may be seen in other diseases as well.
- No other disease has had so many different classification and diagnostic criteria; there are currently 17 published sets of criteria.

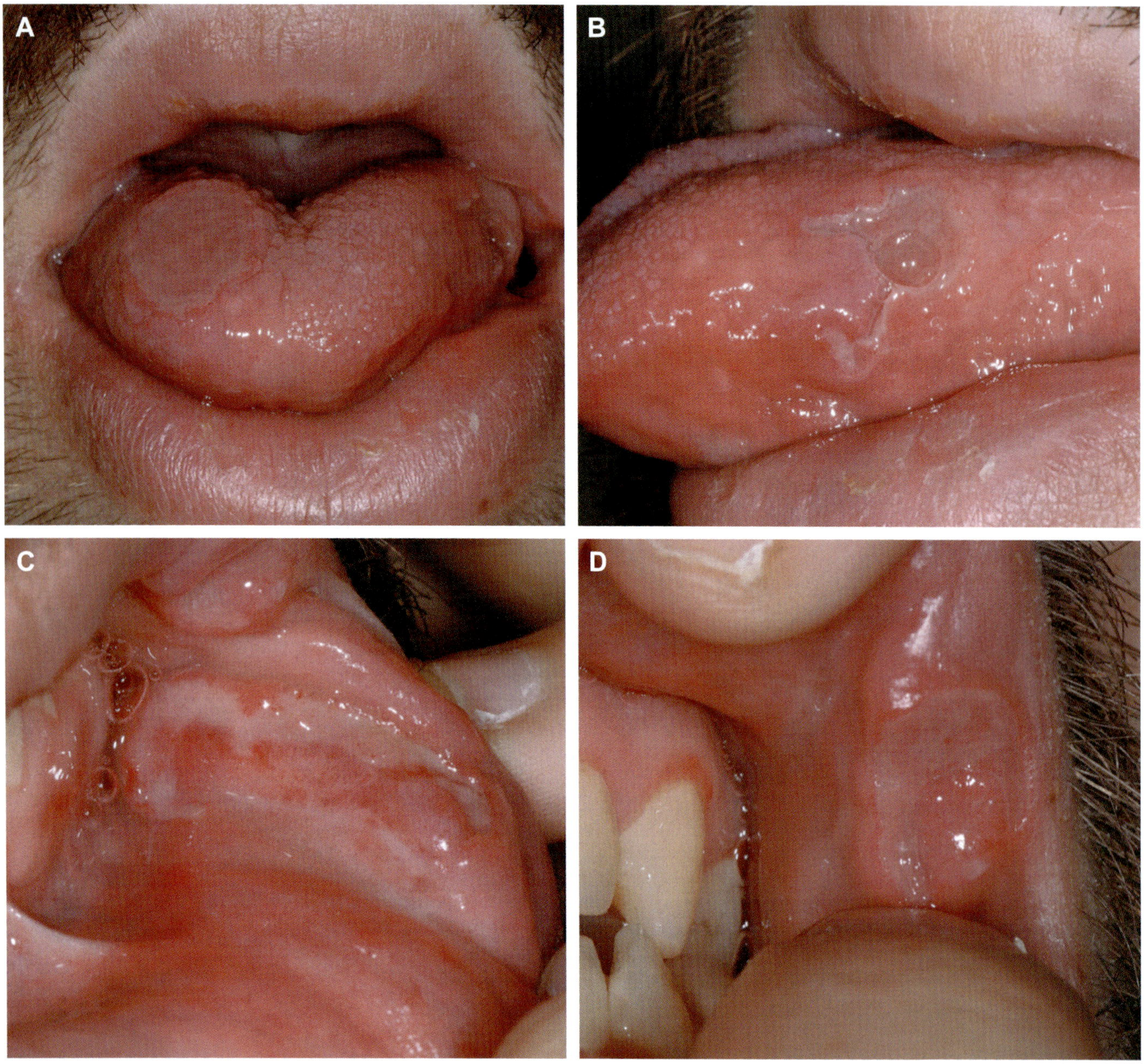

Fig. 8 (*A–D*) Behçet disease. A 26-year-old male of Turkish descent with multiple large ulcers of the dorsal and lateral tongue, labial and buccal mucosa. The patient has a history of recurrent oral ulcers since childhood associated with pustular lesions of the skin and genital ulcers.

- The international criteria for BD were revised in 2014 and state that a patient must get 4 points from a list of symptoms:
  - Oral aphthosis (2 points),
  - Genital aphthosis (2 points),
  - Ocular manifestations (2 points),
  - Skin manifestations (1 point),
  - Vascular manifestations (1 point),
  - Neurologic manifestations (1 point), and
  - Positive pathergy test (1 point).
- BD must be differentiated from other systemic conditions presenting with oral ulcerations (see Table 3 in Recurrent Aphthous Stomatitis section).

Treatment

- Symptomatic treatment for oral ulcers, such as topical or intralesional corticosteroids.
- No treatment or medication has been found to be universally effective for BD; different patient groups have responded to systemic antiinflammatory and immunosuppressive medications such as azathioprine, colchicine, corticosteroids, cyclosporine, dapsone, methotrexate, thalidomide, and tumor necrosis factor-alpha inhibitors.[12–14]

Erythema multiforme

Description

- Self-limiting condition that presents with an acute onset of erythema, erosions, vesicles, and ulcers affecting the skin and mucous membranes.
- Clinical and microscopic features suggest that this is an immunologically mediated condition but the pathogenesis is not well-understood.
- Approximately 50% of cases are associated with a preceding infection, in particular herpes simplex infection;

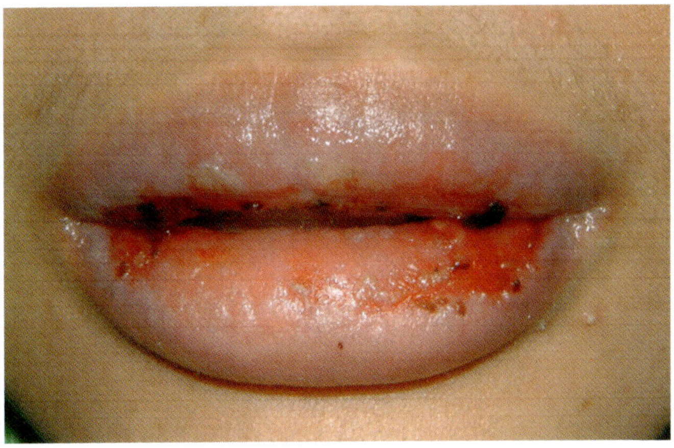

Fig. 9 Hemorrhagic, crusting lesions of the lips in a patient with erythema multiforme.

mycoplasmal infection, histoplasmosis, coccidioidomycosis and Epstein–Barr virus have also been implicated.
- May also be triggered by use of medications, in particular sulfonamides, penicillin, barbiturates, salicylates and antimalarial drugs (see Kentaro Ikeda's article, "Drug-Induced Oral Complications," in this issue).
- Controversial whether erythema multiforme (EM) is a separate condition from Stevens–Johnson syndrome and toxic epidermal necrolysis; the latter 2 conditions are characterized by more severe and extensive lesions of the skin and multiple mucosal sites and displays epithelial necrosis upon biopsy; the majority of cases of Stevens–Johnson syndrome and toxic epidermal necrolysis are triggered by medications (see Kentaro Ikeda's article, "Drug-Induced Oral Complications," in this issue).
- May also present in association with cancer, in particular carcinomas and lymphomas, and in patients with collagen vascular diseases, such as systemic lupus erythematosus and polyarteritis nodosa.

Prevalence
- Presents in the second to fifth decades of life, with no sex predilection.
- In comparison, toxic epidermal necrolysis presents in older adults with a female predilection, whereas Stevens–Johnson syndrome occurs more commonly in children.

Clinical presentation
- Acute onset with lesions appearing over a few days.
- Self-limiting course with resolution after 2 to 6 weeks.
- Flulike symptoms consisting of low-grade fever, malaise, headache, and sore throat may precede the onset of EM by 1 week.
- EM associated with a precipitating infection (eg, recurrent herpetic labialis) usually presents 10 to 14 days after the infection.
- Skin lesions typically include symmetric targetoid lesions on the hands and feet.
- Hemorrhagic crusting of the lips is a characteristic finding (Fig. 9).
- Erythematous patches and irregular shallow ulcers on any oral mucosal surface, most commonly on the labial and buccal mucosa; often sparing the gingiva and palate (Fig. 10A, B).
- Exclusive oral involvement is not uncommon; alternatively oral involvement may precede worsening of disease severity.
- Oral lesions are painful and cause difficulty with eating and drinking.
- More severe presentation (EM major) involves extensive skin lesions, conjunctival, nasal, and genital lesions.
- Recurrent episodes may occur in a minority of cases, often after recurrent herpetic labialis.
- Differential diagnosis includes:
  - Pemphigus vulgaris,
  - Paraneoplastic pemphigus,

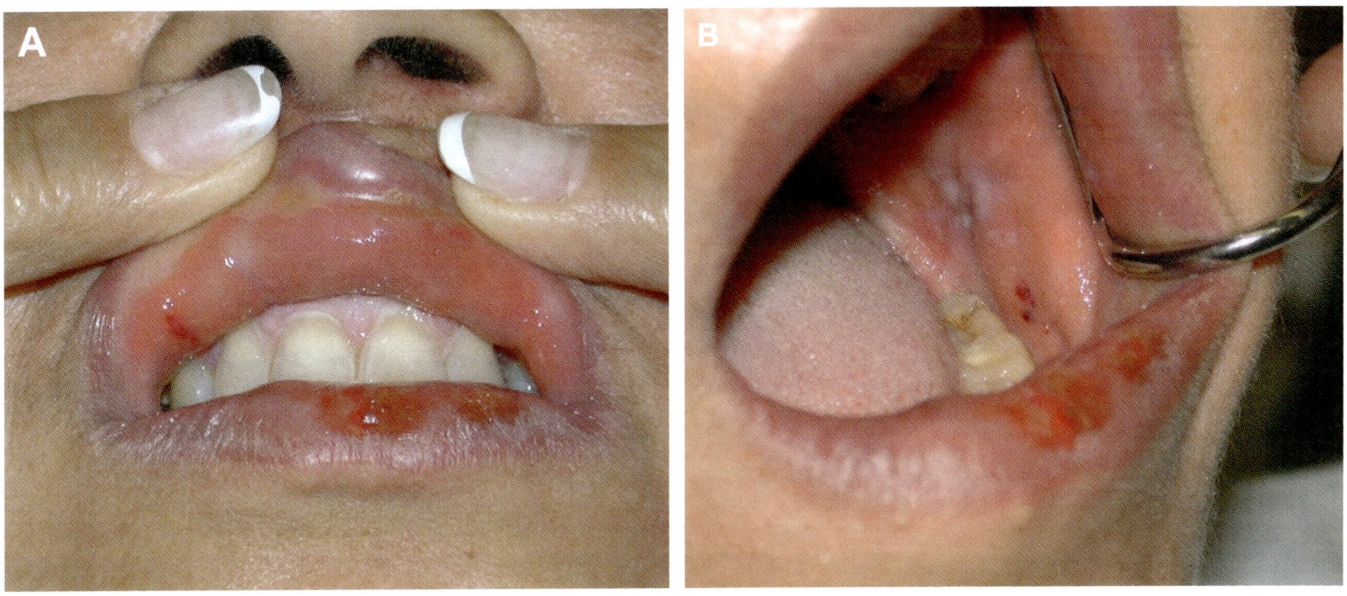

Fig. 10 A 55-year-old female with diffuse erythema and ulcers of the lips (*A*) and buccal mucosa (*B*) of 2 weeks' duration. The lesions had a sudden onset, with no history of use of medications or viral infection in the preceding month. There were no associated skin lesions. Topical corticosteroids and prednisone (10 mg/d) were not helpful. The clinical diagnosis of erythema multiforme was confirmed at the 4-week follow-up appointment when the lesions had completely resolved.

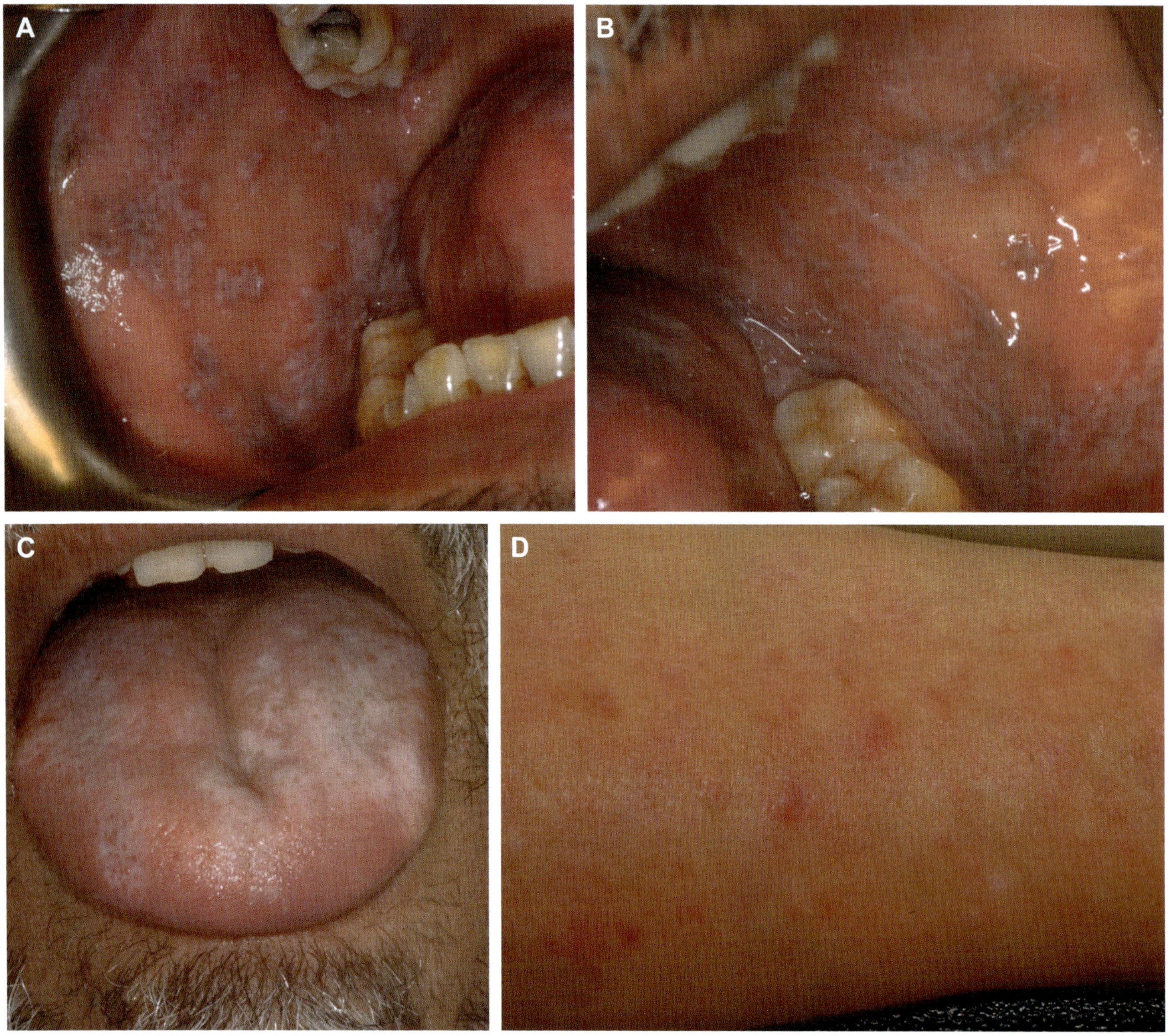

Fig. 11 Oral mucosal and skin lesions of a patient with lichen planus. (*A, B*) Reticular white lesions associated with mucosal pigmentation in a symmetric presentation on both buccal mucosa. (*C*) White plaques and a small area of white reticular appearance on the dorsum of the tongue. (*D*) Pruritic, purplish-red papules on the skin of the forearm.

- ○ Erosive lichen planus,
- ○ Fixed drug reaction, and
- ○ Infections, including human immunodeficiency virus, primary herpetic gingivostomatitis, and fungal infections.

Histopathology

- Biopsy of perilesional tissue may show subepithelial or intraepithelial vesicle formation with necrosis of the basal cell layer.
- A mixed inflammatory infiltrate is seen in the connective tissue, composed of lymphocytes, neutrophils, and eosinophils, often with a perivascular distribution.
- The histologic findings are not diagnostic, but are useful for excluding mucocutaneous diseases with a similar clinical presentation, particularly pemphigus vulgaris and paraneoplastic pemphigus.
- Direct immunofluorescence is negative for the presence of autoantibodies.

Diagnosis

- Diagnosis of EM is initially a presumptive diagnosis based on clinical history and the characteristic appearance of skin and mucosal lesions.
- Diagnosis of EM is confirmed by seeing complete resolution of lesions in 2 to 6 weeks.
- In cases where the clinical findings are nonspecific, biopsy, and direct and indirect immunofluorescence assays can be used to exclude other skin and mucosal diseases.
- Determine if there is a precipitating factor such as viral infection or use of systemic medication; this is particularly important for patients with recurrent EM.

Treatment

- Supportive care including soft diet, plenty of fluids, topical anesthetics, and rest.
- Use of topical or systemic corticosteroids has not been shown to be highly effective.

- Discontinuation of any medication that is suspected to be the trigger.
- Monitor the patient until all lesions have resolved.
- Prophylactic antiviral medication is indicated in cases of recurrent EM triggered by herpes simplex infection.[14–17]

Red and white lesions

Lichen planus

Description
- Lichen planus is a chronic inflammatory disorder of skin and/or mucosa characterized by immunologically mediated reactions to basal keratinocytes. The etiology and triggering factors are poorly understood and there is currently no cure.

Prevalence
- Oral lichen planus is common, affecting 0.1% to 2.2% of the population.
- Usually presents in the fifth and sixth decades.
- Occurs twice as commonly in women than in men.

Clinical presentation
- Skin lesions are characterized by 4 *P*s: purplish, pruritic, polygonal papules, most commonly on the arms and legs (Fig. 11D).
- Oral lesions are multiple, bilateral, and often symmetric (see Fig. 11A–C).
- Oral lichen planus often presents with a waxing and waning course.
- There are 2 major forms of oral lichen planus: reticular and erosive.
- Reticular lichen planus is more common and usually asymptomatic.
- Lesions of reticular lichen planus appear as white striae and as an annular and/or lacelike pattern of hyperkeratosis that most commonly affects the bilateral buccal mucosa, but other oral sites may also be affected, including lateral and dorsal tongue, gingivae, palate and vermilion border (see Fig. 11A–C).
- Erosive lichen planus is usually symptomatic with patients complaining of pain and/or sensitivity, especially with spicy or acidic foods.
- Erosive lichen planus is characterized by multiple erythematous lesions, erosions and shallow irregularly shaped ulcers that may be bordered by fine radiating white striae (Fig. 12A, B).
- Gingival involvement may present as desquamative gingivitis.

Histopathology
- The mucosal epithelium shows hyperkeratosis and saw-toothed rete ridges with hydropic degeneration of the basal layer.
- Colloid (cytoid, hyaline, or Civatte) bodies are degenerating keratinocytes near the epithelial–connective tissue interface.
- The connective tissue contains a bandlike infiltrate of lymphocytes that is immediately beneath the epithelium.
- A fibrinogen band may be seen at the basement membrane zone with direct immunofluorescence studies.
- The histopathologic features of lichen planus are shared with other conditions, such as lichenoid drug reaction and lichenoid amalgam reaction (please see section on Oral Lichenoid Lesions); clinical correction is required to differentiate among them.

Diagnosis
- Diagnosis of oral lichen planus can be made from the clinical presentation if the oral lesions are sufficiently characteristic.
- Biopsy may be required to confirm the diagnosis and to exclude dysplasia and malignancy.

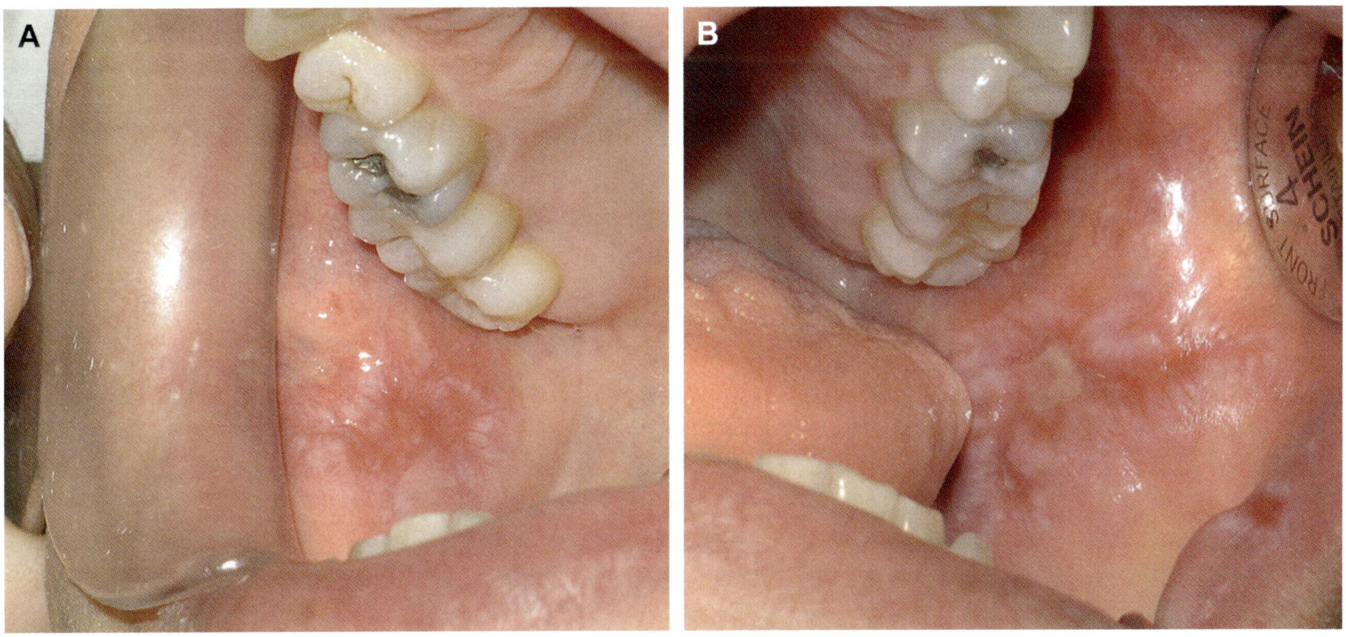

Fig. 12 Erosive lichen planus. A 59-year-old male with a 4-year history of ulceration and erythema with peripheral white striations on the buccal mucosa (*A, B*) and lip mucosa. He was taking hydrochlorothiazide to control hypertension and it was not feasible to alter his medication. The lesions were partly responsive to topical corticosteroids, which provided symptomatic relief.

Treatment

- Reticular lichen planus is not treated because it is usually asymptomatic; however, periodic monitoring is recommended.
- Erosive lichen planus is usually managed with topical corticosteroids delivered in the form of gels, ointments, mouth rinses, or adhesive pastes.
- Midpotency topical corticosteroids such as triamcinolone acetonide, potent fluorinated corticosteroids such as fluocinonide, and super-potent corticosteroids such as clobetasol propionate are effective on most patients; the choice of topical steroid type and formulation depends on the distribution and clinical severity of the lesions.
- Although there are few adrenal suppressive effects associated with use of topical corticosteroids, secondary candidiasis may occur in up to one-third of cases and can be treated with topical antifungal agents.
- Maintenance of good oral hygiene and removal of local mechanical sources of trauma such as sharp dental cusps, rough dental restorations, and poorly fitting dentures will help to prevent exacerbation of lesions.
- Intralesional corticosteroid injections, immunomodulatory agents such as topical tacrolimus, and systemic corticosteroids may be considered in cases of erosive lichen planus refractory to treatment with topical corticosteroids, however, use of these less conventional therapies is best restricted to oral medicine specialty practice.
- Patients with erosive lichen planus should be periodically monitored every 3 to 6 months; a repeat biopsy may be considered for persistent and/or progressive lesions that do not respond to topical steroids.[18–20]

Oral lichenoid lesions

Oral lichen planus is a chronic inflammatory mucosal disease that is associated with a cell-mediated immune reaction to basal keratinocytes. The etiology and pathogenesis are not well-understood (see elsewhere in this article and also Paolo G. Arduino's article, "Oral Complications of Dermatologic Disorders," in this issue). Lesions of the oral mucosa may also present with a clinical appearance similar to lichen planus, as white reticular patches, plaques, and papules, and erosions or ulcerations, but are associated with a causative factor or underlying disease. These are referred to as oral lichenoid lesions, and are managed by removal of the causative factor or treatment of the underlying disease.

Oral lichenoid lesions can be classified into the following categories:

- Contact reaction to dental materials (discussed elsewhere in this article),
- Mucosal reaction to systemic medications (see Kentaro Ikeda's article, "Drug-Induced Oral Complications," in this issue),
- Oral lesions of chronic graft versus host disease (see Elizabeth Waring and Alessandro Villa's article, "Oral Manifestations of Immunodeficiencies and Transplantation Medicine," in this issue), and
- Oral lesions of discoid or systemic lupus erythematosus (see Vidya Sankar and Marcel Noujeim's article, "Oral Manifestations of Autoimmune and Connective Tissue Disorders," in this issue).

Lichenoid contact reaction to dental materials, particularly amalgam

Description

- A chronic mucosal lesion with clinical appearance similar to lichen planus, located in direct contact with a dental material, most commonly an amalgam restoration.
- Most cases represent a type IV, or delayed type hypersensitivity reaction, which is a cell-mediated response.

Prevalence

- Rare.
- Occurs in a minority of the population but the basis of individual susceptibility is unknown.

Clinical presentation

- White reticular patch or white plaque that may be associated with erythema or ulceration.
- Develops in an area of mucosa in direct contact with an amalgam restoration (Fig. 13).
- The amalgam restoration may have been present for months or years.
- Predilection for buccal mucosa and lateral border of the tongue; other areas of the mucosa such as gingiva or palate are unlikely to have direct surface contact with a restoration.
- Migration of the lesion does not occur.
- Pain is uncommon, but may develop when there is erosion or ulceration.

Patch testing for allergy to amalgam or mercury

- Best done in a specialized dermatology clinic or oral medicine center.
- An array of dental materials, including amalgam and mercuric compounds is placed on the skin of the back or arm and held in place for 48 hours.
- Test is read at 48 and 72 hours, plus a late reading at 10 to 14 days for increased sensitivity.
- A positive reaction consists of erythema with or without vesicles.
- False positives and false negatives occur, so the patch test should be used only where there is a strong clinical indication of a contact reaction to amalgam, and interpreted in the context of clinical and biopsy findings.

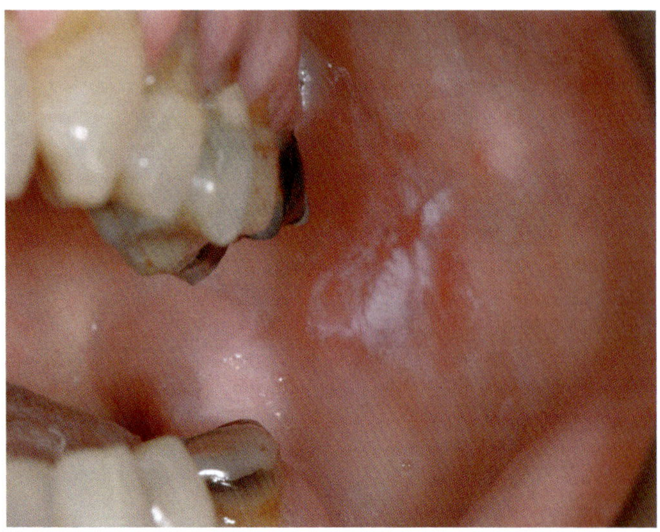

Fig. 13 Lichenoid reaction to amalgam. Erythematous patch associated with white striations on the left buccal mucosa opposite a large amalgam restoration on the left maxillary first molar. There were no other oral lesions.

Histopathology

- Similar to lichen planus with hyperkeratosis, liquefactive degeneration of the basal cell layer with a bandlike, predominately lymphocytic inflammatory infiltrate in the superficial connective tissue.
- May be distinguished from lichen planus by the presence of a deeper, perivascular inflammatory infiltrate in addition to the subepithelial infiltrate, and the presence of plasma cells and neutrophils in addition to lymphocytes and histiocytes in the infiltrate.
- The majority of cases of lichenoid reaction to amalgam cannot be distinguished from lichen planus by histopathologic examination alone (Fig. 14A–D).

Diagnosis

- The strongest diagnostic feature is the clinical demonstration of contact of the mucosal lesion with an amalgam restoration.
- There are conflicting reports on the usefulness of patch testing.
- Biopsy should be done to rule out epithelial dysplasia.

Differential diagnosis

- Lichen planus.
- Lichenoid drug reaction.
- Chronic graft-versus-host disease.
- Chronic discoid lupus erythematosus.
- Oral lesion of systemic lupus erythematosus.
- Dysplasia or squamous cell carcinoma (Table 4).

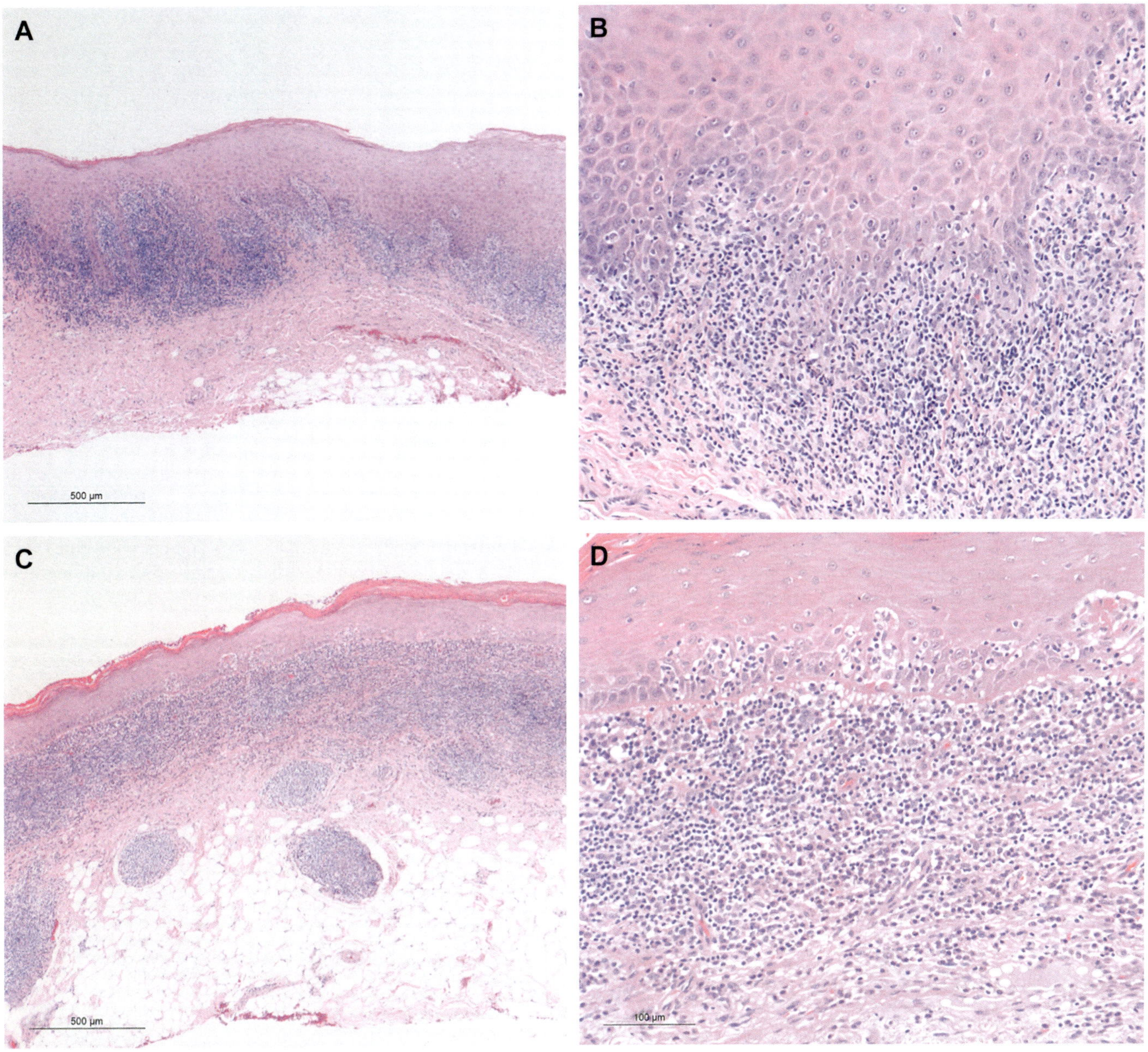

Fig. 14 Histologic similarity between lichen planus and lichenoid reaction to amalgam. (*A, B*) Biopsy of lichen planus of the buccal mucosa showing hyperkeratosis, dense chronic inflammatory infiltrate beneath the epithelium that is predominantly lymphocytic and liquefactive degeneration of basal epithelial cells. (*C, D*) Biopsy of lichenoid reaction to amalgam (clinical photograph in Fig. 13) showing hyperkeratosis, dense chronic inflammatory infiltrate beneath the epithelium, and liquefactive degeneration of basal epithelial cells. There is also a perivascular inflammatory infiltrate in the deeper connective tissue. The high-power view shows that the inflammatory infiltrate consists of lymphocytes and plasma cells.

Table 4 Differentiation of lichenoid contact reaction to amalgam from lesions with a similar clinical appearance

Diagnosis	Clinical and laboratory findings
Lichenoid contact reaction to amalgam	Location in direct contact with amalgam restoration; typically unilateral, not symmetric; positive patch test to amalgam and/or mercuric compounds; resolution of lesion upon removal of the amalgam restoration
Lichen planus	Multiple lesions that are bilateral and symmetric; lesions may be present on skin and other mucosal surfaces
Lichenoid drug reaction	Associated with use of systemic medications
Chronic graft-versus-host disease	History of bone marrow transplantation
Oral discoid lupus erythematosus	Lesions on sun-exposed skin; histologic findings of edema and extravasation of blood in lamina propria, perivascular inflammatory infiltrate; Periodic acid-Schiff diastase (PASD)-positive eosinophilic material along basement membrane zone and perivascular space; direct immunofluorescence examination shows the eosinophilic deposits to contain IgG
Oral lesion of SLE	Clinical manifestations of SLE in skin, joints, kidneys, lungs, heart, central nervous system; laboratory findings
Epithelial dysplasia	Histologic findings of epithelial dysplasia; not related to contact with amalgam or other dental material; does not resolve with removal of dental restorations in the area of the lesions

Abbreviation: SLE, systemic lupus erythematosus.

Treatment

- Remove the amalgam restoration; if this is not possible, cover the amalgam with a crown.
- Diagnosis of lichenoid contact reaction to amalgam is confirmed if resolution occurs within 4 to 5 weeks after elimination of contact with the amalgam.
- Only the amalgam restorations in contact with a lichenoid lesion require removal; a rubber dam, copious water, and high-speed suction should be used during the procedure.[21–23]

Contact stomatitis—cinnamon reaction

Description

- Delayed type, cell-mediated hypersensitivity reaction may occur in the oral mucosa in response to a diverse array of substances including food and food additives, oral hygiene products, and dental materials.
- Should be distinguished from nonallergic mucosal inflammation that occurs in response to physical and/or chemical irritation of the mucosa
- Two common types of allergens, cinnamon (cinnamon essential oil or cinnamaldehyde) and dental restorative materials are known for their distinctive reaction patterns seen clinically. (Lichenoid contact reaction to dental materials, particularly amalgam, is discussed elsewhere in this article.)
- Cinnamon essential oil is widely used as a flavoring agent at concentrations of up to 100 time that of the natural spice.
- Prolonged and frequent contact with artificially flavored cinnamon products, such as candy and chewing gum, lead to a delayed hypersensitivity T-cell–mediated immune response and subsequent inflammatory reaction.

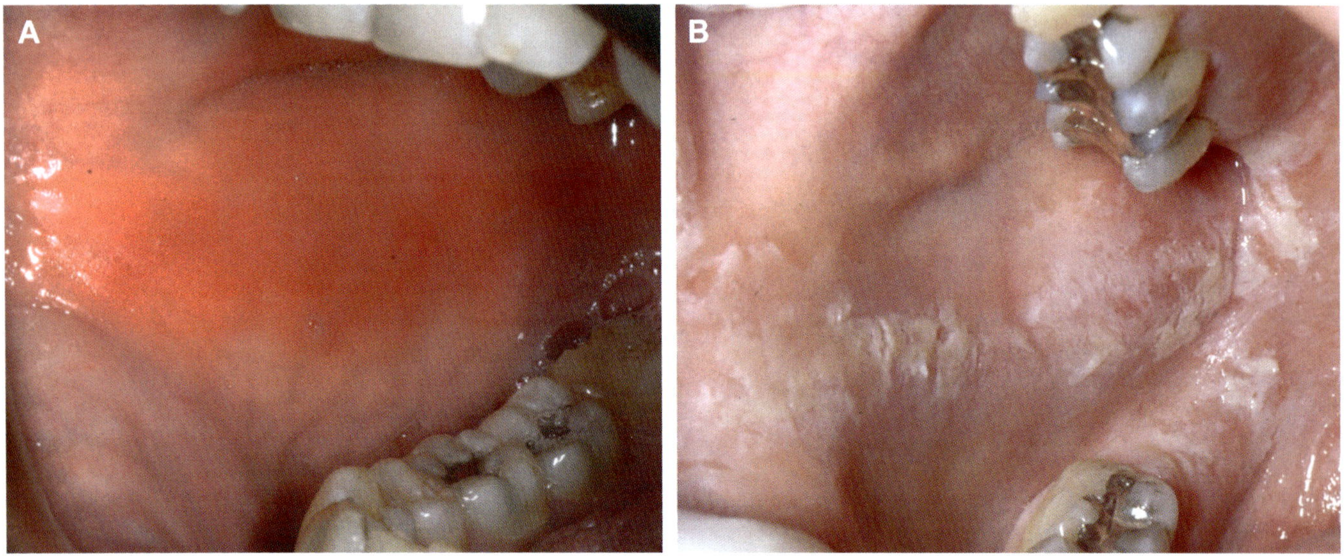

Fig. 15 Contact stomatitis from cinnamon flavoring. (*A*) Diffuse erythema of the buccal mucosa associated with use of cinnamon-flavored gum. The lesion cleared completely when the patient stopped using the cinnamon-containing product. (*B*) Shaggy hyperkeratosis associated with erythema on the buccal mucosa and retromolar mucosa.

Prevalence

- Contact stomatitis is less commonly seen than contact dermatitis; a number of physiologic mechanisms, including the action of saliva, are thought to limit the development of a contact allergic response in the oral mucosa.
- Factors determining susceptibility are unknown.

Clinical presentation

- Tissue involvement is directly related to the surfaces most in contact with the cinnamon allergen.
  - Toothpaste would create a more diffuse reaction involving the gingiva.
  - Chewing gum and candy results in a more focal presentation, often on the buccal mucosa.
- Affected mucosa is often erythematous and may show patches and plaques of hyperkeratosis with or without sloughing, associated edema, erosions, and ulcerations (Fig. 15A, B).
- Painful burning sensation is the most common complaint.

Histopathology

- Hyperkeratosis, atrophic or acanthotic epithelium with neutrophilic exocytosis and a dense inflammatory infiltrate in the superficial lamina propria, consisting predominantly of lymphocytes intermixed with plasma cells, histiocytes, and eosinophils.
- Perivascular inflammatory infiltrates may be seen within the connective tissue.
- Histopathologic appearance is not specific for contact stomatitis to cinnamon.

Diagnosis

- Clinical appearance of the lesions and a history of contact of the affected mucosa with cinnamon-flavored products.
- Diagnosis can be confirmed by withdrawal of the product containing the cinnamon followed by resolution of the lesions (observing a recurrence of the lesions with reintroduction of the offending product would further confirm the diagnosis, although rarely carried out).
- A biopsy may be required to rule out mucocutaneous diseases such as lichen planus, hairy leukoplakia, hyperplastic candidiasis, and epithelial dysplasia.
- Cutaneous patch testing may help with the diagnosis, although false positives and false negatives are common.

Treatment

- Lesions usually resolve within 1 to 2 weeks after elimination of the allergenic agent/cinnamon-flavored product.
- If the lesions are slow to resolve or the patient is experiencing some discomfort then short-term use of topical corticosteroids may be beneficial.[24,25]

References

1. Al Johani KA, Moles DR, Hodgson TA, et al. Orofacial granulomatosis: clinical features and long-term outcome of therapy. J Am Acad Dermatol 2010;62(4):611–20.
2. Campbell H, Escudier M, Patel P, et al. Distinguishing orofacial granulomatosis from Crohn's disease: two separate disease entities? Inflamm Bowel Dis 2011;17(10):2109–15.
3. Fitzpatrick L, Healy CM, McCartan BE, et al. Patch testing for food-associated allergies in orofacial granulomatosis. J Oral Pathol Med 2011;40(1):10–3.
4. Lazzerini M, Martelossi S, Cont G, et al. Orofacial granulomatosis in children: think about Crohn's disease. Dig Liver Dis 2015;47(4): 338–41.
5. McCartan BE, Healy CM, McCreary CE, et al. Characteristics of patients with orofacial granulomatosis. Oral Dis 2011;17(7): 696–704.
6. Miest R, Bruce A, Rogers RS 3rd. Orofacial granulomatosis. Clin Dermatol 2016;34(4):505–13.
7. Mignogna MD, Pollio A, Leuci S, et al. Clinical behaviour and long-term therapeutic response in orofacial granulomatosis patients treated with intralesional triamcinolone acetonide injections alone or in combination with topical pimecrolimus 1%. J Oral Pathol Med 2013;42(1):73–81.
8. Patel P, Brostoff J, Campbell H, et al. Clinical evidence for allergy in orofacial granulomatosis and inflammatory bowel disease. Clin Transl Allergy 2013;3(1):26.
9. Baccaglini L, Lalla RV, Bruce AJ, et al. Urban legends: recurrent aphthous stomatitis. Oral Dis 2011;17(8):755–70.
10. Scully C. Clinical practice. Aphthous ulceration. N Engl J Med 2006; 355(2):165–72.
11. Stoopler ET, Sollecito TP. Recurrent oral ulcers. JAMA 2015; 313(23):2373–4.
12. Davatchi F, Chams-Davatchi C, Shams H, et al. Behcet's disease: epidemiology, clinical manifestations, and diagnosis. Expert Rev Clin Immunol 2017;13(1):57–65.
13. Rokutanda R, Kishimoto M, Okada M. Update on the diagnosis and management of Behcet's disease. Open Access Rheumatol 2015;7:1–8.
14. Neville B, Allen C, Damm D, et al. Oral and maxillofacial pathology. 4th edition. St. Louis (MO): Elsevier; 2016.
15. Kumar V, Abbas A, Fausto N, et al. Pathologic basis of disease. 8th edition. Philadelphia: Saunders/Elsevier; 2010.
16. Celentano A, Tovaru S, Yap T, et al. Oral erythema multiforme: trends and clinical findings of a large retrospective European case series. Oral Surg Oral Med Oral Pathol Oral Radiol 2015;120(6):707–16.
17. Staikuniene J, Staneviciute J. Long-term valacyclovir treatment and immune modulation for Herpes-associated erythema multiforme. Cent Eur J Immunol 2015;40(3):387–90.
18. Thongprasom K, Carrozzo M, Furness S, et al. Interventions for treating oral lichen planus. Cochrane Database Syst Rev 2011;(7). CD001168.
19. van der Meij EH, Mast H, van der Waal I. The possible premalignant character of oral lichen planus and oral lichenoid lesions: a prospective five-year follow-up study of 192 patients. Oral Oncol 2007; 43(8):742–8.
20. Lodi G, Scully C, Carrozzo M, et al. Current controversies in oral lichen planus: report of an international consensus meeting. Part 2. Clinical management and malignant transformation. Oral Surg Oral Med Oral Pathol Oral Radiol Endod 2005;100(2):164–78.
21. McParland H, Warnakulasuriya S. Oral lichenoid contact lesions to mercury and dental amalgam—a review. J Biomed Biotechnol 2012; 2012:589569.
22. Thornhill MH, Sankar V, Xu XJ, et al. The role of histopathological characteristics in distinguishing amalgam-associated oral lichenoid reactions and oral lichen planus. J Oral Pathol Med 2006;35(4): 233–40.
23. van der Waal I. Oral lichen planus and oral lichenoid lesions; a critical appraisal with emphasis on the diagnostic aspects. Med Oral Patol Oral Cir Bucal 2009;14(7):E310–4.
24. Tremblay S, Avon SL. Contact allergy to cinnamon: case report. J Can Dent Assoc 2008;74(5):445–61.
25. Vivas AP, Migliari DA. Cinnamon-induced oral mucosal contact reaction. Open Dent J 2015;9:257–9.

Oral Complications of Multiorgan Disorders

Leah Bowers, BSc, DMD [a,*], Michael Brennan, DDS, MHS [b]

KEYWORDS

• Multiorgan • Systemic disease • Immunosuppresants

KEY POINTS

- Oral manifestations of multiorgan disorders may be the first clinical signs of systemic disease or may signify a new sign of established, recurrent, or refractory disease.
- Stigmata of some of these disorders, such as the "strawberry gingivitis" of granulomatosis with polyangiitis, are pathognomonic, allowing for early detection and intervention. Other disorders, such as IgG4-related disease, require a comprehensive evaluation to establish a definitive diagnosis.
- Clinical manifestations of these diseases are diverse, ranging from isolated mucosal nodules to salivary gland masses. Histopathologic examination, serologic analyses, and other investigations may be necessary to rule out the differential diagnoses.
- Treatment of many of these disorders involves immunosuppressive therapy and the use of biologic agents or adjuvants, many of which have oral side effects.

Amyloidosis

Brief description

Amyloidosis represents a group of acquired or hereditary diseases involving a systemic or localized accumulation of insoluble fibrillar proteins. Modern classification uses an abbreviation of the protein that composes most deposits, prefixed by the letter "A." AL amyloidosis, for example, the most common form of the disease, is caused by deposition of protein derived from immunoglobulin light chain fragments.

AL amyloidosis can occur alone or in association with multiple myeloma, Waldenström macroglobulinemia, or non-Hodgkin lymphoma. AA (serum amyloid A protein) amyloidosis may complicate chronic diseases, such as rheumatoid arthritis or inflammatory bowel disease. Dialysis-related amyloidosis (Aβ_2-microglobulin) may be seen in those on long-term dialysis. Transthyretin-related amyloidosis (ATTR) is a hereditary form. Alzheimer disease and orofacial amyloidosis are examples of localized amyloidoses.

Amyloid involvement of the tongue, appearing as macroglossia, is almost universally secondary to systemic disease.[1] In contrast, most cases of amyloidosis affecting the head and neck are localized AL amyloidosis, the most common sites being the larynx, oropharynx, trachea, orbit, and nasopharynx.[2]

The authors have nothing to disclose.

[a] Oral and Maxillofacial Surgery, UCSF School of Dentistry, 533 Parnassus Avenue, PO Box 0404, UB-10, San Francisco, CA 94143, USA

[b] Department of Oral Medicine, Carolinas Medical Center, Carolinas HealthCare System, 1000 Blythe Boulevard, Charlotte, NC, 28203, USA

* Corresponding author.

E-mail address: leah.bowers@ucsf.edu

Clinical features

Systemic clinical manifestations can include signs and symptoms of heart failure, hepatomegaly, nephrotic syndrome, peripheral and/or autonomic neuropathy (eg, carpal tunnel syndrome), impaired coagulation, and muscular pseudohypertrophy (eg, macroglossia).

Macroglossia can result in indentations from the teeth and protrusion of the teeth resulting in an anterior open bite. Amyloid deposition within the tongue and suprahyoid muscles can result in hypogeusia, dysarthria, dysphagia, dysphonia, dyspnea, and obstructive sleep apnea.[3]

Other manifestations include yellowish, red, blue, or purple papules, nodules, and plaques, petechiae, bullous lesions, vesicles, and ulcers of the oral mucosa; periodontal destruction; and sclerotic lips.[3–7] Infiltration of the salivary glands can result in glandular hypertrophy and xerostomia. Rarely, amyloidosis can present with jaw claudication, temporal area headaches, and visual disturbances.

Dermal involvement in systemic amyloidosis may manifest as a waxy thickening; easy bruising; and subcutaneous nodules, plaques, or purpura developing after minor trauma (characteristically in a periorbital distribution). Localized cutaneous amyloidosis can have a macular, lichenoid, biphasic, or nodular pattern.[8]

Incidence, predilection, genetics

The global annual incidence of amyloidosis is estimated at five to nine cases per million, is highest among adults aged 60 to 80 years, and there is a male preponderance.[9–13]

Hereditary amyloidoses (ATTR and non-TTR) are caused by inheritance of genetic mutations in an autosomal-dominant fashion causing misfolding of amyloid proteins. Some of the

Atlas Oral Maxillofacial Surg Clin N Am 25 (2017) 187-195

http://dx.doi.org/10.1016/j.cxom.2017.04.010

acquired amyloidoses may also be affected by genetically determined factors.

Histopathology

Tissue biopsy is necessary to confirm the diagnosis in all suspected cases of amyloidosis. The amyloid subtype must then be identified and the extent of systemic involvement determined.

On hematoxylin-eosin examination, amyloid appears as acellular, amorphous, eosinophilic material that accumulates in the lamina propria and in a perivascular manner. Amyloid may also infiltrate and replace minor salivary gland parenchyma and there may be a variable foreign body reaction.[7] Congo red–stained amyloid, examined using polarized light, shows anomalous colors including "apple-green birefringence" (Fig. 1).[14]

In AL amyloidosis, plasma cells may have a normal or atypical morphology; the latter warrants suspicion for multiple myeloma. Further investigation employs immunohistochemical stains, such as in an amyloid panel (ie, kappa and lambda light chains, prealbumin, β_2-microglobulin, and SAA1). The normal kappa/lamba ratio is 2:1. Restricted expression of either kappa or lambda suggests monoclonality and a neoplastic process, such as multiple myeloma.[15]

Differential diagnoses

Consideration for the following differential diagnoses should be entertained based on the shared presenting clinical signs and symptoms:

- Sjögren syndrome (SS): hyposalivation, xerostomia, glandular swelling, or hypertrophy.
- Giant cell arteritis: headaches and visual disturbances, weight loss, fatigue, muscle pain and vascular symptoms including jaw claudication, elevated erythrocyte sedimentation rate, and anemia. Congo red staining of the temporal artery biopsy specimen should be performed to rule out amyloidosis if the initial findings are negative for giant cell arteritis.[16]
- Granulomatosis with polyangiitis (GPA): gingivitis, jaw claudication, airway involvement.
- Macroglossia: neoplasms; acromegaly; idiopathic, traumatic, and iatrogenic causes; tongue enlargement following tooth loss; advanced amyotrophic lateral sclerosis; and lymphangioma or lingual vascular malformations.[17]

Treatment considerations

Treatment of systemic amyloidosis addresses the cause of excess fibril production and ranges from use of high-dose chemotherapy with possible stem cell transplant for multiple myeloma associated with AL amyloidosis, to organ transplant in some hereditary amyloidoses. Localized amyloidosis may be managed symptomatically, depending on the organ involved and the grade of functional impairment.[3]

Surgical intervention may be considered for macroglossia caused by systemic amyloidosis, where there are functional or aesthetic problems; however, tongue enlargement and lesions are likely to recur if cessation of deposition of amyloid is not achieved.[6]

Sarcoidosis including Heerfordt syndrome

Brief description

Sarcoidosis is a nonnecrotizing granulomatous disease of unknown cause that most commonly affects the lungs, skin, lymphatic system, and eyes.

Incidence, predilection, genetics

There is wide geographic and ethic variation in incidence, with increased incidence among persons of Scandinavian, Irish, German, West Indian, African-American, and Afro-Caribbean origin.[18–24]

In the United States, the annual incidence rate among white persons is approximately 10.9 cases per 100,00 but is threefold higher in black patients of African descent at 35.5 cases per 100,000 and is especially high in black women of African descent between the ages of 30 and 39 years at 107 cases per 100,000.[18,19]

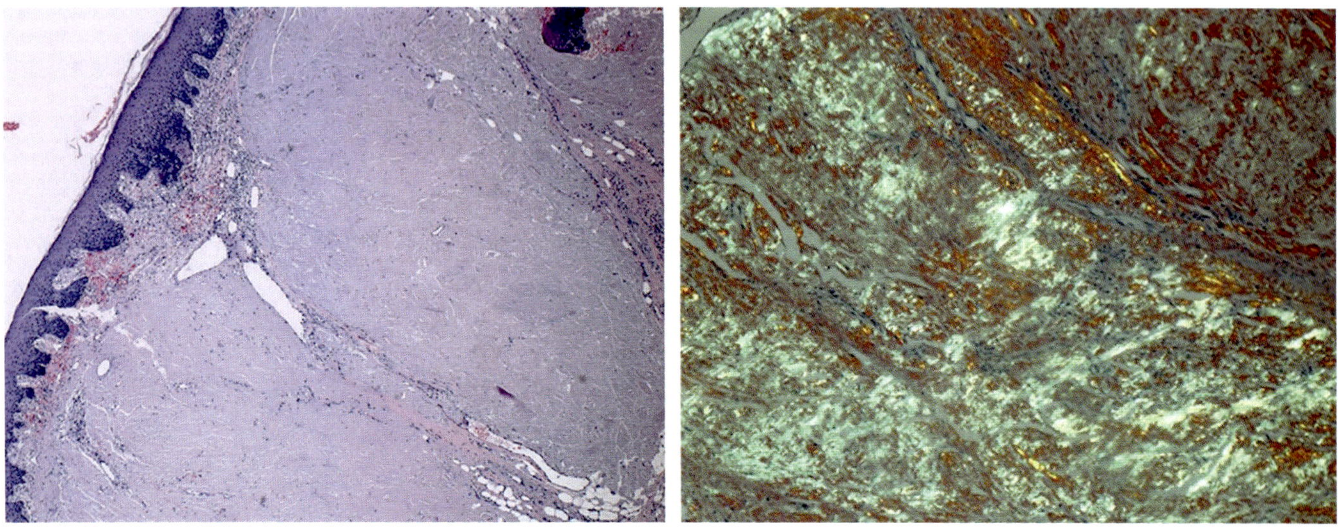

Fig. 1 (*Left*) Oral mucosa demonstrating accumulation of amorphous, eosinophilic material in the lamina propria consistent with amyloid deposition (hematoxylin-eosin, original magnification ×100). (*Right*) Congo red–stained amyloid examined under polarized light showing "apple-green birefringence" (original magnification ×200). (*Courtesy of* Richard Jordan, DDS, PhD, University of California, San Francisco, CA.)

There is a slight female predilection and a bimodal age distribution; the first peak arises between ages 25 and 35 years and the second peak between ages 45 and 65 years.[25]

Most cases of sarcoidosis are sporadic, but familial and ethnic group clusters connote a possible role of genetic factors. Polymorphism of genes encoding HLA class II proteins may determine susceptibility to, or may confer protection against, sarcoidosis.[26–29]

Clinical features

The clinical manifestations of sarcoidosis are highly variable and depend on the organs affected and the extent and severity of granulomatous involvement. Sarcoidosis may present asymptomatically (eg, detected during routine chest radiograph), with nonspecific constitutional symptoms (eg, fever, fatigue, malaise, and weight loss) or with symptoms related to specific organ involvement (eg, dyspnea).

The most common clinical presentation in the oral soft tissues is that of a localized swelling or nodules (typically on the buccal mucosa), but it may present as ulcers, gingivitis, gingival hyperplasia, or gingival recession (Fig. 2).[18]

Parotid gland involvement, presenting as a firm, persistent, and nontender tumescence, most often bilaterally, occurs in up to 10% of cases of sarcoidosis, and is often accompanied by xerostomia, giving a clinical picture redolent of SS.[30] The submandibular and sublingual glands are similarly affected, albeit less frequently. The triad of parotid gland involvement with facial nerve palsy, uveitis, and fever is known as Heerfordt syndrome (uveoparotid fever) and represents 0.3% of all cases of sarcoidosis.[31]

In the gnathic bones, sarcoidosis may present radiographically as lytic and permeative (ie, "moth-eaten") lesions. Clinical manifestations of osseous involvement have been reported as tooth mobility, pain radiating to the ears, nasal obstruction, swelling, maxillary bone loss, and nonhealing of extraction sockets.[18]

Lupus pernio (violaceous or erythematous indurated papules, plaques, or nodules of the nose, ears, cheeks, lips, and forehead) is pathognomonic for sarcoidosis and is associated with more severe systemic disease.[32]

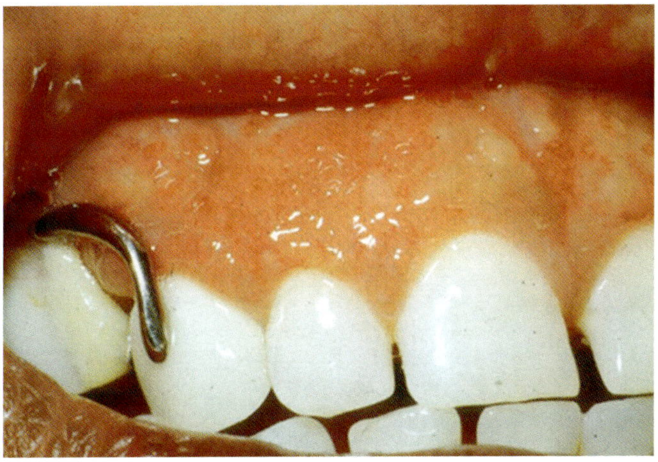

Fig. 2 Biopsy-proven gingival sarcoidosis. (*Courtesy of* Gretchen Folk, DDS, MS, Scripps Oral Pathology Service, San Diego, CA and Archives of the Armed Forces Institute of Pathology, Washington, DC.)

Histopathology

Histologic findings described in sarcoidosis involve multiple, discrete, nonnecrotizing ("noncaseating") granulomas replete with Langerhans giant cells and a rim of lymphocytes (Fig. 3).[20] Inclusion bodies (eg, asteroid bodies, Schaumann bodies) are commonly seen.

No histopathologic finding is pathognomonic for sarcoidosis. The presence of granulomas should prompt the use of special histochemical stains to rule out the presence of infectious microorganisms.

Differential diagnosis

Sarcoidosis and SS can present clinically with salivary gland enlargement and xerostomia. Histopathologic findings consistent with sarcoidosis are reported in palatal or labial salivary gland biopsies from clinically normal mucosa in patients with sarcoidosis in 19% to 58% of cases. A minor salivary gland biopsy, therefore, may be useful in differentiating sarcoidosis from SS.[18,33–35]

Clinical differential diagnoses for similar parotid gland swelling includes obstruction from neoplasms (eg, Warthin tumor), sialolithiasis, infection (eg, viral parotitis [mumps], human immunodeficiency virus), granulomatous diseases (see below), lymphoproliferative diseases (eg, lymphoma, Castleman disease), sialadenosis caused by endocrinopathy (eg, diabetes mellitus, hypothyroidism), nutritional disturbances (eg, bulimia nervosa, alcoholism), medications, and Kimura's disease.

The presence of nonnecrotizing granulomas requires further clinical investigation to rule out other granulomatous diseases, particularly orofacial granulomatosis: a group of related conditions including bacterial infections (eg, tuberculosis, syphilis, cat-scratch disease, leprosy), fungal infections (eg, histoplasmosis, coccidiodomycosis), foreign body granulomas, and Crohn's disease.[18,36]

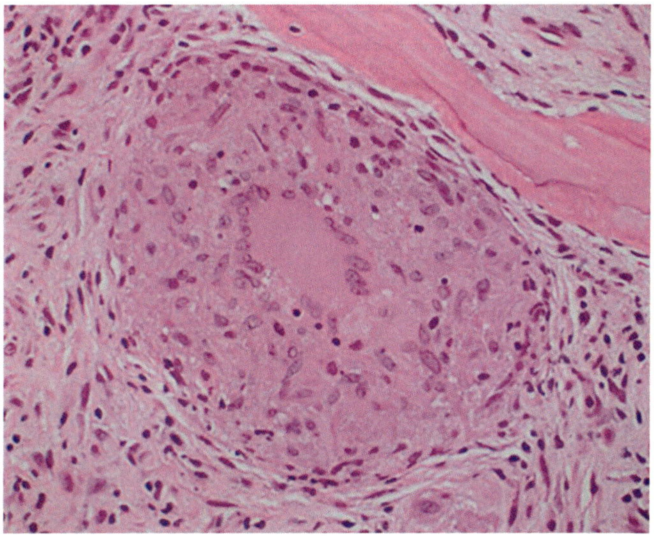

Fig. 3 Non-necrotizing granuloma in sarcoidosis composed of epithelioid histiocytes and a central multinucleated Langerhans giant cell (hematoxylin-eosin, original magnification ×400). (*Courtesy of* Lee Slater, DDS, MS, Scripps Oral Pathology Service, San Diego, CA.)

Treatment considerations

Appropriate treatment of sarcoidosis is dependent on the extent and severity of disease. Spontaneous regression can occur particularly in those with mild and focal disease.

In patients requiring systemic disease management, glucocorticoids are the most common treatment used.[18] Adjuvant agents include methotrexate, azathioprine, leflunomide, and the antimalarial drugs chloroquine and hydroxychloroquine. The tumor necrosis factor-α antagonist infliximab may be used in those with refractory disease.

Surgical excision of isolated, accessible oral lesions is appropriate. If the oral lesions are widespread, systemic medications may be used to control the disease.[18,29,37] Jaw lesions should be curetted and mobile teeth splinted.[18]

In patients with hyposalivation and/or xerostomia caused by sarcoid infiltration of the salivary glands, caries and oral fungal infection prevention, dry mouth management, and frequent recall examination are advised.

Granulomatosis with polyangiitis

Brief description

GPA (formerly Wegener granulomatosis) represents an immune-mediated vasculitis of small and medium-sized vessels, which most commonly presents as necrotizing granulomatous inflammation, affecting the upper and lower respiratory tracts, and glomerulonephritis.

The "limited" form of the disease is restricted to the upper and or/lower respiratory tract, whereas the "generalized" form includes renal involvement and/or imminent organ failure. Most patients with the localized form progress to generalized disease. The average life expectancy for a patient with GPA without treatment is 5 months.

The American College of Rheumatology 1990 criteria for classification requires the presence of at least two of the four following criteria: (1) oral ulcers or purulent or bloody nasal discharge; (2) chest radiograph showing the presence of nodules, fixed infiltrates, or cavities; (3) microhematuria or urinary red cell casts; and (4) granulomatous inflammation on biopsy.[38]

The presence of anti-neutrophil cytoplasmic antibodies (ANCA) is the most important serologic test in the diagnosis of vasculitis.[39] A total of 80% to 95% of cases of GPA are associated with cytoplasmic ANCA with autoantibodies directed against proteinase 3; the remainder is perinuclear-ANCA-positive with autoantibodies against myeloperoxidase.[40–42] A combination of clinical presentation, biopsy, and ANCA results, therefore, provides an effective approach for diagnosis.[39]

Incidence, predilection, genetics

The reported annual incidence of GPA ranges from 2 to 12 cases per million.[39,43] Peak incidence is observed between 64 and 75 years of age.[42] GPA appears more commonly in white patients but shows no gender predilection.

Although the definitive cause of GPA is unknown, the disease may be triggered by an environmental agent in genetically susceptible individuals (ie, those with an exaggerated Th1-type response). Previously identified autoimmune disease susceptibility loci in genes *HLA-DPB*,[44] *CTLA4*,[45] and *PTPN22*[46] and the null allele α_1-antitrypsin have been found to be statistically significantly associated with GPA.[45]

Exposure to inhaled environmental triggers (silica and dust[47–49]) and antigens associated with gardening and farming are thought to increase the risk of GPA.[49] Nasal carriage of *Staphylococcus aureus* has also been implicated.[50]

Clinical features

Oral involvement has been observed in 5% to 13% of patients with GPA.[39,51,52] The presence of a "strawberry" gingivitis (granular-appearing, hyperplastic anterior gingiva with petechiae) is pathognomonic for GPA (Fig. 4). Additional manifestations include oral or oropharyngeal aphthous-like ulcers,[53] mucosal nodules,[54] increased tooth mobility, alveolar bone loss[55] or exposure,[39] delayed healing of extraction sockets, oroantral fistulae,[56] and palatal osteonecrosis.[53]

Major salivary gland involvement (parotid > submandibular > sublingual), presenting as a painful tumescence, usually in conjunction with respiratory signs and symptoms, is suggestive of GPA. Facial nerve neuropathy can accompany GPA-associated parotitis.[57]

The earliest manifestations of GPA usually involve the sinonasal region in the form of sinusitis, rhinitis, epistaxis, nasal obstruction, or discharge. Although any structure in the sinonasal cavity may be affected, the anterior nasal septum supplied by the Kiesselbach plexus is the most common site of sinonasal GPA.[52] Perforation of the septum and subsequent loss of cartilaginous support can result in a "saddle-nose" deformity.

Histopathology

Hematoxylin-eosin examination of specimens consistent with GPA demonstrates granulomas with multinucleated giant cells, a mixed inflammatory cell infiltrate, epithelioid histiocytes with ulceration, necrotizing vasculitis, and (often pseudoepitheliomatous) hyperplasia of the overlying epithelium. The presence of granulomas should prompt application of special stains to help in identification of microorganisms to rule out an infectious cause.

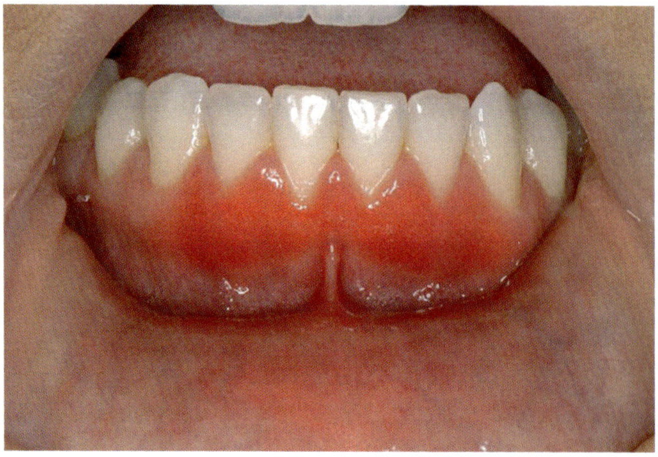

Fig. 4 Biopsy-proven GPA of the mandibular anterior gingiva. (*Courtesy of* Tina Woods, DMD, University of Mississippi Medical Center, Jackson, MS.)

Differential diagnosis

Although "strawberry" gingivitis is pathognomonic, consideration should be made for a multitude of additional conditions that can affect the gingiva similarly, such as squamous cell carcinoma, leukemic infiltrate, lymphoma, pyogenic granuloma, peripheral giant cell granuloma, peripheral ossifying fibroma, drug-induced gingival hyperplasia, plaque- and calculus-associated gingivitis/periodontitis, foreign-body reaction, orofacial granulomatosis, sarcoidosis, inflammatory bowel disease, infectious causes (fungal, bacterial, viral, parasitic), and Langerhans cell histiocytosis.

Additional causes with a similar palatal ulcerative presentation include trauma, necrotizing sialometaplasia, extranodal natural killer cell/T-cell lymphoma (nasal type), and neoplasms of the minor salivary glands. Both cocaine abuse and GPA can present with necrosis of the anterior nasal septum and palate.

Treatment considerations

Treatment of GPA is dependent on the extent of disease. A glucocorticoid regimen with additional immunosuppressant drugs is the current standard. Patients with limited GPA typically respond favorably to less-toxic regimens of methotrexate and glucocorticoids; severe GPA often requires aggressive therapy with glucocorticoids and the addition of cyclophosphamide.[58] B-cell depletion with rituximab and the anti-tumor necrosis factor-α drug infliximab used in conjunction with cyclophosphamide and methotrexate have also been used with success.[52]

IgG4-related disease

Brief description

IgG4-related disease (IgG4-RD) is an immune-mediated condition first recognized in 2001 with the following features[59]: tumefactive lesions often affecting multiple organs synchronously or metachronously, an elevated level of IgG4-secreting plasma cells, a characteristic histopathologic appearance, and a swift response to immunosuppressive therapy.

The pseudotumor conditions formerly known as Mikulicz disease, Küttner tumor, and Riedel thyroiditis are now attributed to IgG4-RD. IgG4-RD has now been described in virtually all organ systems. Additional diseases ascribed to IgG4-RD include type 1 autoimmune pancreatitis (IgG-related pancreatitis) and IgG4-related sclerosing cholangitis.

Prevalence, predilection, genetics

The definitive epidemiology of IgG4-RD has not been fully elucidated. Because most studies originate in Asia, particularly Japan, it is unclear whether Asian patients are at an increased susceptibility to the disease.[60]

The estimated annual incidence of IgG4-RD is 0.28 to 1.08 cases per 100,000 and, according to a nationwide survey conducted in Japan, the mean age at diagnosis is 61.67 years (age range, 11–89 years).[60–64] IgG4-related sialadenitis and dacryoadenitis may appear more frequently in females in contrast to many of the other conditions classified as IgG4-RD, such as autoimmune pancreatitis.

Although the decisive pathogenesis of IgG4-RD remains elusive, it is apparent that inflammation and subsequent fibrosis occur because of excess cytokine production from T helper and regulatory T cells. A study by Nakajima and colleagues[65] found that expression of genes involved in allergy development and innate immunity were lower in patients with IgG4, whereas the remarkable efficacy of B-cell depletion therapy for IgG4-RD supports a pathogenic role of a B-cell/T-cell collaboration.[66] Current research, therefore, is focused on the interaction between components of the innate and adaptive immune response.

Presenting features

IgG4-RD has no pathognomonic findings; its diagnostic work-up involves clinical examination, imaging, histologic, and serologic analyses.[60] Internal organ involvement may precede, occur simultaneously, or follow presentation of IgG4-RD in the head and neck. The head and neck region, especially the orbit and submandibular glands, is the second most common site of presentation after the pancreas.[59]

Bilateral, painless, symmetric, and persistent swelling of the major salivary glands, which may or may not be accompanied by xerostomia, xerophthalmia, and hyposalivation, accompanied by lacrimal gland involvement (dacryoadenitis) (previously described as Mikulicz disease) is a common presentation. Isolated swelling of the submandibular gland (previously given the eponym Küttner tumor) has also been reported. Cervical lymphadenopathy is common and is often accompanied by distant site lymphadenopathy (eg, mediastinal and retroperitoneal).

Histopathology

The presence of defining histopathologic findings represents the gold standard for diagnosis of IgG4-RD. These include storiform (whorling or cartwheel) fibrosis, a dense lymphoplasmacytic infiltrate, and obliterative phlebitis.[67] Smaller specimens, or those from the minor salivary glands, however, may not demonstrate all of these characteristic histopathologic features.

An unequivocal diagnosis of IgG4-RD in salivary gland tissue requires documentation of greater than 100 IgG4-positive cells per high powered field and an IgG4/IgG ratio of greater than 40% (Fig. 5).[68]

Differential diagnoses

The clinical presentation of IgG4-RD may mimic several other diseases and conditions, namely other forms of chronic sialadenitis, SS, and lymphoma. Similar bilaterally occurring tumescent parotitis may be caused by obstruction from neoplasms (eg, Warthin tumor), infection (eg, viral parotitis [paramyxovirus], human immunodeficiency virus), sialolithiasis, granulomatous diseases (eg, sarcoidosis, Heerfordt syndrome, GPA), lymphoproliferative diseases (eg, lymphoma, Castleman disease); sialadenosis caused by endocrinopathy (eg, diabetes mellitus, hypothyroidism); nutritional disturbances (eg, bulimia nervosa, alcoholism); medications; and Kimura's disease.

SS is more likely to present with significant sicca symptoms and hyposalivation. Glandular swelling in SS is less likely to be symmetric and more likely to be recurrent. Minor salivary gland

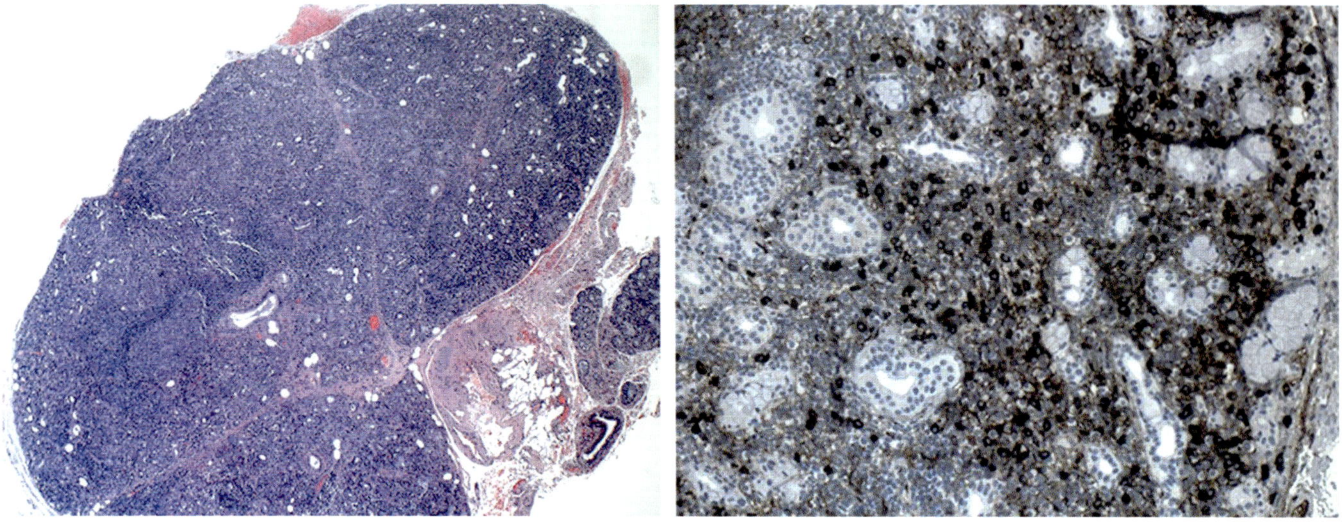

Fig. 5 (*Left*) Lymph node biopsy in IgG4-related disease showing a dense lymphoplasmacytic infiltrate. (*Right*) Immunohistochemistry staining demonstrating >100 IgG4-positive cells per high powered field. (*Courtesy of* Richard Jordan, DDS, PhD, University of California, San Francisco, CA.)

biopsy in SS does not show the defining histopathologic features of IgG4-RD and there is no increase in IgG4-positive plasma cells.

Treatment considerations

Glucocorticoids are first-line therapy for active disease. Steroid-sparing agents, such as azathioprine, have also been used. B-cell depletion using rituximab has also been shown to be effective. Watchful waiting with close clinical follow-up may be considered for patients who are asymptomatic or with mild symptoms, no signs of organ dysfunction, or involvement of areas not likely to cause major complications.[60]

In patients with hyposalivation and/or xerostomia, caries and oral fungal infection prevention, dry mouth management, and frequent recall examination are advised.

Systemic sclerosis (systemic scleroderma) including CREST syndrome

Brief description

Systemic sclerosis (SSc) is an autoimmune fibroproliferative vasculopathy in which there is a deposition of surplus collagen (types I and III), and other extracellular matrix components, in the skin and internal organs.

SSc is classified by the extent of skin involvement. Limited cutaneous SSc refers to involvement distal to the elbows and knees, whereas diffuse cutaneous SSc indicates skin involvement of the upper arms, anterior chest, abdomen, and/or thighs. Facial skin may or may not be effected in either form.

Patients with diffuse cutaneous SSc are at greater risk for developing significant cardiac, lung, and renal fibroses.[69] Cardiopulmonary involvement is the leading cause of death in patients with SSc. Scleroderma renal crisis, leading to renal failure, is a feared complication of SSc.[70]

CREST syndrome (calcinosis cutis, Raynaud's phenomenon [RP], esophageal dysmotility, sclerodactyly, and telangiectasias) (Fig. 6) can manifest with either limited cutaneous SSc or long-standing diffuse cutaneous SSc.[70]

SSc is a clinical diagnosis. The presence of SSc-specific autoantibodies (anti-centromere, anti-topoisomerase I, anti-RNA polymerase III), nailfold capillary abnormalities, and skin thickening are among the classification criteria established by the American College of Rheumatology and the European League Against Rheumatism.[71]

Incidence, predilection, genetics

The annual incidence of SSc is approximately 20 cases per million.[72,73] The female to male ratio is 4:1 and the peak age of onset is between 30 and 50 years.[74] Black women of African descent have higher incidence and diffuse disease rates.[74] There is also an exceptionally high prevalence rate among Choctaw Native Americans.

SSc is a complex, multifactorial, and polygenic disease with currently undefined contributory environmental and epigenetic factors.

Clinical features

Facial fibrosis may result in perioral radial furrows, a pinched, beak-like nose and atrophy and contracture of the upper lip ("mouse-facies") or a "mask-like" visage.

Hyposalivation or sicca syndrome, caused by glandular fibrosis, is common. SS occurs in conjunction with SSc in 17% to 29% of cases.[75–79] Oral mucosal atrophy may be present secondary to micronutrient deficiency (eg, vitamin B complex, iron, and zinc) because of difficulty with oral alimentation.

Esophageal dysmotility predisposes patients to gastroesophageal reflux disease. The resultant acidic oral environment promotes erosion of dental hard tissue and caries. Patients with SSc have higher indices of periodontal inflammation and loss of gingival attachment.[80,81] Maintenance of oral hygiene may be hindered by microstomia, trismus, and finger contractures.

Periodontal ligament space widening with, an intact lamina dura and absence of pathologic mobility, can be regional (eg, molars and premolars) or affect the entire dentition. It can affect the coronal or periapical regions, and appear on one or both sides of the root.[73]

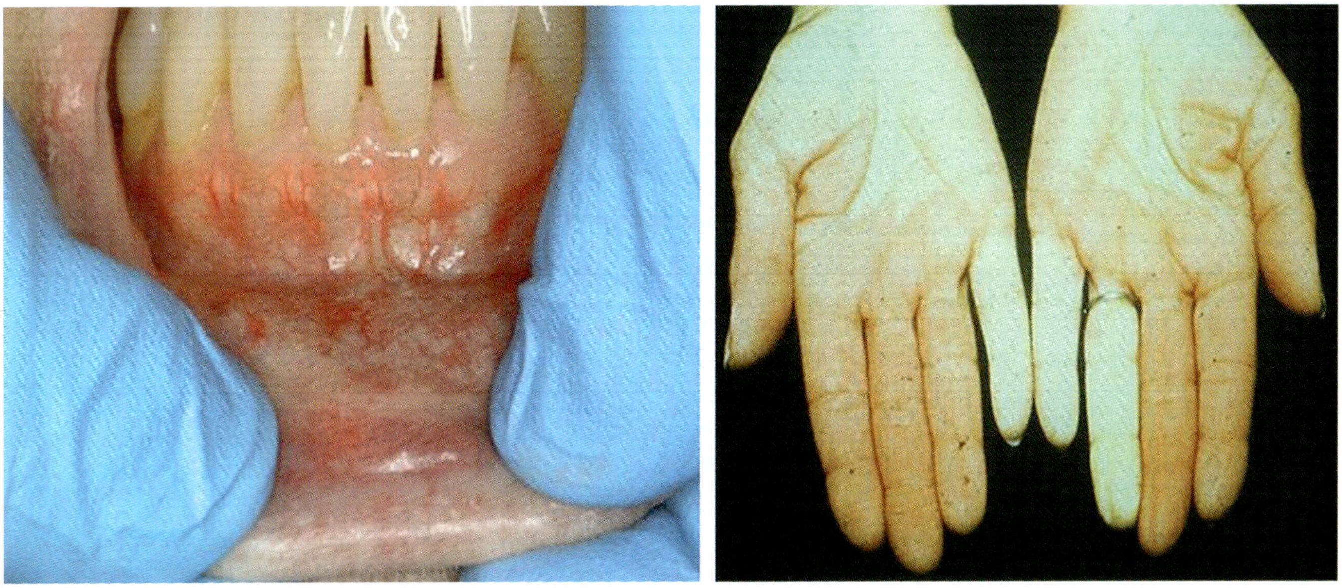

Fig. 6 (*Left*) Intraoral telangiectasias in CREST syndrome. (*Courtesy of* Dr Michael Brennan, DDS, MHS, Carolinas Medical Center, Charlotte, NC.) (*Right*) Raynaud's phenomenon showing well-demarcated regions of variegated color. (*Courtesy of* Gretchen Folk, DDS, MS, Scripps Oral Pathology Service, San Diego, CA and Archives of the Armed Forces Institute of Pathology, Washington, DC.)

Mandibular resorption occurs most frequently (in descending order) at the mandibular angle, the condyle, the coronoid process, the posterior border of the ascending ramus, and the zygomatic arches.[82–84] Resorption appears as well-demarcated and symmetric, often bilateral, erosions at the sites of muscle attachments.[85,86] Severe resorption can lead to mandibular fractures and trigeminal sensory complaints.[87]

Histopathology

A skin biopsy may be performed when a scleroderma-like disorder is suspected. Histopathologic changes consistent with scleroderma include dermal thickening with copious dense collagen accumulation and atrophy of adnexal structures. Luminal narrowing of vascular structures is seen with variable dystrophic calcification.

Differential diagnosis

Most conditions considered among the clinical differential diagnoses for SSc lack additional supporting stigmata, such as RP, skin manifestations, or elevated levels of anti-nuclear antibodies. Graft-versus-host disease and rare cases of multiple myeloma–associated amyloidosis have initially presented with sclerodermoid skin lesions.[88] Widening of the PDL may also be seen in periodontal or periapical disease, occlusal trauma, orthodontic movement, and malignancy.

Treatment considerations

Patients with SSc may be treated with methotrexate, mycophenolate mofetil, cyclophosphamide, azathioprine, etanercept, infliximab, or tocilizumab.[89,90] Intravenous immunoglobulin or rituximab may be considered for refractory disease. Patients with early progressive disease may also be offered autologous hematopoietic stem cell transplant.[70,91]

Patients may benefit from an increased frequency of recall appointments, referral to periodontal specialists, the use of adaptive toothbrushes and interdental devices, and physical and occupational therapy.[92] Patients are at an increased risk of oral candidiasis because of hyposalivation, suboptimal oral hygiene, and medication-related immunosuppression. Frequently sipping water and the use of topical agents can palliate oral dryness. Side effects of methotrexate include an ulcerative stomatitis and a lymphoproliferative disorder. Corticosteroid agents should be used judiciously because of the risk of precipitation of scleroderma renal crisis.

Attention should be paid to operatory temperature and patient comfort to prevent cold- or stress-induced vasospasm. RP is most commonly treated with calcium channel blockers and topical nitrates. Calcium channel blocker–associated gingival hyperplasia, however, has rarely been reported in patients with SSc.[93,94]

References

1. Fahrner KS, Black CC, Gosselin BJ. Localized amyloidosis of the tongue: a review. Am J Otolaryngol 2004;25(3):186–9.
2. Glenner GG. Amyloid deposits and amyloidosis: the beta-fibrilloses (second of two parts). N Engl J Med 1980;302(24):1333–43.
3. Kaushik R, Pushpanshu K, Punyani SR. Orofacial amyloidosis-unusual presentation of a rare condition: a case report. Spec Care Dentist 2016;36(2):104–7.
4. Aono J, Yamagata K, Yoshida H. Local amyloidosis in the hard palate: a case report. Oral Maxillofac Surg 2009;13:119–22.
5. Reichart PA, Philipsen HP. Color atlas of dental medicine: oral pathology. New York: Thieme Stuttgart; 2000.
6. Elad S, Czerninski R, Fischman S, et al. Exceptional oral manifestations of amyloid light chain protein (AL) systemic amyloidosis. Amyloid 2010;17(1):27–31.
7. Gouvêa AF, Ribeiro AC, León JE, et al. Head and neck amyloidosis: clinicopathological features and immunohistochemical analysis of 14 cases. J Oral Pathol Med 2012;41(2):178–85.
8. Gorevic, PD. Overview of amyloidosis. In: Schur PH, Romain PL, editors. UpToDate. Waltham (MA): UpToDate. Available at: https://www.uptodate.com/contents/overview-of-amyloidosis. Accessed June 12, 2016.

9. Real de Asúa D, Costa R, Galván JM, et al. Systemic AA amyloidosis: epidemiology, diagnosis, and management. Clin Epidemiol 2014;6: 369–77.
10. Kyle RA, Linos A, Beard CM, et al. Incidence and natural history of primary systemic amyloidosis in Olmsted County, Minnesota, 1950 through 1989. Blood 1992;79(7):1817–22.
11. Kyle RA, Bayrd ED. Amyloidosis: review of 236 cases. Medicine (Baltimore) 1975;54:271–99.
12. Kerner MM, Wand MB, Angier G, et al. Amyloidosis of the head and neck. A clinicopathologic study of the UCLA experience 1955-1991. Arch Otolaryngol Head Neck Surg 1995;121:778–82.
13. Xavier SD, Bussoloti IF, Müller H. Macroglossia secondary to systemic amyloidosis: case report and literature review. Ear Nose Throat J 2005;84(6):358–61.
14. Howie AJ, Brewer DB, Howell D, et al. Physical basis of colors seen in Congo red-stained amyloid in polarized light. Lab Invest 2008; 88(3):232–42.
15. Pernick N. Stains-kappa. PathologyOutlines.com; 2015. Available at: http://www.pathologyoutlines.com/topic/stainskappa.html. Accessed June 16, 2016.
16. Churchill CH, Abril A, Krishna M, et al. Jaw claudication in primary amyloidosis: unusual presentation of a rare disease. J Rheumatol 2003;30(10):2283–6.
17. Matsuda C, Shimizu T, Nakayama Y, et al. Macroglossia in advanced amyotrophic lateral sclerosis. Muscle Nerve 2016;54(3):386–90.
18. Suresh L, Radfar L. Oral sarcoidosis: a review of literature. Oral Dis 2005;11(3):138–45.
19. Dastoori M, Fedele S, Leao JC, et al. Sarcoidosis: a clinically orientated review. J Oral Pathol Med 2013;42(4):281–9.
20. Govender P, Berman J. The diagnosis of sarcoidosis. Clin Chest Med 2015;36(4):585–602.
21. Thomas KW, Hinninghake GW. Sarcoidosis. JAMA 2003;289:3300–3.
22. Rybicki BA, Major M, Popovich J Jr, et al. Racial differences in sarcoidosis incidence: a 5-year study in a health maintenance organization. Am J Epidemiol 1997;145:234–41.
23. Du Bois RM, Goh N, McGrath P, et al. Is there a role for microorganisms in the pathogenesis of sarcoidosis? J Intern Med 2003;253: 4–17.
24. Poate TWJ, Sharma R, Moutasim KA, et al. Orofacial presentations of sarcoidosis – a case series and review of the literature. Br Dent J 2008;205:437–42.
25. Hillerdal G, Nöu E, Osterman K, et al. Sarcoidosis: epidemiology and prognosis. A 15-year European study. Am Rev Respir Dis 1984; 130(1):29–32.
26. Marchell RM, Thiers B, Judson MA. Sarcoidosis. In: Wolff K, Goldsmith L, Katz S, et al, editors. Fitzpatrick's dermatology in general medicine. 7th edition. New York: McGraw-Hill; 2008. p. 1484–93.
27. Baughman RP, Lower EE, du Bois RM. Sarcoidosis. Lancet 2003;361: 1111–8.
28. Rybicki BA, Maliarik MJ, Poisson LM, et al. Sarcoidosis and granuloma genes: a family-based study in African-Americans. Eur Respir J 2004;24:251–7.
29. Motswaledi MH, Khammissa RAG, Jadwat Y, et al. Oral sarcoidosis: a case report and review of the literature. Aust Dent J 2014;59:389–94.
30. Nunes H, Bouvry D, Soler P, et al. Sarcoidosis. Orphanet J Rare Dis 2007;2:46.
31. Darlington P, Tallstedt L, Padyukov L, et al. HLA-DRB1* alleles and symptoms associated with Heerfordt's syndrome in sarcoidosis. Eur Respir J 2011;38(5):1151–7.
32. Mana J, Marcoval J, Graells J, et al. Cutaneous involvement in sarcoidosis. Relationship to systemic disease. Arch Dermatol 1997; 133:882–8.
33. Giotaki H, Constantopoulus SH, Papadimimitriou CS, et al. Labial minor salivary gland biopsy: a highly discriminatory diagnostic method between sarcoidosis and Sjögren's syndrome. Respiration 1986;50:102–7.
34. Nessan VJ, Jacoway JR. Biopsy of minor salivary glands in the diagnosis of sarcoidosis. N Engl J Med 1979;301:922–4.
35. Drosos AA, Constantopoulos SH, Psychos D, et al. The forgotten cause of sicca complex; sarcoidosis. J Rheumatol 1989;16:1548–51.
36. Sciubba JJ, Said-Al-Naief N. Orofacial granulomatosis: presentation, pathology and management of 13 cases. J Oral Pathol Med 2003;32:576–85.
37. Bouaziz A, Le Scanff J, Chapelon-Abric C, et al. Oral involvement in sarcoidosis: report of 12 cases. QJM 2012;105(8):755–67.
38. Leavitt RY, Fauci AS, Bloch DA, et al. The American College of Rheumatology 1990 criteria for the classification of Wegener's granulomatosis. Arthritis Rheum 1990;33:1101–7.
39. Sung IY, Kim YM, Cho YC, et al. Role of gingival manifestation in diagnosis of granulomatosis with polyangiitis (Wegener's granulomatosis). J Periodontal Implant Sci 2015;45(6):247–51.
40. Venning MC, Quinn A, Broomhead V, et al. Antibodies directed against neutrophils (c-ANCA and p-ANCA) are of distinct diagnostic value in systemic vasculitis. Q J Med 1990;77:1287–96.
41. Savige JA, Gallicchio M, Georgiou T, et al. Diverse target antigens recognized by circulating antibodies in antineutrophil cytoplasm antibody-associated renal vasculitides. Clin Exp Immunol 1990;82: 238–43.
42. Kubaisi B, Samra KA, Foster CS. Granulomatosis with polyangiitis (Wegener's disease): an updated review of ocular disease manifestations. Intractable Rare Dis Res 2016;5(2):61–9.
43. Guidelli GM, Tenti S, Pascarelli NA, et al. Granulomatosis with polyangiitis and intravenous immunoglobulins: a case series and review of the literature. Autoimmun Rev 2015;14:659–64.
44. Heckmann M, Holle JU, Arning L, et al. The Wegener's granulomatosis quantitative trait locus on chromosome 6p21. 3 as characterised by tag SNP genotyping. Ann Rheum Dis 2008;67(7):972–9.
45. Chung SA, Xie G, Roshandel D, et al. Meta-analysis in granulomatosis with polyangiitis reveals shared susceptibility loci with rheumatoid arthritis. Arthritis Rheum 2012;64(10):3463–71.
46. Jagiello P, Aries P, Arning L, et al. The PTPN22 620W allele is a risk factor for Wegener's granulomatosis. Arthritis Rheum 2005;52(12): 4039–43.
47. Mahr A, Neogi T, Merkel P. Epidemiology of Wegener's granulomatosis: lessons from descriptive studies and analyses of genetic and environmental risk determinants. Clin Exp Rheumatol 2006;24:S82–91.
48. Lane S, Watts R, Bentham G, et al. Are environmental factors important in primary systemic vasculitis? A case-controlled study. Arthritis Rheum 2003;48:814–23.
49. Stamp LK, Chapman PT, Francis J, et al. Association between environmental exposures and granulomatosis with polyangiitis in Canterbury, New Zealand. Arthritis Res Ther 2015;17:333.
50. Tadema H, Heeringa P, Kallenberg CG. Bacterial infections in Wegener's granulomatosis: mechanisms potentially involved in autoimmune pathogenesis. Curr Opin Rheumatol 2011;23(4):366–71.
51. Ponniah I, Shaheen A, Shankar KA, et al. Wegener's granulomatosis: the current understanding. Oral Surg Oral Med Oral Pathol Oral Radiol Endod 2005;100:265–70.
52. Wojciechowska J, Krajewski W, Krajewski P, et al. Granulomatosis with polyangiitis in otolaryngologist practice: a review of current knowledge. Clin Exp Otorhinolaryngol 2016;9(1):8–13.
53. Carter LM, Brizman E. Lingual infarction in Wegener's granulomatosis: a case report and review of the literature. Head Face Med 2008;4:19.
54. Bachymeyer B, Petitjean B, Testart F, et al. Lingual necrosis as the presenting sign of Wegener's granulomatosis. Clin Exp Dermatol 2006;31:321–2.
55. Brooke RI. Wegener's granulomatosis involving the gingiva. Br Dent J 1965;118:30–2.
56. Edwards MB, Buckerfield JP. Wegener's granulomatosis: a case with primary mucocutaneous lesions. Oral Surg Oral Med Oral Pathol 1978;46:53–63.
57. Green I, Szyper-Kravitz M, Shoenfeld Y. Parotitis as the presenting symptom of Wegener's granulomatosis: case report and meta-analysis. Isr Med Assoc J 2013;15(3):188–92.
58. Stone JHWegener's Granulomatosis Etanercept Trial Research Group. Limited versus severe Wegener's granulomatosis: baseline data on patients in the Wegener's granulomatosis etanercept trial. Arthritis Rheum 2003;48(8):2299–309.

59. Mulholland GB, Jeffery CC, Stija P, et al. Immunoglobulin G4-related diseases in the head and neck: a systematic review. Head Neck Surg 2015;44:24.
60. Lang D, Zwerina J, Pieringer H. IgG4-related disease: current challenges and future prospects. Ther Clin Risk Manag 2016;12: 189–99.
61. Uchida K, Masamune A, Shimosegawa T, et al. Prevalence of IgG4-related disease in Japan based on nationwide survey in 2009. Int J Rheumatol 2012;2012:358371.
62. Cheuk W, Tam FK, Chan AN, et al. Idiopathic cervical fibrosis-a new member of IgG4-related sclerosing diseases: report of 4 cases, 1 complicated by composite lymphoma. Am J Surg Pathol 2010; 34(11):1678–85.
63. Melo JC, Kitsko D, Reyes-Múgica M. Pediatric chronic sclerosing sialadenitis: Küttner tumor. Pediatr Dev Pathol 2012;15(2):165–9.
64. Hong X, Li W, Su JZ, et al. Internal organ involvement in IgG4-related sialadenitis: a systemic review. Chin J Dent Res 2015;18(2): 85–94.
65. Nakajima A, Masaki Y, Nakamura T, et al. Decreased expression of innate immunity-related genes in peripheral blood mononuclear cells from patients with IgG4-related disease. PLoS One 2015; 10(5):e0126582.
66. Della-Torre E, Lanzillotta M, Doglioni C. Immunology of IgG4-related disease. Clin Exp Immunol 2015;181(2):191–206.
67. Deshpande V, Zen Y, Chan JK, et al. Consensus statement on the pathology of IgG4-related disease. Mod Pathol 2012;25(9):1181–92.
68. Stone JH, Zen Y, Deshpande V. IgG4-related disease. N Engl J Med 2012;366:539–51.
69. Albilia JB, Lam DK, Blanas N, et al. Small mouths...big problems? A review of scleroderma and its oral health implications. J Can Dent Assoc 2007;73(9):831–6.
70. Young A, Khanna D. Systemic sclerosis: commonly asked questions by rheumatologists. J Clin Rheumatol 2015;21(3):149–55.
71. van den Hoogen F, Khanna D, Fransen J, et al. 2013 classification criteria for systemic sclerosis: an American College of Rheumatology/European League against Rheumatism collaborative initiative. Arthritis Rheum 2013;65(11):2737–47.
72. Mayes MD. Epidemiology of systemic sclerosis and related diseases. Curr Opin Rheumatol 1997;9:557–61.
73. Dagenais M, MacDonald D, Baron M, et al. The Canadian systemic sclerosis oral health study IV: oral radiographic manifestations in systemic sclerosis compared with the general population. Oral Surg Oral Med Oral Pathol Oral Radiol 2015;120(2):104–11.
74. Mayes MD. Scleroderma epidemiology. Rheum Dis Clin North Am 2003;29(2):239–54.
75. Coll J, Rives A, Grino MC, et al. Prevalence of Sjögren's syndrome in autoimmune diseases. Ann Rheum Dis 1987;46:286–9.
76. Cipoletti JF, Buckingham RB, Barnes EL, et al. Sjögren's syndrome in progressive systemic sclerosis. Ann Intern Med 1977;87:535–41.
77. Osial TA Jr, Whiteside TL, Buckingham RB, et al. Clinical and serologic study of Sjögren's syndrome in patients with progressive systemic sclerosis. Arthritis Rheum 1983;26:500–8.
78. Drosos AA, Andonopoulos AP, Costopoulos JS, et al. Sjögren's syndrome in progressive systemic sclerosis. J Rheumatol 1988;15: 965–8.
79. Salliot C, Mouthon L, Ardizzone M, et al. Sjögren's syndrome is associated with and not secondary to systemic sclerosis. Rheumatology (Oxford) 2007;46(2):321–6.
80. Eversole LR, Jacobsen PL, Stone CE. Oral and gingival changes in systemic sclerosis (scleroderma). J Periodontol 1984;55(3):175–8.
81. Elimelech R, Mayer Y, Braun-Moscovici Y, et al. Periodontal conditions and tumor necrosis factor-alpha level in gingival crevicular fluid of scleroderma patients. Isr Med Assoc J 2015;17(9):549–53.
82. Rout PG, Hamburger J, Potts AJ. Orofacial radiological manifestations of systemic sclerosis. Dentomaxillofac Radiol 1996;25: 193–6.
83. Hopper FE, Giles AD. Orofacial changes in systemic sclerosis-report of a case of resorption of mandibular angles and zygomatic arches. Br J Oral Surg 1982;20:129–34.
84. Chu CH, Yeung CM, Lai IA, et al. Oral health of Chinese people with systemic sclerosis. Clin Oral Investig 2011;15(6):931–9.
85. Haers PE, Sailer HF. Mandibular resorption due to systemic sclerosis. Case report of surgical correction of a secondary open bite deformity. Int J Oral Maxillofac Surg 1995;24(4):261–7.
86. Delantoni A, Matziari E. Osteolysis affecting the jaws in systemic sclerosis: clinical and osseous changes based on a case presentation. Clin Med Insights Arthritis Musculoskelet Disord 2015;18(8): 65–7.
87. Doucet JC, Morrison AD. Bilateral mandibular condylysis from systemic sclerosis: case report of surgical correction with bilateral total temporomandibular joint replacement. Craniomaxillofac Trauma Reconstr 2011;4(1):11–8.
88. Reyes CM, Rudinskaya A, Kloss R, et al. Scleroderma-like illness as a presenting feature of multiple myeloma and amyloidosis. J Clin Rheumatol 2008;14(3):161–5.
89. Phumethum V, Jamal S, Johnson SR. Biologic therapy for systemic sclerosis: a systematic review. J Rheumatol 2011;38(2):289–96.
90. Young A, Khanna D. Systemic sclerosis: a systematic review on therapeutic management from 2011 to 2014. Curr Opin Rheumatol 2015;27(3):241–8.
91. Daoussis D, Liossis SN, Tsamandas AC, et al. Experience with rituximab in scleroderma: results from a 1-year, proof-of-principle study. Rheumatology (Oxford) 2010;49(2):271–80.
92. Yuen HK, Weng Y, Bandyopadhyay D, et al. Effect of a multifaceted intervention on gingival health among adults with systemic sclerosis. Clin Exp Rheumatol 2011;29(2 Suppl 65):S26–32.
93. Shah AA, Wigley FM. Often forgotten manifestations of systemic sclerosis. Rheum Dis Clin North Am 2008;34:221–38.
94. Alantar A, Cabane J, Hachulla E, et al. Recommendations for the care of oral involvement in patients with systemic sclerosis. Arthritis Care Res (Hoboken) 2011;63(8):1126–33.

Further readings

Amyloidosis

Pau M, Reinbacher KE, Feichtinger M, et al. Surgical treatment of macroglossia caused by systemic primary amyloidosis. Int J Oral Maxillofac Surg 2013;42(2):294–7.

IgG4-related disease

Deshpande V. IgG4 related disease of the head and neck. Head and Neck Pathol 2015;9:24–31.
Yamamoto M, Takahashi H, Ohara M, et al. A new conceptualization for Mikulicz's disease as an IgG4-related plasmacytic disease. Mod Rheumatol 2006;16:335–40.

Granulomatosis with polyangiitis

Greco A, Marinelli C, Fusconi M, et al. Clinic manifestations in granulomatosis with polyangiitis. Int J Immunopathol Pharmacol 2016; 29(2):151–9.
Pakalniskis MG, Berg AD, Policeni BA, et al. The many faces of granulomatosis with polyangiitis: a review of the head and neck imaging manifestations. AJR Am J Roentgenol 2015;205(6):W619–29.

Systemic sclerosis (systemic scleroderma) including CREST syndrome

Cazal C, Sobral APV, Neves RFN, et al. Oral complaints in progressive systemic sclerosis: two cases report. Med Oral Patol Oral Cir Bucal 2008;13(2):E114–8.

Head and Neck Manifestations of Endocrine Disorders

Arwa M. Farag, BDS, DMSc, FDS RCSEd [a,b,*]

KEYWORDS

• Endocrine disorders • Pituitary • Thyroid • Parathyroid • Adrenal • Diabetes

KEY POINTS

- The endocrine system produces hormones that regulate essential body functions.
- Endocrine dysfunctions can lead to various forms of disease that negatively impact the patients' well-being and quality of life.
- Endocrine disorders have distinguishable manifestations, especially in the head and neck region, in which the dentist should be familiar with.
- Dental management of patients with endocrine disorders requires special knowledge and considerations.

Introduction

The endocrine system is a collection of glands that synthesizes and releases its hormones directly into the bloodstream. These hormones are responsible for fundamental and essential body processes, such as metabolism, tissue growth, homeostasis, sexual development, reproduction, immune regulation, cognitive function, and emotional stabilization. The endocrine glands are highly controlled by the nervous system and by the sensitive biofeedback mechanism that maintain well-balanced levels of hormones throughout the body. Any shift in this balance can significantly disturb body function and lead to disease manifestation that can negatively impact the individual's health and well-being.

Pituitary gland disorders

The pituitary gland is commonly referred to as the '"master gland" owing to its essential involvement in the functions of several organs. It occupies the sella turcica, a bony compartment of the sphenoid bone, and receives its stimulation directly from the hypothalamus.[1]

The intermediate and posterior lobes of the pituitary have limited function of storing and secreting melanocyte-stimulating hormone and antidiuretic hormone, respectively. In contrast, the anterior pituitary lobe is responsible for synthesizing and secreting several hormones:

- Growth hormone (GH),
- Puberty hormones (gonadotropins),
- Thyroid-stimulating hormone,
- Prolactin, and
- Adrenocorticotrophic hormone (ACTH).

Hypopituitarism

Etiology and epidemiology

Several etiologic factors can be responsible for pituitary hormone deficiency. Conditions affecting the pituitary gland itself (eg, genetic, neoplastic, infectious, iatrogenic, and traumatic) evolve into primary hypopituitarism, whereas dysfunction of the hypothalamus leads to secondary hypopituitarism.[2] Owing to the multifunctional activity of this gland, hypopituitarism can affect individuals' growth, puberty, thyroid, and adrenal functions. GH and gonadotropins have the highest susceptibility for deficiency among all pituitary hormones with the former being highly linked to head and neck manifestations.[3] Several earlier studies have estimated the prevalence of GH deficiency in pediatric population to fall between 1:1800 and 1:30,000.[4–7]

Clinical manifestations

GH deficiency during childhood is known as pituitary dwarfism. The condition is known for the low growth velocity, short stature, and abundant clinical features. In contrast, GH deficiency during adulthood has been associated with less dramatic effect and nonspecific clinical features. The manifestations of hypopituitarism in the head and neck region are summarized in Table 1.[8–14]

Differential diagnosis

Idiopathic short stature, hypothyroidism, osteogenesis imperfecta, and other skeletal dysplasia are included in the differential diagnosis of hypopituitarism.

[a] Division of Oral Medicine, Department of Diagnostic Sciences, Tufts University School of Dental Medicine, 1 Kneeland Street, DHS #638, Boston, MA 02111, USA
[b] Department of Oral Medicine, Faculty of Dentistry, King AbdulAziz University, 1 Umm Al Muminin Road, Jeddah 21589, Kingdom of Saudi Arabia
* Division of Oral Medicine, Department of Diagnostic Sciences, Tufts University School of Dental Medicine, 1 Kneeland Street, DHS #638, Boston, MA 02111.
E-mail address: arwa.farag@tufts.edu

Atlas Oral Maxillofacial Surg Clin N Am 25 (2017) 197-207
1061-3315/17/
http://dx.doi.org/10.1016/j.cxom.2017.04.011

Table 1 Head and neck manifestations of the onset of hypopituitarism during childhood and adulthood

Childhood hypopituitarism	Adulthood hypopituitarism
Hypognathic maxilla and mandible that run proportionally with smaller facial features	Immobile expression
Smaller size of the jaws with normal sized teeth. This results in dental crowding and malocclusion.	Thin lips, scant eye brows, and loss of eyelashes
Exfoliation pattern of deciduous dentition is delayed with consequent retardation in the eruption of permanent teeth.	No specific oral manifestations have been described.
Agenesis of third molars (common) and maxillary incisors (rare).	
Amelogenesis imperfecta (very rare).	

Hyperpituitarism

Etiology and epidemiology

Excessive production of GH is the most abundant form of hyperpituitarism. The disorder is known as acromegaly if it occurs during adulthood (around the age of 40), whereas gigantism is the childhood counterpart of the same disorder (Figs. 1 and 2). The incidence of acromegaly is estimated to be 3 to 4 cases per million per year,[15] although there have been only 100 reported cases of gigantism in medical literature.[16] GH hypersecretion may be caused by:

- Primary pituitary adenomas, and
- Secondary pituitary hypersecretion owing to excessive production of hypothalamic GH releasing hormones or genetic disorders, such as multiple endocrine neoplasia type-1, McCune-Albright syndrome or Carney complex.

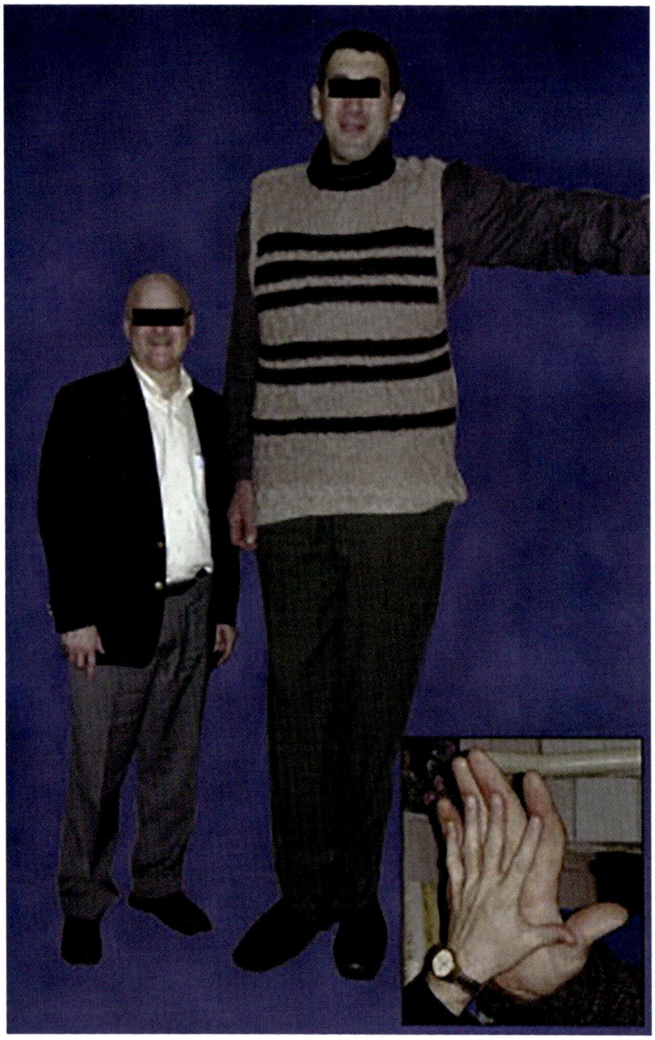

Fig. 1 Head and neck manifestations of pituitary gigantism. (*From* Kleinschmidt-DeMasters K. Pituitary gland. In: Rosai J, editor. Rosai & Ackerman's surgical pathology. 10th edition. Elsevier; 2011:2441–65; with permission.)

Clinical manifestations

Gigantism is characterized by generalized overgrowth of body parts while maintaining symmetry and proportionality. Acromegaly, in contrast, is characterized by progressive acquired disfigurement involving the face and extremities. The craniofacial characteristics of both conditions are summarized in Table 2.[17–22]

Differential diagnosis

Familial tall stature, cerebral gigantism (Sotos syndrome owing to NSD1 gene mutation), estrogen receptor mutation, and Weaver syndrome are included in the differential diagnosis for hyperpituitarism.

Treatment considerations

Early intervention by endocrinologists to correct the underlying hormonal disorder is required to prevent further growth

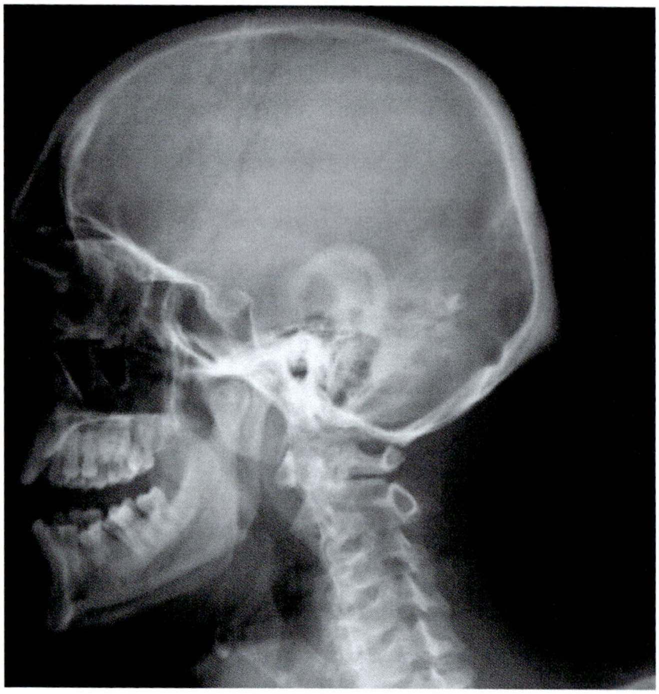

Fig. 2 Lateral skull radiograph in a patient with acromegaly. Note the prognathism of the mandible and the increased and interdental spacing between teeth. (*From* Farishta F, Hadi MS. Acromegaly: a case study. J Diabetes Metab 2015;6:621; with permission.)

Table 2 Oral and maxillofacial manifestation of gigantism and acromegaly

Gigantism	Acromegaly
Frontal bossing	Glabellar protrusion and face height increase
Mandibular prognathism	Mandibular prognathism
Interdental spacing	Interdental spacing and open bite
Root hypercementosis	Enlarged pulp chambers (taurodontism) and roots hypercementosis
	Facial skin and lips thickening (owing to collagen and glycosaminoglycan deposition)
	Macroglossia and mucosal hypertrophy of the oropharyngeal tissues (may contribute to sleep apnea)

deterioration or imbalance. In some cases, surgical intervention is needed to eliminate the causative factor (such as pituitary tumors) or correct disfigurement.

Orthodontic consultations for correction of hypognathia or hypergnathia and malocclusion should be pursued as early as possible. Prosthodontic work and dental implants can help those with teeth agenesis and amelogenesis imperfecta. Those with signs and symptoms of sleep apnea should be referred for pulmonology or ear, nose, and throat examination and, if required, sleep test (polysomnography) can be performed. Dentist can help those with mild to moderate sleep apnea by constructing dental sleep appliances.

Thyroid gland disorders

The thyroid gland is responsible for metabolic functions in the body including oxygen consumption and energy production through the release of triiodothyronine and thyroxine. Thyroid-stimulating hormone, produced by the pituitary gland, is responsible for regulating the secretion of triiodothyronine and thyroxine through a negative feedback mechanism. Calcitonin, another product of thyroid gland, interacts with parathyroid hormone (PTH) and vitamin D to regulate serum calcium and phosphorus and modulate bone remodeling.[23,24]

Hypothyroidism

Etiology and epidemiology

Hypothyroidism is defined as deficiency in thyroid hormones that can be either congenital or acquired in nature. The condition is known as cretinism if it presents during early childhood, whereas myxedema is the term used to describe severe hypothyroidism acquired during adulthood.[24–27]

Congenital hypothyroidism is among the conditions commonly seen in newborns, with an annual incidence of 1 in 4000. However, a severe form of the disease that can evolve to cretinism is pretty rare. Adult hypothyroidism is a more common disorder, especially in middle-age females with a prevalence of 1% to 2%.[28]

Etiologic factors

- Congenital factors include thyroid agenesis and other genetic disease (eg, Turner and Down syndromes).
- Acquired
  - Primary: autoimmune (eg, Hashimoto thyroiditis), irradiation, surgical removal, and neoplastic destruction.
  - Secondary: hypothalamic dysfunction and pituitary dysfunction.

Clinical manifestations

Severe congenital hypothyroidism can evolve to cretinism, in which physical and mental retardation are the hallmarks. Signs of the disorder involves bradycardia, dyspnea, and decreased activity. Characteristics features in the head and neck region include large head, short neck, broad nose, lack of facial expressions, hypertelorism, and thick, dry, and wrinkled skin (Fig. 3).

The onset of hypothyroidism during adulthood is associated with diminished metabolic activities that is manifested as overweight, slower respiratory rate, bradycardia, and generalized edema (myxedema). A summary of the head and neck manifestations is listed in Table 3.[24,26,27] A severe form of hypothyroidism can evolve to myxedematous crisis, a rare and life-threatening condition that can be precipitated by infection, medications, trauma, cerebrovascular disease, or heart failure. Signs and symptoms include significant hypothermia, hypotension, hypoglycemia, and disoriented mental status.

Differential diagnosis

Anemia, hypopituitarism, chronic fatigue syndrome, and polyglandular autoimmune syndrome are included in the differential diagnosis of hypothyroidism.

Hyperthyroidism

Etiology and epidemiology

Hyperthyroidism is the excess production of thyroid hormone (thyrotoxicosis). All thyroid disorders have a greater female predilection and the most common etiologic factors include Graves disease, toxic thyroid adenoma, toxic multinodular or diffuse goiter, ectopic thyroid tissue (eg, lingual thyroid), and subacute thyroiditis.[23,27]

Graves disease is the most common form of hyperthyroidism causing 60% to 80% of thyrotoxicosis cases in the United States.[29] The annual incidence is approximately 0.5 cases per 1000 people and the peak occurrence is usually found in people aged 20 to 40 years.[29]

Toxic multinodular goiter comes as the second most common and constitutes 15% to 20% of thyrotoxicosis cases followed by thyroid adenoma, which causes only 3% to 5% of the cases. Majority of these patients are diagnosed at the age of 50 and older.

Clinical manifestations

Generally, signs of hyperthyroidism are manifested as weight loss regardless of an increased appetite, warm sweaty skin, brittle hair and nails, tachycardia, irritability, and heat intolerance. Manifestations of the head and neck region are summarized in Table 3.[23,27]

Differential diagnosis

Anxiety disorders, cocaine toxicity, and drug-induced thyroiditis (eg, interferon-alfa and amiodarone) are included in the differential diagnosis of thyrotoxicosis.

Treatment considerations

Treatment of thyrotoxicosis may involve antithyroid agents (eg, propylthiouracil) or glucocorticosteroids to inhibit

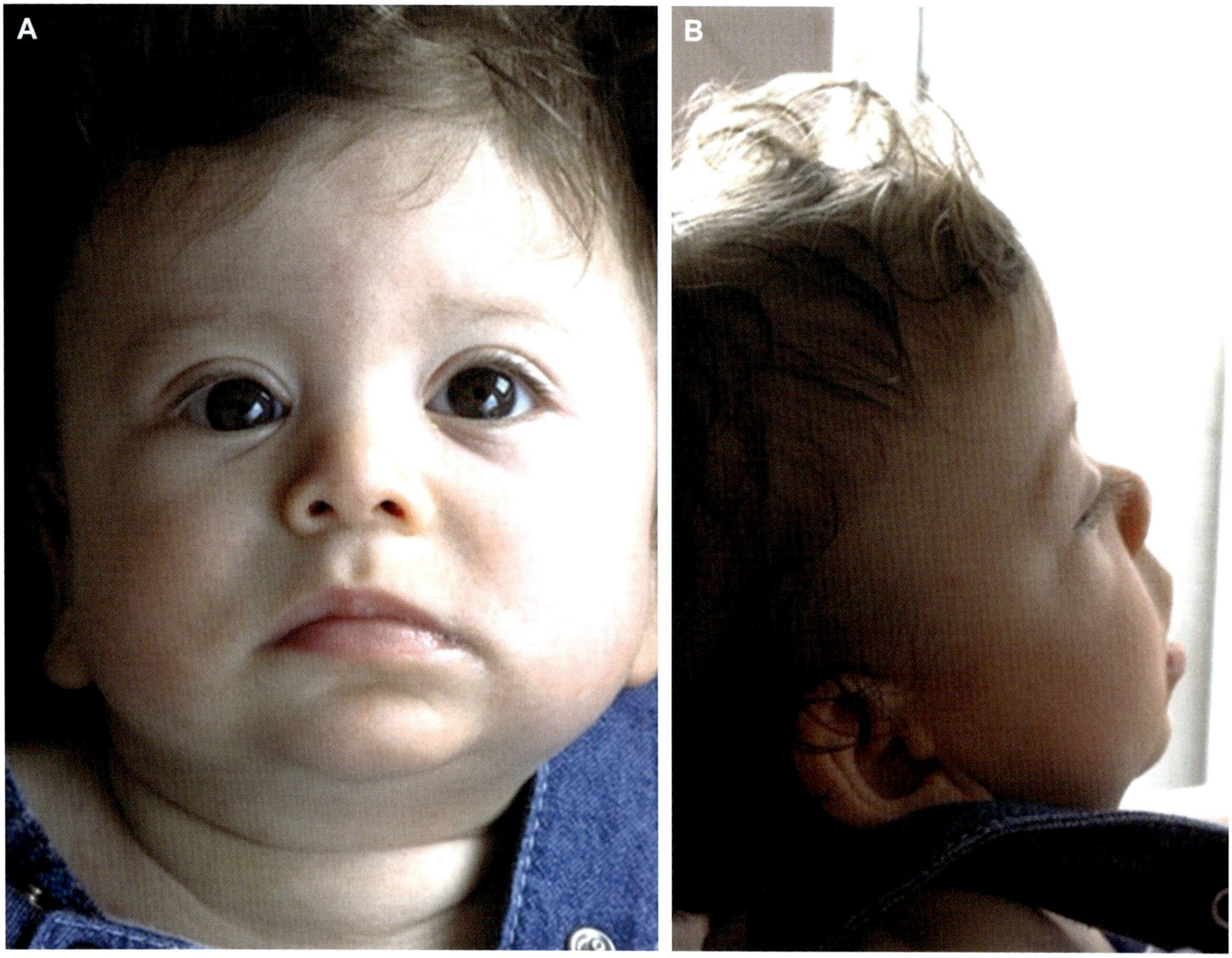

Fig. 3 Head and neck manifestation of cretinism. (*A*). Frontal view. (*B*). Lateral view. Note the large head, short neck, flat nasal bridge, periorbital and cheek fullness, epicanthal folds thickening, and thin upper lip with downturned corners of the mouth. (*From* Dimitriadou M, Christoforidis A, Sarri C, et al. Congenital hypothyroidism as the initial presentation that led to the diagnosis of Williams syndrome. Gene 2012;494(1):103; with permission.)

hormone synthesis and release. Ipodate sodium is also prescribed to inhibit the conversion of thyroxine to triiodothyronine. Beta-blockers are used to control the disease manifestation such as tachycardia, anxiety, tremors, and sweating.[23,27]

Dental management of patients with thyrotoxicosis should start with a treatment plan that is based on a comprehensive medical history and, if necessary, an endocrinology consultation. Well-controlled cases can be treated in an ordinary manner after paying extra precautions to stress and pain management. Challenges are usually anticipated in cases of uncontrolled thyrotoxicosis and the following precautions should be followed.

1. Avoid the use of epinephrine-containing local anesthetics or retraction cords.[24]
2. Avoid invasive surgical procedures and acute oral infections because they may precipitate thyrotoxic crisis.

Table 3 Head and neck manifestations of thyroid dysfunction

Hypothyroidism	Hyperthyroidism
Facial swelling (especially nose, ears, and lips)	Exophthalmos
Thickened dry skin	Enlarged thyroid and extraglandular thyroid tissue (eg, lingual thyroid)
Brittle scalp and scant eyebrows	Maxillomandibular osteoporosis
Hoarseness	Burning mouth
Delayed tooth eruption	Periodontal disease
Enamel hypoplasia of primary and permanent dentitions	Increased susceptibility to dental caries owing to increased carbohydrate consumption
Micrognathia/open bite owing to retarded mandibular and condylar growth (only if present during childhood)	
Macroglossia, glossitis, and dysgeusia in patients with myxedema	

Generally, periodic monitoring of complete blood count, chemistry, and coagulation panel is a must in patients using propylthiouracil to rule out agranulocytosis, hypoproteinemia, or bleeding disorders.[24] Discontinuation of any dental procedure should immediately take place if signs or symptoms of a thyrotoxicosis develop (tachycardia, hypertension, sweating, tremor, nausea, vomiting, and/or coma) and emergency medical services should be activated.[24]

Hypothyroidism is mostly managed by levothyroxine, sodium liothyronine, or 1-throixine, a synthetic thyroid hormone. Dental management of these patients should not differ from the management of healthy patients. In uncontrolled cases of hypothyroidism, central nervous system depressants, the presence of oral infection, and invasive surgical procedures can precipitate a myxedematous crisis that is manifested as hypothermia, hypotension, bradycardia, and epileptic seizure. Dental treatment should be discontinued and emergency medical services should be pursued.[25]

Parathyroid gland disorders

PTH is the regulator of calcium absorption from the intestine and bone and phosphorus excretion by the kidney. The hormone is involved in tooth development, bone mineralization and resorption, and vitamin D transformation.

Hyperparathyroidism

Etiology and epidemiology

Hyperparathyroidism is defined as the hypersecretion of PTH that can be[30,31]:

1. Primary—such as parathyroid neoplasia or hyperplasia. This accounts for more than 85% of the cases and results in hypercalcemia and hypophosphatemia.
2. Secondary—owing to renal failure or intestinal malabsorption that causes subsequent hypocalcemia and hyperphosphatemia. This positive feedback effect stimulates excessive production of the PTH.
3. Tertiary—this is a secondary hyperparathyroidism that persists after renal transplantation. It is characterized by autonomous hypersecretion of PTH and subsequent hypercalcemia. The etiology is unknown, but may be related to monoclonal expansion of parathyroid cells or hyposensitivity of the calcium-sensing mechanism. This condition is found in only 8% of the patients with hyperparathyroidism.

Table 4 Head and neck manifestations of hyperparathyroidism and hypoparathyroidism

Hyperparathyroidism	Hypoparathyroidism
Loss of jawbone density (unilocular or multilocular well-defined radiolucency)	Enamel and dentin hypoplasia and/or hypocalcification and shortened roots
Fragile teeth with widened pulp chambers	Widening of pulp chambers and/or pulpal calcifications
	Hypodontia and dental growth delay
Loss of lamina dura	Maxillary and mandibular tori
Malocclusions	Orofacial paresthesia
Brown tumor of hyperparathyroidism	Facial muscles aching/twitching
Soft tissue calcifications	Susceptibility to oral candidiasis

Clinical manifestations

Loss of bone density, kidney stones, abdominal pain, proximal myopathy and depression are the most common manifestations of hyperparathyroidism. The head and neck manifestations of hyperparathyroidism are summarized in Table 4.

Brown tumor of hyperparathyroidism (giant cell tumor)

Brown tumor is a rare, localized, benign, osteolytic lesion that is not neoplastic in nature. It is mainly owing to increased osteoclastic activity secondary to increased PTH production (Fig. 4). The brown color is a result of localized hemosiderin

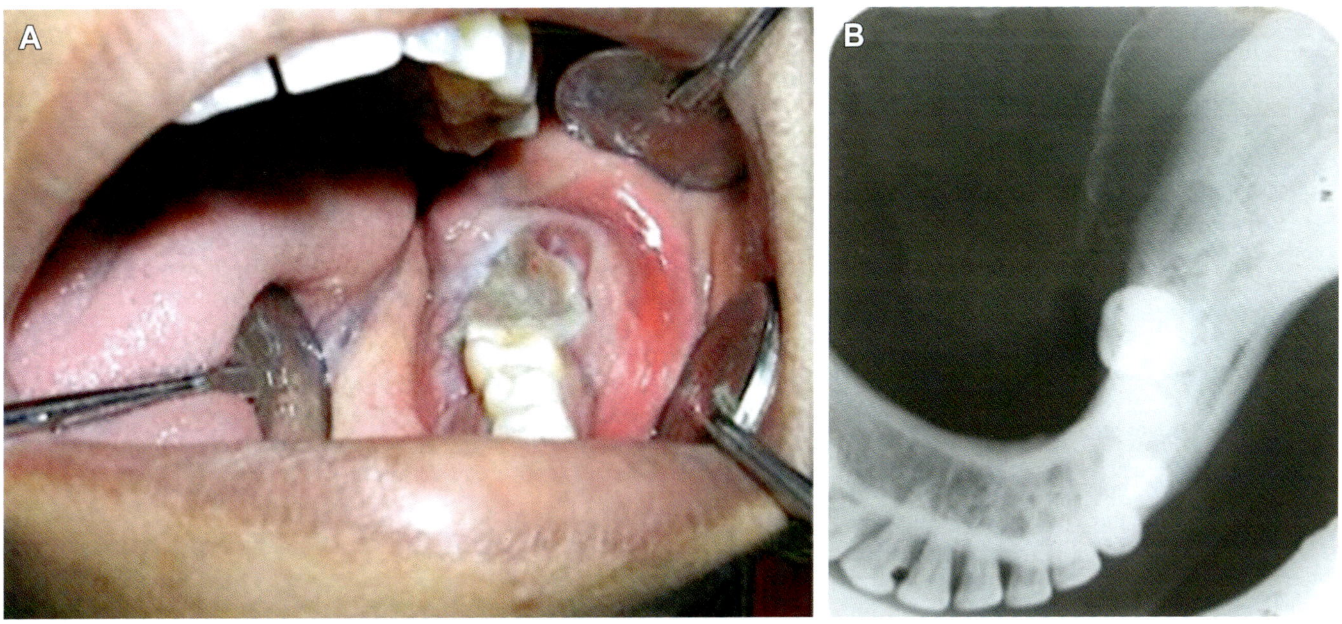

Fig. 4 Brown tumor of hyprtparathyroidism. (*A*) Clinical presentation of the lesion in the mandible. (*B*) Occlusal radiograph showing structural and morphologic bony changes secondary to Brown tumor. (*From* Nair PP, Gharote HP, Thomas S, et al. Brown tumour of the jaw. BMJ Case Rep 2011;2011:bcr0720114465; with permission.)

deposition and the lesion may cause bone swelling, pain, and pathologic fracture. Histologically, it is characterized by an abundant stroma consisting of several multinucleated osteoclast-like giant cells. Calcified material can be found, as well as areas of red blood cells, extravasation, and hemosiderin pigmentation.

Differential diagnosis

The histologic findings of Brown tumor are not pathognomonic and may overlap with the features of aneurysmal bone cyst, central giant cell granuloma, and cherubism. Correlation with clinical findings and spiking of PTH levels are the keys for proper diagnosis.

Hypoparathyroidism

Etiology and epidemiology

Hypoparathyroidism is the state of hypocalcemia and hypophosphatemia owing to absence or deficiency of PTH. Etiologic factors can be:

- Iatrogenic (eg, surgical removal of the parathyroid gland),
- Congenital (eg, agenesis or hypoplasia of the parathyroid gland),
- Autoimmune (eg, type 1 autoimmune polyglandular syndrome), or
- Metal overload such as hemochromatosis, thalassemia, and Wilson disease.

In the United States, the estimated prevalence of hypoparathyroidism is 37 per 100,000 person-years.[32]

Clinical manifestations

The state of hypocalcemia can lead to tetany, paresthesia, and seizures.[33] In the head and neck region, tissues of ectodermal origin can be affected and alopecia and scaling of the skin are commonly reported.[33] Other head and neck manifestations are summarized in Table 4.[33]

Differential diagnosis

Hypoalbuminemia-induced hypocalcemia, pseudohypoparathyroidism, and renal failure are included in the differential diagnosis of hypoparathyroidism.

Treatment considerations

In patients with hyperparathyroidism, Brown tumor, if existent, should be investigated, recognized, and not mixed with other oral lesions. Management of the excessive production PTH leads to spontaneous regression of the lesion is most instances.[30,34] Persistent tumors, even after normalization of PTH levels, can be surgically resected.[30,34] When it comes to dental management of patients with hyperparathyroidism, no specific considerations need to be taken into account, except for gentle mechanical manipulation owing to an increased risk of bone fractures.

Patient with hypoparathyroidism have greater susceptibility to dental caries and teeth fracture owing to structural defects of teeth. Periodic dental visits with shorter intervals, prophylaxis, fluoridation, and dietary counseling are all essential strategies in preventing dental complications. Recent serum calcium level should be confirmed to be at 8 mg/100 mL or above to ensure patients do not face complications of hypocalcemia such as cardiac arrhythmias, bronchospasms, or seizures.

Adrenal glands disorders

The adrenal glands, residing on the upper pole of the kidneys, consist of 2 portions: the medulla (internal portion) and the cortex (external portion). The adrenal medulla is responsible for the production of adrenaline, noradrenaline, dopamine and progesterone, and the adrenal cortex releases corticosteroids (glucocorticoids, mineralocorticoids, and androgens).[35]

Corticosteroids are involved in stress adaptation, antiinflammation, immunosuppression, liver neoglycogenesis, hyperglycemia, adipose tissue deposition, inhibition of osteogenesis, inhibition of tissue healing, and impairment of cognitive function. The release of corticosteroids is regulated via feedback mechanism of the hypothalamic–pituitary–adrenal axis. The reduced level of blood corticosteroids stimulates the release of corticotropin-releasing hormone from the hypothalamus that, in turn, stimulates the anterior lobe of the pituitary to synthesize and release the adrenocorticotropic hormone (ACTH) and stimulate the production of corticosteroid from the adrenal cortex.[35]

Adrenocortical insufficiency or hypoadrenocorticism (Addison disease)

Etiology and epidemiology

Primary adrenocortical insufficiency is the deficiency of glucocorticoid and mineralocorticoid hormones and is known as Addison's disease. Etiologic factors can be:

- Primary, whether idiopathic, or owing to destructive effect of surgical procedures, infections, neoplasms, or granulomatous diseases; or
- Secondary, owing to dysfunction of the hypothalamus or pituitary glands in which the release of ACTH and/or corticotropin-releasing hormone is compromised.[35]

In the United States, the prevalence of Addison disease is low, ranging between 40 and 60 cases per 1 million populations.[36]

Clinical manifestations

Generally, corticosteroids deficiency manifests as muscle weakness, hypoglycemia, hypotension, anorexia, nausea, weight loss, and anxiety. Hyperpigmentation is characteristic, especially in the elbows, folds of the hands, or areolas of the breasts. This hyperpigmentation is owing to the increase in ACTH levels that directly stimulates the production of melanocyte-stimulating hormone. In the perioral and intraoral tissues, black–bluish plaques are very characteristic (Fig. 5).

Differential diagnosis

Hemochromatosis, Peutz-Jeghers syndrome, and heavy metal ingestion (eg, iron and silvers) are associated with skin and mucosal pigmentations and therefore included in the differential diagnosis of Addison disease.

Hyperadrenocorticism (Cushing syndrome)

Etiology and epidemiology

Cushing syndrome refers to the state of hyperadrenocorticism owing to excessive production of endogenous glucocorticoids from the adrenal cortex or prolonged administration of

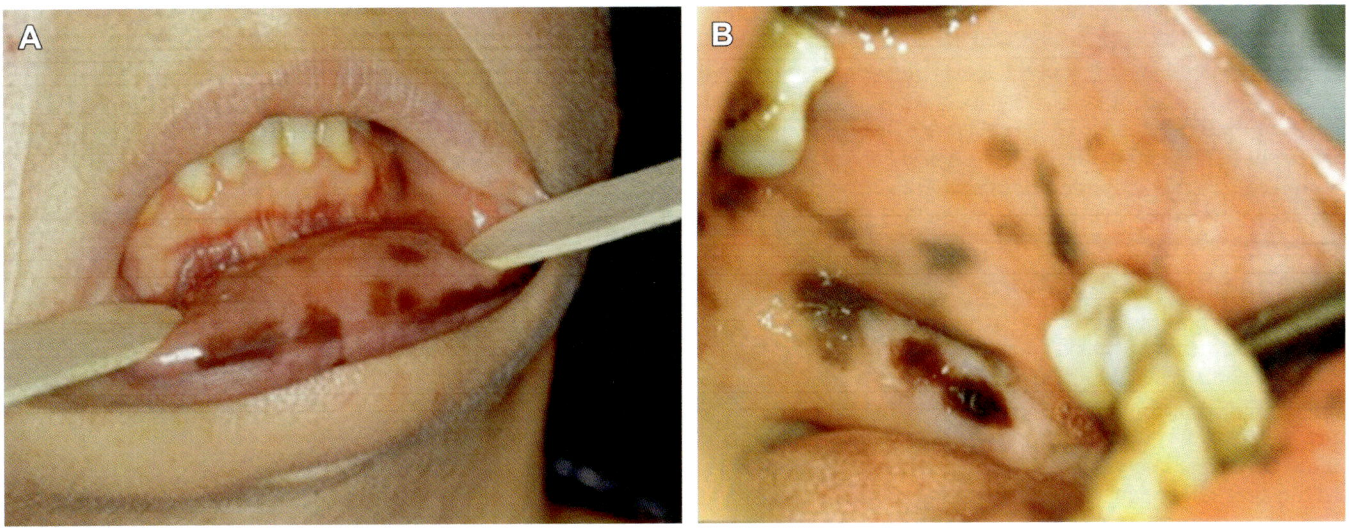

Fig. 5 Hyperpigmentation in patient with Addison disease. (*A*) Perioral pigmentation. (*B*) Intraoral pigmented macules of the buccal mucosa and alveolar ridge. (*From* Lanza A, Heulfe I, Perillo L, et al. Pigmentation as a sign of Addison's disease: a brief reappraisal. Open Dermatol J 2009;3:4; with permission.)

exogenous corticosteroids (iatrogenic Cushing syndrome). In clinical practice, iatrogenic Cushing syndrome is the most commonly encountered form of the disease. Estimating the prevalence of this condition is difficult and relies mainly on the frequency of prolonged steroid prescription in certain populations.[37] Endogenous Cushing syndrome, in contrast, is rare, with a reported incidence of 1.2 to 1.7 per million per year.[37]

Cushing disease is a form of Cushing syndrome in which the excessive release of ACTH hormone is the driver for glucocorticoid overproduction. It is the second most common etiology of Cushing syndrome and is seen in patients with pituitary adenoma and small cell lung cancer. Other less commonly reported etiologic factors include adrenal adenoma, adrenal carcinoma, and adrenal hyperplasia.[37]

Clinical manifestations

Cushing syndrome is characterized by obesity, hump back, hypertension, hyperglycemia, osteoporosis, thinned skin, muscle atrophy, immunosuppression, emotional disturbance, and cognitive dysfunction.[38,39] In the head and neck region the disease is manifested as:

- Moon face, acne breakout, and hirsutism (Fig. 6); and
- Susceptibility to oral infection and bone fractures.

Differential diagnosis

Pseudo-Cushing syndrome can be induced by depression, obesity, uncontrolled diabetes, and chronic alcoholism and is therefore included in the differential diagnosis of Cushing syndrome.

Treatment considerations

Corticosteroids are the standard treatment for patients with Addison disease. The exogenous administration of corticosteroids may inhibit the hypothalamic–pituitary–adrenal axis via negative biofeedback and significantly diminish the release of endogenous corticosteroids. This will, theoretically, compromise the patients' ability to manage acute physiologic stressors such as sepsis, surgical procedures, and postoperative pain. Patients maybe predisposed to adrenal crisis manifested as sudden and severe hypotension, hypothermia or hyperthermia, abdominal pain, nausea, and vomiting.

In the early 1950s, the concept of corticosteroid supplementation emerged in an attempt to prevent perioperative complications.[40–42] This concept has been recently challenged

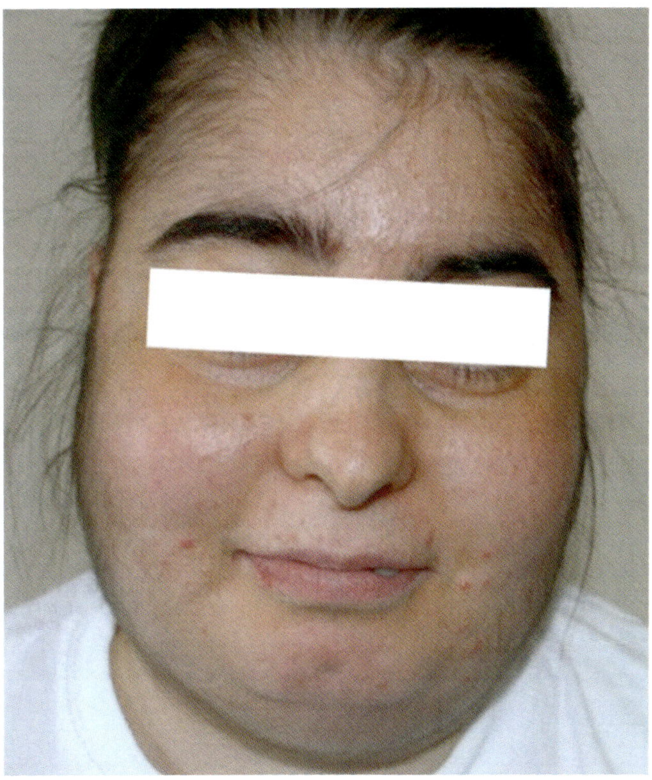

Fig. 6 Patient with features of Cushing syndrome, including moon face, acne vulgaris breakout, and hirsutism. (*From* Celik O, Niyazoglu M, Soylu H, et al. Iatrogenic Cushing's syndrome with inhaled steroid plus antidepressant drugs. Multidiscip Respir Med 2012;7(1):26; with permission.)

and several investigations have questioned the evidence of this approach.[43–46] It is now agreed that no supplemental steroid doses are required in most routine dental procedures, including minor surgeries, performed under local anesthesia.[47] Steroid supplementation, although lacking evidence, may be considered only for patients undergoing major surgeries requiring general anesthesia.[47] Other considerations in dental management of patients with adrenal insufficiency are included in Box 1.[35]

Endocrine pancreatic disorders

Diabetes mellitus (DM) is an endocrine metabolic disorder characterized by a state of hyperglycemia owing to compromised insulin secretion by the pancreas or insulin use by the body cells.[48] It is a major cause of kidney failure, blindness, nontraumatic lower limb amputations, heart disease, and strokes and the seventh leading cause of death in the United States.[48]

Etiology and epidemiology

In the United States, the prevalence of DM is steadily increasing. According to the statistics published in 2011 by the Centers for Disease Control and Prevention, approximately 8.3% of the population is affected.[49] According to the American Diabetes Association's DM is classified as[50]:

- Type 1 DM, which constitutes 5% to 10% of all DM cases and is commonly found in pediatric population. The etiology is autoimmune, in which insulin-producing beta islets are majorly destroyed.
- Type 2 DM, which constitutes 90% to 95% the cases and is highlighted by cellular resistance to insulin. The etiology is unknown, but has been strongly linked to genetic predisposition. The risk of the disease increases with age.
- Gestational DM, is the onset of hyperglycemia during pregnancy that normalizes after delivery. Its prevalence is approximately 4% of all pregnancies in the United States and it indicates higher susceptibly of the women to develop type 2 DM later in life.
- Others, which is relatively uncommon and includes genetic, infectious, traumatic, or iatrogenic factors affecting beta islets.

Box 1. Special considerations in dental management of patients with adrenal insufficiency

1. Prevention and treatment of oral infections such as candidiasis and periodontitis.
2. Conducting treatment during the morning when the cortisol level is the highest.
3. Monitoring patient's blood pressure and hemoglobin A1C level before any dental procedure.
4. Establishing good pain control techniques: long-acting local anesthetic preoperatively and good analgesic regimen postoperatively.
5. Implementing good anxiety control strategies, including conscious sedation.
6. Counseling with the patient's endocrinologist in case of prolonged steroids therapy to make decisions in regard to steroid supplementation before major maxillofacial surgeries.
7. Prevention of iatrogenic bone fracture during dental procedures requiring heavy mechanical manipulation.
8. Avoid prescribing medications with potential interaction with corticosteroids such as phenytoin, barbiturates, and rifampicin.

Clinical manifestations

Polyuria, polydipsia, polyphagia, and weight loss are the classic signs of DM. If the disease remained untreated or poorly controlled, vasculopathy, retinopathy, nephropathy, and neuropathy may become significant and can negatively influence the patient's quality of life. The most common oral complications in patients with DM are gingivitis and periodontitis (Fig. 7). Compromised host immune function and healing capacity in addition to reduced salivary flow are the main etiologic factors. Other complications of DM affecting the orofacial region are included in Box 2.

Treatment considerations

1. A thorough medical history and consultation with the primary care physician or endocrinologist if needed.
2. Frequent dental visits to treat and prevent periodontal disease, dental caries, and oral candidiasis.
3. Periodic monitoring of hemoglobin A1C levels before dental procedures.
4. Avoid performing dental procedures during peak activity periods of DM medications.
5. Recognition of signs and symptoms of hypoglycemic state and prompt delivery of glucose if required.
6. Consideration of postoperative antibiotic in patients with poorly controlled DM (only after surgical procedures).

Pregnancy

Etiology

Several physical and physiologic changes occur during pregnancy owing to increased levels of estrogen, progesterone, and

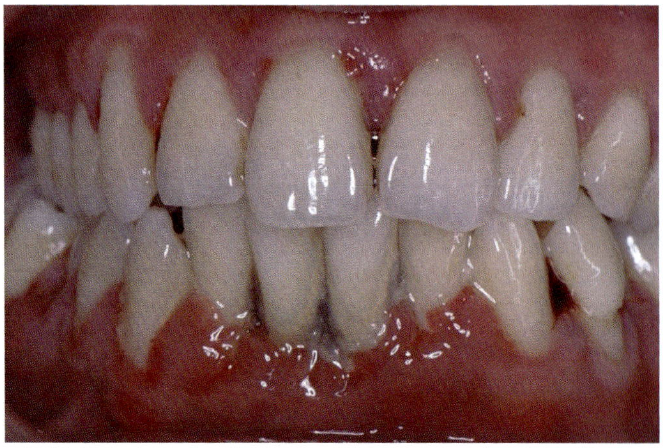

Fig. 7 Diabetic patient with periodontitis. Note the gingival inflammation, bleeding, and attachment loss of gingival tissues. (*From* Preshaw PM, Alba AL, Herrera D, et al. Periodontitis and diabetes: a two-way relationship. Diabetologia 2012;55(1):23; with permission.)

Box 2. Complications affecting the orofacial region in patients with DM

1. Periodontal disease.
2. Salivary gland dysfunction
   a. Hyposalivation that affects up to 80% of DM patients.
   b. Sialadenosis, a bilateral hypertrophy of the parotid glands that is asymptomatic and frequently linked to uncontrolled type 2 DM.[51]
3. Fungal infections owing to suboptimal immune function and hyposalivation
   a. Oral candidiasis.[52]
   b. Mucormycosis, although rare, can evolve to serious systemic infection.
4. Oral burning sensation and taste dysfunction
   a. This results from hyposalivation, peripheral neuropathy, and oral fungal infection.
   b. OLP and OLR. Few studies[53,54] reported an increased prevalence of OLP in type 1 DM patients, whereas others have documented the causal and effect relationship between OLR and anti-hyperglycemic medication.[55,56]
5. Dental caries: owing to hyposalivation, immune suppression, and elevated salivary glucose.
6. Oral ulceration and irritation fibroma especially in type 1 DM patients.[54] The increase prevalence maybe correlated to compromised immune function and wound healing.

Abbreviations: DM, diabetes mellitus; OLP, Oral lichen planus; OLR, oral lichenoid reactions.

human chorionic gonadotropin that significantly influences several body organs, including the oral cavity.

Oral manifestations during pregnancy

Several oral manifestations can be seen during the different stages of pregnancy. (Box 3) summarizes the most commonly reported oral findings and complications.

Consideration during dental management of pregnant women

1. Maintenance of optimal oral hygiene and periodontal health. Recent studies have shown the correlation between periodontal disease and low birth weight.[61,62]
2. Limit dental treatment to periodontal prophylaxis and emergency treatments. Elective treatment is safe during second trimester, but better postponed until after parturition.
3. Avoid routine dental radiographs unless urgently needed and use protective shielding.
4. Limit medication usage to US Food and Drug Administration (FDA) classes A and B, if required.
5. If local anesthetics are to be used, they should be limited to FDA class B anesthetics such as lidocaine. Avoid mepivacaine and bupivacaine, which are FDA class C.
6. If treatment is required during the third trimester, ensure maintaining a semisupine position to avoid hypotension/syncope owing to uterine pressure on the inferior vena cava.
7. Persistent gingival hyperplasia or pyogenic granuloma can be surgically excised after delivery.

Box 3. The most commonly reported oral complications during pregnancy

1. Pregnancy gingivitis owing to peaking levels of estrogen and progesterone and alteration host–immune response.
2. Periodontitis and tooth mobility owing to ongoing hormone-mediated inflammatory response and progression of gingivitis.
3. Gingival hyperplasia and pyogenic granuloma (pregnancy tumor) affects approximately 1% to 5% of pregnant women. It occurs toward the end of the first trimester with regression occurring spontaneously after delivery, in most cases (Fig. 8).[57]
4. Dental erosion owing frequent vomiting, especially during the first trimester. Hyperemesis gravidarium (excessive vomiting) occurs in 1% of all pregnancies, lasts throughout the 3 trimesters, and causes significant enamel erosion.[58]
5. Gastroesophageal reflux that increases toward the third trimester owing to increased fetus size and decreased strength of the stomach sphincter secondary to high levels of estrogen.
6. Chloasma or pregnancy mask: bilateral brown patches that appear on the face, trunk, and extremities owing to direct stimulation of melanocyte by estrogen and progesterone. It is seen in up to 73% of pregnant women and in those using hormonal oral contraceptives (especially women with tanned complexions).[59] Chloasma resolves spontaneously after parturition in most cases.
7. Salivary flow disturbance and changes in oral pH.[60]
8. Increased susceptibility to dental caries owing to an increase carbohydrate craving.

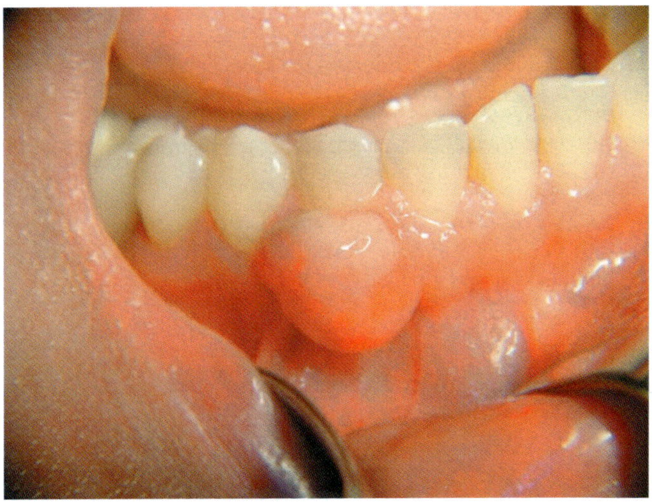

Fig. 8 Pregnancy pyogenic granuloma of the gingiva. Note the ulcerated surface of the nodule. (*From* Cardoso JA, Spanemberg JC, Cherubini K, et al. Oral granuloma gravidarum: a retrospective study of 41 cases in Southern Brazil. J Appl Oral Sci 2013;21(3):216; with permission.)

References

1. Mancall ELB, David G, editors. Cranial fossae. Gray's clinical anatomy. Philadelphia: Elsevier Saunders; 2011. p. 154. ISBN 9781437735802.
2. Melmed S. Pathogenesis of pituitary tumors. Nat Rev Endocrinol 2011;7(5):257–66.
3. Smith JC. Hormone replacement therapy in hypopituitarism. Expert Opin Pharmacother 2004;5(5):1023–31.
4. Vimpani GV, Vimpani AF, Lidgard GP, et al. Prevalence of severe growth hormone deficiency. Br Med J 1977;2(6084):427–30.
5. Bao XL, Shi YF, Du YC, et al. Prevalence of growth hormone deficiency of children in Beijing. Chin Med J (Engl) 1992;105(5): 401–5.
6. Tani N. Epidemiologic study of dwarfism in Niigata prefecture. Nihon Naibunpi Gakkai Zasshi 1985;61(12):1295–309 [in Japanese].
7. de Mel T, Warnasooriya N, Fonseka C. Growth hormone deficiency in Sri Lanka: a preliminary study. Ceylon Med J 1991; 36(3):95–7.
8. Atreja G, Atreja SH, Jain N, et al. Oral manifestations in growth hormone disorders. Indian J Endocrinol Metab 2012;16(3):381–3.
9. Kosowicz J, Rzymski K. Abnormalities of tooth development in pituitary dwarfism. Oral Surg Oral Med Oral Pathol 1977;44(6): 853–63.
10. Sarnat H, Kaplan I, Pertzelan A, et al. Comparison of dental findings in patients with isolated growth hormone deficiency treated with human growth hormone (hGH) and in untreated patients with Laron-type dwarfism. Oral Surg Oral Med Oral Pathol 1988;66(5):581–6.
11. Bigeard L, Sommermater J. Dental delay and microdontia in children with somatotropin hormone deficiency. J Biol Buccale 1991; 19(4):291–6 [in French].
12. Breteche F, Delaire J, Ginguene Y. Agenesis of the superior central incisor. Its relation to pituitary nanism. Rev Stomatol Chir Maxillofac 1984;85(1):72–4 [in French].
13. Lo FS, Lee YJ, Lin SP, et al. Solitary maxillary central incisor and congenital nasal pyriform aperture stenosis. Eur J Pediatr 1998; 157(1):39–44.
14. Parentin F, Perissutti P. Solitary median maxillary central incisor, Duane retraction syndrome, growth hormone deficiency and duplicated thumb phalanx: a case report. Clin Dysmorphol 2003; 12(2):141–2.
15. Etxabe J, Gaztambide S, Latorre P, et al. Acromegaly: an epidemiological study. J Endocrinol Invest 1993;16(3):181–7.
16. Sotos JF. Overgrowth. Hormonal causes. Clin Pediatr (Phila) 1996; 35(11):579–90.
17. Neville B, Damm D, Allen MC, editors. Oral and maxillofacial pathology. 3rd edition. St Louis (MO): Saunders Elsevier; 2010. p. 831–3.
18. Chanson P, Salenave S. Acromegaly. Orphanet J Rare Dis 2008;3:17.
19. Lima DL, Montenegro RM Jr, Vieira AP, et al. Absence of periodontitis in acromegalic patients. Clin Oral Investig 2009;13(2):165–9.
20. Cohen RB, Wilcox CW. A case of acromegaly identified after patient complaint of apertognathia. Oral Surg Oral Med Oral Pathol 1993; 75(5):583–6.
21. Sugata T, Myoken Y, Tanaka S. Acromegaly identified in a patient with a complaint of malocclusion. Oral Surg Oral Med Oral Pathol Oral Radiol Endod 1998;85(1):44–6.
22. Silvertone FS. Endocrine disease. In: Greenberg SM, Glick M, Ship JA, editors. Burket's oral medicine. 11th edition. Shelton (CT): BC Decker Inc; 2007. p. 521–4.
23. Little JW. Thyroid disorders. Part I: hyperthyroidism. Oral Surg Oral Med Oral Pathol Oral Radiol Endod 2006;101(3):276–84.
24. Pinto A, Glick M. Management of patients with thyroid disease: oral health considerations. J Am Dent Assoc 2002;133(7):849–58.
25. Little JW. Thyroid disorders. Part II: hypothyroidism and thyroiditis. Oral Surg Oral Med Oral Pathol Oral Radiol Endod 2006;102(2):148–53.
26. Roberts CG, Ladenson PW. Hypothyroidism. Lancet 2004; 363(9411):793–803.
27. Woeber KA. Update on the management of hyperthyroidism and hypothyroidism. Arch Fam Med 2000;9(8):743–7.
28. Canaris GJ, Manowitz NR, Mayor G, et al. The Colorado thyroid disease prevalence study. Arch Intern Med 2000;160(4):526–34.
29. Larsen R, Kronenberg H, Melmed S, et al, editors. Williams textbook of endocrinology. 10th edition. Philadelphia: Saunders; 2003. p. 374–421.
30. Magalhaes DP, Osterne RL, Alves AP, et al. Multiple brown tumours of tertiary hyperparathyroidism in a renal transplant recipient: a case report. Med Oral Patol Oral Cir Bucal 2010;15(1):e10–3.
31. Ionescu O, Sonnet E, Roudaut N, et al. Oral manifestations of endocrine dysfunction. Ann Endocrinol (Paris) 2004;65(5):459–65 [in French].
32. Clarke BL, Brown EM, Collins MT, et al. Epidemiology and diagnosis of hypoparathyroidism. J Clin Endocrinol Metab 2016;101(6): 2284–99.
33. Yamazaki H, Ota Y, Aoki T, et al. Brown tumor of the maxilla and mandible: progressive mandibular brown tumor after removal of parathyroid adenoma. J Oral Maxillofac Surg 2003; 61(6):719–22.
34. Triantafillidou K, Zouloumis L, Karakinaris G, et al. Brown tumors of the jaws associated with primary or secondary hyperparathyroidism. A clinical study and review of the literature. Am J Otolaryngol 2006;27(4):281–6.
35. Lorenzo-Calabria J, Grau D, Silvestre FJ, et al. Management of patients with adrenocortical insufficiency in the dental clinic. Med Oral 2003;8(3):207–14.
36. Olafsson AS, Sigurjonsdottir HA. Increasing prevalence of Addison disease: results from a nationwide study. Endocr Pract 2016;22(1): 30–5.
37. Lindholm J, Juul S, Jorgensen JO, et al. Incidence and late prognosis of Cushing's syndrome: a population-based study. J Clin Endocrinol Metab 2001;86(1):117–23.
38. Gibson N, Ferguson JW. Steroid cover for dental patients on long-term steroid medication: proposed clinical guidelines based upon a critical review of the literature. Br Dent J 2004;197(11):681–5.
39. Bertagna X, Guignat L, Groussin L, et al. Cushing's disease. Best Pract Res Clin Endocrinol Metab 2009;23(5):607–23.
40. Fraser CG, Preuss FS, Bigford WD. Adrenal atrophy and irreversible shock associated with cortisone therapy. J Am Med Assoc 1952; 149(17):1542–3.
41. Lewis L, Robinson RF, Yee J, et al. Fatal adrenal cortical insufficiency precipitated by surgery during prolonged continuous cortisone treatment. Ann Intern Med 1953;39(1):116–26.
42. Plumpton FS, Besser GM, Cole PV. Corticosteroid treatment and surgery. 1. An investigation of the indications for steroid cover. Anaesthesia 1969;24(1):3–11.
43. Bromberg JS, Alfrey EJ, Barker CF, et al. Adrenal suppression and steroid supplementation in renal transplant recipients. Transplantation 1991;51(2):385–90.
44. Salem M, Tainsh RE Jr, Bromberg J, et al. Perioperative glucocorticoid coverage. A reassessment 42 years after emergence of a problem. Ann Surg 1994;219(4):416–25.
45. Shaw M, Mandell BF. Perioperative management of selected problems in patients with rheumatic diseases. Rheum Dis Clin North Am 1999;25(3):623–38. ix.
46. de Lange DW, Kars M. Perioperative glucocorticosteroid supplementation is not supported by evidence. Eur J Intern Med 2008; 19(6):461–7.
47. Napenas JJ, Kujan O, Arduino PG, et al. World workshop on oral medicine VI: controversies regarding dental management of medically complex patients: assessment of current recommendations. Oral Surg Oral Med Oral Pathol Oral Radiol 2015;120(2): 207–26.
48. American Diabetes Association. Diagnosis and classification of diabetes mellitus. Diabetes Care 2006;29(Suppl 1):S43–8.
49. Centers for Disease Control and Prevention. National diabetes fact sheet: national estimates and general information on diabetes and prediabetes in the United States, 2011. Atlanta (GA): U.S. Department of Health and Human Services, Centers for Disease Control and Prevention; 2011. Available at: https://www.cdc.gov/diabetes/pubs/pdf/ndfs_2011.pdf. Accessed December 11, 2016.

50. American Diabetes Association. Diagnosis and classification of diabetes mellitus. Diabetes Care 2010;33(Suppl 1):S62–9.
51. Russotto SB. Asymptomatic parotid gland enlargement in diabetes mellitus. Oral Surg Oral Med Oral Pathol 1981;52(6):594–8.
52. Guggenheimer J, Moore PA, Rossie K, et al. Insulin-dependent diabetes mellitus and oral soft tissue pathologies: II. Prevalence and characteristics of Candida and Candidal lesions. Oral Surg Oral Med Oral Pathol Oral Radiol Endod 2000;89(5):570–6.
53. Petrou-Amerikanou C, Markopoulos AK, Belazi M, et al. Prevalence of oral lichen planus in diabetes mellitus according to the type of diabetes. Oral Dis 1998;4(1):37–40.
54. Guggenheimer J, Moore PA, Rossie K, et al. Insulin-dependent diabetes mellitus and oral soft tissue pathologies. I. Prevalence and characteristics of non-candidal lesions. Oral Surg Oral Med Oral Pathol Oral Radiol Endod 2000;89(5):563–9.
55. Van Dis ML, Parks ET. Prevalence of oral lichen planus in patients with diabetes mellitus. Oral Surg Oral Med Oral Pathol Oral Radiol Endod 1995;79(6):696–700.
56. Romero MA, Seoane J, Varela-Centelles P, et al. Prevalence of diabetes mellitus amongst oral lichen planus patients. Clinical and pathological characteristics. Med Oral 2002;7(2):121–9.
57. Yuan K, Wing LY, Lin MT. Pathogenetic roles of angiogenic factors in pyogenic granulomas in pregnancy are modulated by female sex hormones. J Periodontol 2002;73(7):701–8.
58. Evans RD, Briggs PF. Tooth-surface loss related to pregnancy-induced vomiting. Prim Dent Care 1994;1(1):24–6.
59. Kauh YC, Zachian TF. Melasma. Adv Exp Med Biol 1999;455:491–9.
60. Laine M, Tenovuo J, Lehtonen OP, et al. Pregnancy-related changes in human whole saliva. Arch Oral Biol 1988;33(12):913–7.
61. Lopez NJ, Smith PC, Gutierrez J. Periodontal therapy may reduce the risk of preterm low birth weight in women with periodontal disease: a randomized controlled trial. J Periodontol 2002;73(8):911–24.
62. da Rocha JM, Chaves VR, Urbanetz AA, et al. Obstetricians' knowledge of periodontal disease as a potential risk factor for preterm delivery and low birth weight. Braz Oral Res 2011;25(3): 248–54.

Oral Complications of Systemic Bacterial and Fungal Infections

Amr Bugshan, BDS, PhD [a,b,*], Arwa M. Farag, BDS, DMSc, FDS RCSEd [a,c], Bhavik Desai, DMD, PhD [a]

KEYWORDS

• Bacterial infections • Fungal infections • Oral lesions • Ulcers

KEY POINTS

- Infections of the oral cavity can be primary and caused by pathogenic oral microflora or secondary and caused by dissemination of the infections from other systemic organs.
- Disseminated infections should be listed in the differential diagnoses of solitary deep mucosal ulcerative lesions.
- Ulcerative lesions caused by local or systemic infections may be clinically indistinguishable from oral malignancies and other immune-mediated lesions. Additional diagnostic modalities are required to confirm the diagnosis.
- Histopathology and microorganisms staining are helpful in revealing definitive diagnosis.
- The patient's immune status plays a critical role in infection dissemination and majorly affects treatment approaches.

Introduction

The oral cavity is colonized by a variety of microorganisms, beginning shortly after birth. The oral microenvironment provides appropriate nutrients, pH, and temperature for bacterial colonization. Consequently, synergetic and symbiotic polymicrobial communities live in harmony with the surrounding oral environment and form biofilms that adhere to soft and hard oral tissues. Any alterations in the oral microenvironment, by local or systemic factors, may shift this balance and cause proliferation of pathologic microorganisms at the expense of healthy oral microflora.

Dental caries is one of the most common oral diseases attributable to pathogenic microflora, such as streptococcal species, lactobacilli, actinomyces, and prevotellae. The symbiotic relationship between candida and other caries-associated bacteria might also have a role in caries development.[1] Gingivitis, periodontitis, and jaw osteomyelitis are also caused by the pathogenic bacterial oral microflora (mostly anaerobes). Systemic bacterial and fungal infections may also give rise to secondary oral manifestations, especially in individuals with compromised immunity.

[a] Division of Oral Medicine, Department of Diagnostic Sciences, Tufts University School of Dental Medicine, 1 Kneeland Street, 6th Floor, Boston, MA 02111, USA

[b] Collage of Dentistry, Imam Abdulrahman Bin Faisal University, P.O. Box 1982, Dammam 31441, Kingdom of Saudi Arabia

[c] Department of Oral Medicine, Faculty of Dentistry, King AbdulAziz University, 1 Umm Al Muminin Road, Jeddah 21589, Kingdom of Saudi Arabia

* Corresponding author. Division of Oral Medicine, Department of Diagnostic Sciences, Tufts University School of Dental Medicine, 1 Kneeland Street, DHS #644, Boston, MA 02111.

E-mail address: amr.bugshan@tufts.edu

Bacterial infections

Tuberculosis

Tuberculosis (TB) is a systemic bacterial infection that seldom involves the oral cavity. Globally, TB is the second most common death-causing infectious disease after human immunodeficiency virus (HIV).[2] Southeast Asia, Western Pacific Regions, and Africa have the highest prevalence of TB.[2]

Causative pathogen

Mycobacterium tuberculosis is the causative pathogen.[2]

Clinical presentation

TB is known to affect men more than women, mostly adults. Lungs are typically the primary site of infection but other sites may be affected including skin, central nervous system, lymphatic system, kidneys, and gastrointestinal tract.[2,3]

The disease is transmitted by inhalation of contaminated air droplets of a patient with active disease. First-time exposure primarily involves the lungs and may cause nonspecific signs of inflammation, such as fever and pleural effusion (primary TB). This can result in formation of fibrocalcified nodules that are seen on chest radiograph at the primary site of infection (usually at the apex of the lung). Mycobacteria may remain dormant inside these nodules for many years (latent TB). Weakening of the patient's immunity may lead to disease reactivation and spread via vascular and lymphatic systems to other body sites (secondary TB).[3,4]

Oral manifestations

A total of 1% to 5% of affected patients has oral manifestations and 1.33% of the cases are associated with HIV infection.[5] Most oral manifestations of TB are secondary to the primary pulmonary infection. However, primary oral TB may occur from direct inoculation of the organisms in the oral mucosa, in which

Atlas Oral Maxillofacial Surg Clin N Am 25 (2017) 209–220

http://dx.doi.org/10.1016/j.cxom.2017.04.012

younger patients are mostly affected.[3,5] Tongue is the most commonly affected site followed by buccal mucosa, lip, palate, and gingiva (Fig. 1). The lesions are mostly manifested as single chronic ulceration with irregular margins. However, multiple ulcers, swelling, nodular masses, and mandibular osteomyelitis have been reported.[5]

Histopathology

Histopathology shows caseating granulomatous lesion that consists of a mixture of histiocytes, multinucleated giant cells, and lymphocytes with central necrosis (Fig. 2).

Diagnosis

Diagnostic modalities may include tuberculin skin test, special mycobacterial stains of infected tissue (Ziehl-Neelsen stain) (see Fig. 2), culture of infected sputum, and molecular methods (polymerase chain reaction [PCR]).[5]

Differential diagnosis

Oral ulcerative lesion of TB can clinically mimic traumatic ulcer; deep fungal infections; and squamous cell carcinoma.

Treatment

Treatment includes 6-month regimen of pyrazinamide, isoniazid, rifampin, and ethambutol as the first-line treatment of TB. Patients with multiple drug-resistant TB, mainly to isoniazid and rifampicin, require longer treatment regimen for up to 20 months.[2]

Bacterial salivary gland infection

Sialadenitis is inflammation of salivary glands, which can be induced by several etiologic factors including infectious agents (bacterial and viral), radiation, and autoimmune disorders (eg, Sjögren syndrome). Bacterial sialadenitis may be facilitated by hyposalivation. Decreased salivary flow may impede the ability of salivary glands to flush out microorganisms and debris and lead to retrograde spread of the bacterial pathogens from the oral microflora to salivary gland ducts and parenchyma. Less commonly, systemic bacteremia in immunocompromised patients may cause secondary bacterial sialadenitis.[6–8]

Causative pathogens

Acute bacterial sialadenitis

Gram-positive *Staphylococcus aureus* is the most common causative organism in acute bacterial parotitis. However, other bacterial microorganisms, such as other gram-positive cocci (*Streptococcus pyogenes* and *Streptococcus viridans*), gram-negative bacilli (*Prevotella* and *Porphyromonas* species), and gram-negative bacilli (*Escherichia coli*) are also implicated.[6,9]

Chronic bacterial sialadenitis

This is caused by mixed bacterial community. *S viridans* is the most common followed by *S aureus* and *Streptococcus pneumoniae*.[9]

Clinical presentation

Acute bacterial infection

Mucous content of submandibular and sublingual salivary glands acts as protective barrier against bacterial infection. Paucity of mucous secretion renders the parotid glands more susceptible to infection. Acute bacterial parotitis is most commonly seen in elderly and immunocompromised patients. However, neonates and hospitalized patients are also susceptible to this infection. Acute bacterial parotitis is strongly linked to salivary ducts obstruction by sialolith, foreign body, or tumor. Poor oral hygiene, Sjögren syndrome, or drug-induced hyposalivation may also increase the risk of acquiring the acute infection. Clinical manifestations include sudden onset of tender swelling of the auricular area with occasional pus discharge when massaging the infected gland.[8,9]

Chronic bacterial infection

It is characterized by recurrent episodes of painful swelling of salivary glands and chronic purulent discharge (Fig. 3). Both parotid and submandibular glands can be affected. Chronic hyposalivation combined with ascending infection from the oral cavity to the gland ducts/parenchyma is the most common scenario. Congenital malformation of the glands ducts or acini can also impact salivary flow and may be associated with chronic recurrent juvenile parotitis.[9]

Diagnosis

Diagnostic modalities may include bacterial culture, sialography, and biopsy to rule out salivary gland tumors.[9]

Histopathology

Acute bacterial infection

Neutrophils accumulation within salivary gland tissue.

Chronic bacterial infection

Scattered infiltration of lymphocytes and plasma cells with occasional acinar atrophy, dilated ducts and fibrosis are reported.[3]

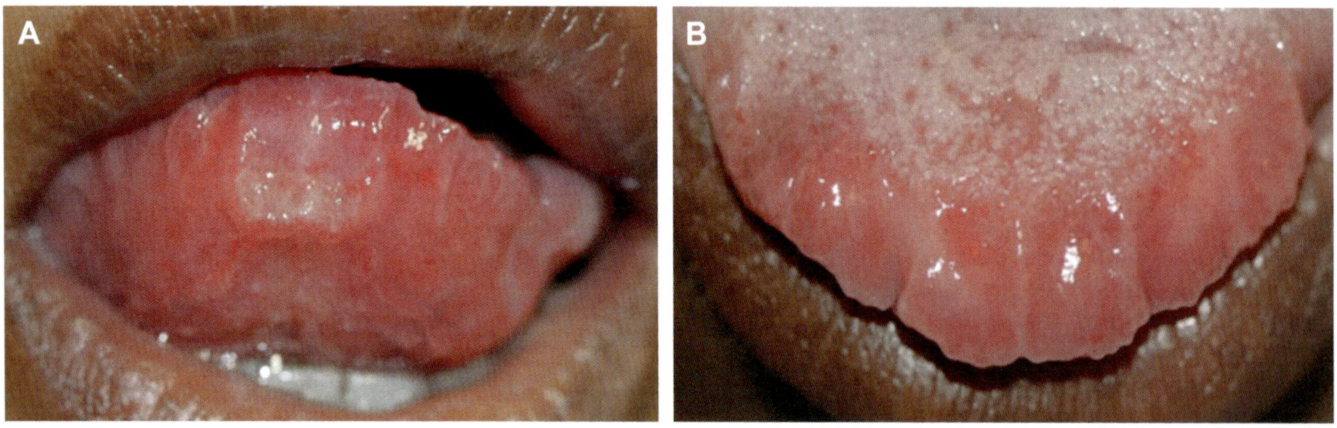

Fig. 1 Primary oral TB. (*A*) Ulcerative lesion on the tongue tip with a surrounded erythematous zone. (*B*) Lobulated erythematous appearance of anterior third of the tongue caused by granulomatous inflammation in the lip submucosa. (*Reproduced from* Khammissa RA, Wood NH, Meyerov R, et al. Primary oral tuberculosis as an indicator of HIV infection. Patholog Res Int 2010;2011:893295.)

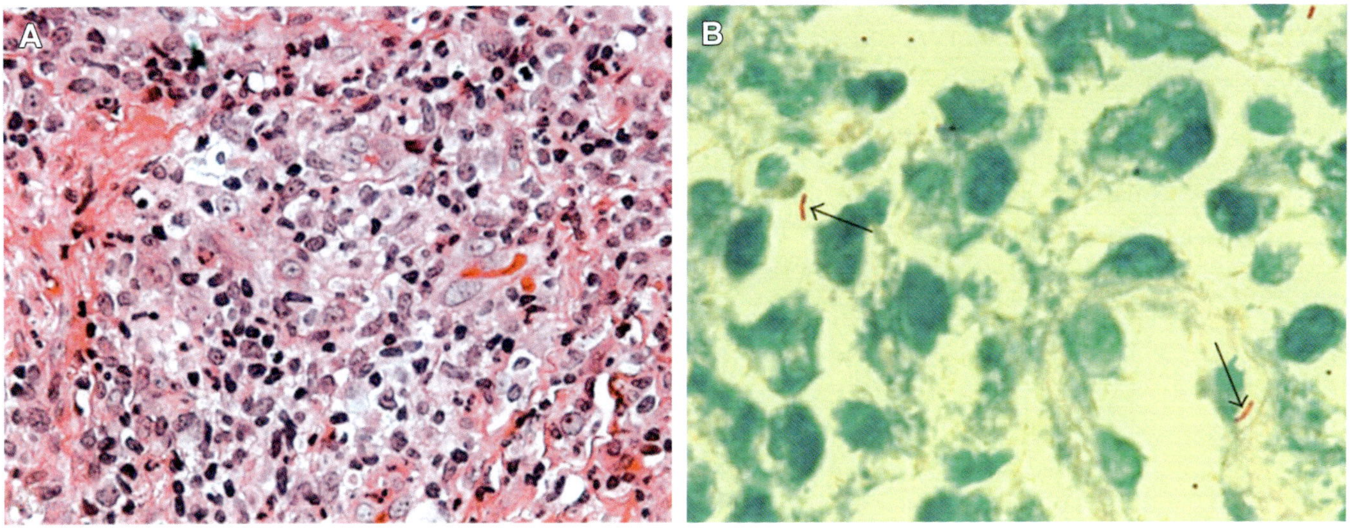

Fig. 2 Oral TB. (*A*) Hematoxylin-eosin stain shows chronic granulomatous inflammation consists of a mixture of histiocytes, multinucleated giant cells, and lymphocytes (original magnification ×300). (*B*) Two mycobacterial organisms (*arrows*) are stained by Ziehl-Neelsen stain (original magnification ×1000). (*Reproduced from* Khammissa RA, Wood NH, Meyerov R, et al. Primary oral tuberculosis as an indicator of HIV infection. Patholog Res Int 2010;2011:893295.)

Differential diagnosis

This includes viral infection (mumps), sialadenosis, Sjögren syndrome, and salivary gland tumors.

Treatment

Massaging the infected gland and using sialogogues can stimulate saliva secretion. Pus drainage and appropriate systemic antibiotics (penicillin and metronidazole, amoxicillin and clavulanate, or cephalexin) based on culture and bacterial sensitivity test are also part of treatment.[9]

Syphilis

Syphilis is a sexually transmitted infectious disease that can evolve to serious complications if left untreated. Based on the mode of transmission, syphilis is categorized as acquired or congenital. Over the past few decades, the incidence of syphilis has sharply declined because of the introduction of penicillin. However, a recent spike has been noticed among young homosexual men and those with HIV.[10]

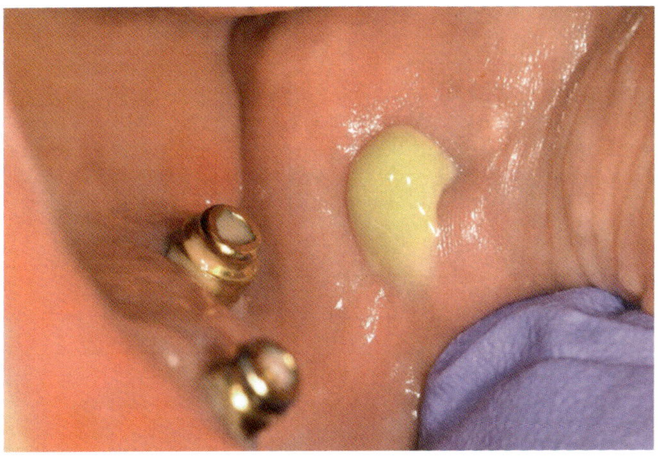

Fig. 3 Chronic suppurative sialadenitis. Pus discharge arising from the Stenson duct during massaging of the infected parotid gland. (*Courtesy of* Dr Mabi Singh, Division of Oral Medicine, Department of Diagnostic Sciences, Tufts University School of Dental Medicine, Boston, MA.)

Causative pathogen

Syphilis is caused by anaerobic filamentous spirochete *Treponema pallidum*.[10]

Clinical presentation

Based on its infectivity, acquired syphilis is classified into four stages, summarized in Tables 1 and 2. Untreated patients with secondary syphilis enter the latent phase where the patients are serology positive for syphilis with no clinical symptoms. Latent phase is divided to early (less than 2 years) or late (more than 2 years).[10] Patients are highly contagious in the first two stages (primary and secondary). However, an infected mother can transmit the disease to her child in the latent stage.[3]

Diagnosis

Diagnosis can be obtained by dark-field microscopy of lesion exudate, direct florescent antibody test of lesion exudate, special microorganism stain of infected tissue specimen (special silver stain), or serologic tests (nontreponemal and treponemal).[14]

Histopathology

Microscopic evaluation shows that surface epithelium may be hyperplastic or ulcerated. The underlying stroma shows chronic inflammatory cells (lymphocytes and plasma cells).[3]

Differential diagnosis

Oral chancre can clinically resemble traumatic ulcer, deep fungal infection, and squamous cell carcinoma. Condylomata lata can mimic squamous papilloma, condyloma acuminatum, or verruca vulgaris.

Treatment

Parenteral administration of penicillin G is the first line treatment for all stages. Alternative antibiotics such as ceftriaxone, doxycycline, tetracycline, and azithromycin may be

Table 1 Stages of acquired syphilis

	Primary Syphilis	Secondary Syphilis	Tertiary Syphilis
Duration	• Develops 3–10 wk after bacterial incubation (9–120 d) at the primary inoculation site • Heals within 7–10 d[10,11]	Begins 4–10 wk after initial infection Spontaneous resolution within 3–12 wk 25% of untreated cases evolves into secondary syphilis[3,11]	25% of untreated patients develop tertiary syphilis up to 30 y or more after infection More serious stage[10]
Transmission mode	• Sexual contact with infectious mucus membrane[10]	• Spread of the untreated primary syphilis pathogen	• Pathogen spreads again after latent phase (if secondary syphilis left untreated)
Clinical presentation	• Most lesions are located on the genital area • Commonly manifests as solitary painless chancre (Fig. 4) • Most chancres begin as plaque raised lesion and then become ulcerated[10]	• Nonspecific symptoms (fever, malaise, and lymphadenopathy) • Generalized mucocutaneous rash (palms and soles) • Condylomata lata: white-gray raised lesions on warm areas (anus and labia) caused by direct spread of pathogen from the primary site	• Cardiosyphilis and neurosyphilis are the most common manifestation of this stage; however, other systems can be affected • Gumma: Scattered foci of granulomatous lesions can affect skin, mucosa, and bone[3,10]
Oral manifestation	• Primary oral lesions result from orogenital or oroanal contact with infection site • Solitary ulcer most commonly on the upper lip in males and lower lip in females • Tongue, tonsils, and pharynx are rarely affected • Oral chancre presents as deep ulcerative area with red or brown base and irregular raised borders[11]	• 30% of patients present with oral manifestation • Macular syphilides: flat red lesions commonly arise in the hard palate • Papular syphilides: Raised red lesions with gray centers arise commonly on buccal mucosa and commissures (Fig. 5). • Mucous patches: shallow ulcer with a red zone covered with mucoid exudate; on the commissures, they look as split papules, whereas they appear as irregular fissure on the tongue (see Fig. 5). • Snail track ulcers: results from coalesce of mucus patches • Lues maligna (ulceronodular disease): patients develop fever and myalgia followed by papulopustular eruptions that rapidly become necrotic on face and scalp (presents intraorally as multiple ulcerative lesions)[3,11–13]	• Gumma may manifest intraorally as single or multiple nodular or ulcerative lesions mostly on tongue and hard palate • May perforate the hard palate and produce oronasal communication • May resemble malignant bony lesions on radiograph • Interstitial glossitis: large lobulated tongue caused by gumma[3,11]

used in patient with penicillin allergies given that no pregnancy or signs of neurpsyphilis present. Penicillin remains the solely effective pahrmacotherapeutic agent in pregnant patient and those with neurosyphilis in which desensitizing therapy should perused prior to penicillin administration.[14]

Actinomycosis

Actinomycosis is a chronic infectious disease caused by a group of bacteria belonging to *Actinomyces* species. They are part of normal microflora in the oral cavity, gastrointestinal tract, and female

Table 2 Congenital syphilis

	Congenital Syphilis
Mode of transmission	• From infected mother to fetus through the placenta (after the sixteenth week of gestation)[10,11]
Clinical presentation	• Fetal loss or premature labor • Early congenital syphilis manifest as bullous rash, rhinitis, laryngitis, lymphadenopathy, hepatosplenomegaly, osteochrondritis, periostitis, meningitis, and chorioretinitis • Late congenital syphilis (child older than 2 y) may present with inflammation of eyes, ears, and joints and skeletal malformation[10]
Oral manifestation	• Hutchinson triad includes interstitial keratitis of the cornea, hearing loss, and dental anomalies (Hutchinson incisors and mulberry molars) • Other manifestations may occur including frontal bossing, short maxilla, and high-arched palate[3]

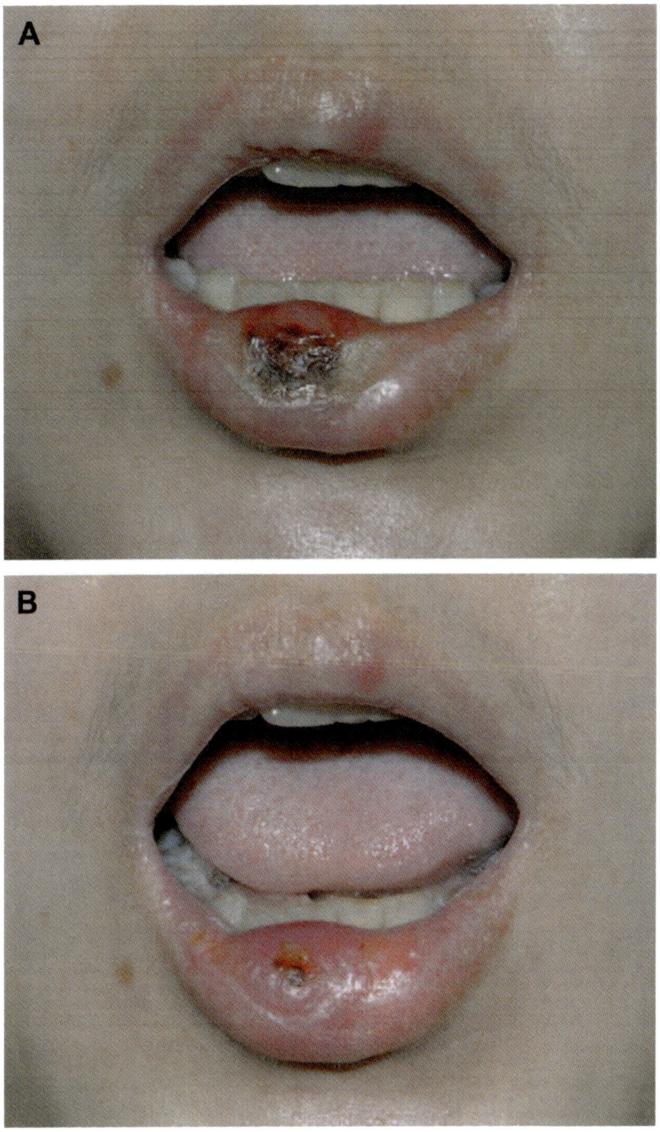

Fig. 4 Chancre of primary syphilis. (*A*) Asymptomatic indurated ulcerative nodule on lower lip with a surrounded erythematous zone. (*B*) Improvement of the lesion after penicillin G benzathine therapy. (*Reproduced from* Yu X, Zheng H. Syphilitic chancre of the lips transmitted by kissing: a case report and review of the literature. Medicine (Baltimore) 2016;95(14):e3303.)

genital tract. They cause opportunistic infections when they penetrate injured mucosa and elicit an inflammatory response.[9]

Causative pathogen

Gram-positive anaerobic bacteria *Actinomyces israelii* is the most common pathogen isolated from human actinomycosis. Less commonly, other species may be involved, such as *Actinomyces odontolyticus*, *Actinomyces naeslundii*, and *Actinomyces meyeri*.[9]

Clinical presentation

Acute local infection may develop at the primary infection site (injured mucosa). If left untreated, the pathogen slowly invades the underlying tissue and develops chronic granulomatous infection. Clinically, it manifests as single or multiple masses with peripheral fibrotic boundaries (wooden area) and central necrotic tissues intermixed with bacterial colonies that may discharge yellowish material known as sulfur granules.

Cervicofacial actinomycosis is the most frequent manifestation of the disease. However, other regions can be affected, such as the lung, abdomen, and pelvis.[9,15,16]

Cervicofacial actinomycosis

Actinomyces is part of healthy oral mucosa, gingival crevices, oropharynx, periodontal pockets, dental plaque, and carious teeth. Tissue injury from traumatic extractions, gingival trauma, or other surgical procedures may trigger actinomycosis infection in the oral cavity. Poor oral hygiene, malnutrition, alcoholism, bisphosphonate-related osteonecrosis of the jaw, radiation, and compromised immunity are predisposing factors that increase the risk of infection. Clinically, actinomycosis typically presents as painless indurated swelling or, in advanced cases, a mass that drain through skin. The mandibular angle is the most frequently affected site (lumpy jaw). Salivary glands, cheeks, and jawbone are also affected (Fig. 6A, B). Persistent infection may drain sulfur granules externally through the skin or intraorally through mucosal sinus tract. Periapical actinomycosis is associated with nonresolving periapical lesion with history of recurrent sinus tract (Fig. 7A, B).[3,9,16,17]

Diagnosis

Actinomycosis may be diagnosed by culture of sulfur granules,using special microorganisms stain for the infected tissue specimen (special silver stain), or by molecular methods (PCR).[9]

Histopathology

Tissue fibrosis enclosed a zone of granulation tissue intermixed with bacterial colonies surrounding by neutrophils.[3]

Differential diagnosis

Other infections, such as botryomycosis, odontogenic abscess, and salivary gland tumors, can be mistaken with cervicofacial actinomycosis.

Treatment

Serious infection should be treated by incision and drainage and intravenous penicillin for 2 to 6 weeks followed by 6 to 12 months of oral penicillin. Dose can be adjusted to a shorter course with less extensive infection.[9]

Cat-scratch disease

Cat-scratch disease is a bacterial infection that occurs following a scratch or a bite by infected cats. Some recent reports have shown that the disease may also be transmitted to human via other infected mammals hosts, such as dogs.[18]

Causative pathogen

It is mainly caused by gram-negative bacterium *Bartonella henselae*. Other organisms such as *Bartonella clarridgeiae* and *Bartonella quintana* have been reported to cause cat-scratch disease.[19-21]

Clinical presentation

Children aged 5 to 9 years are mostly affected with significant female predilection. Three to 10 days after being scratched by infected cat, a red papule develops at the wound site, and a few days later becomes vesiculated and crusted. Regional lymphadenopathy, proximal to the infected site, occurs 1 to 2 weeks after the papule eruption. Axillary lymph nodes are frequently affected. Patients mostly complain of fever, malaise, and nausea, and a few may develop severe complications involving the nervous system, heart, lung, liver, and bone.[19,21,22]

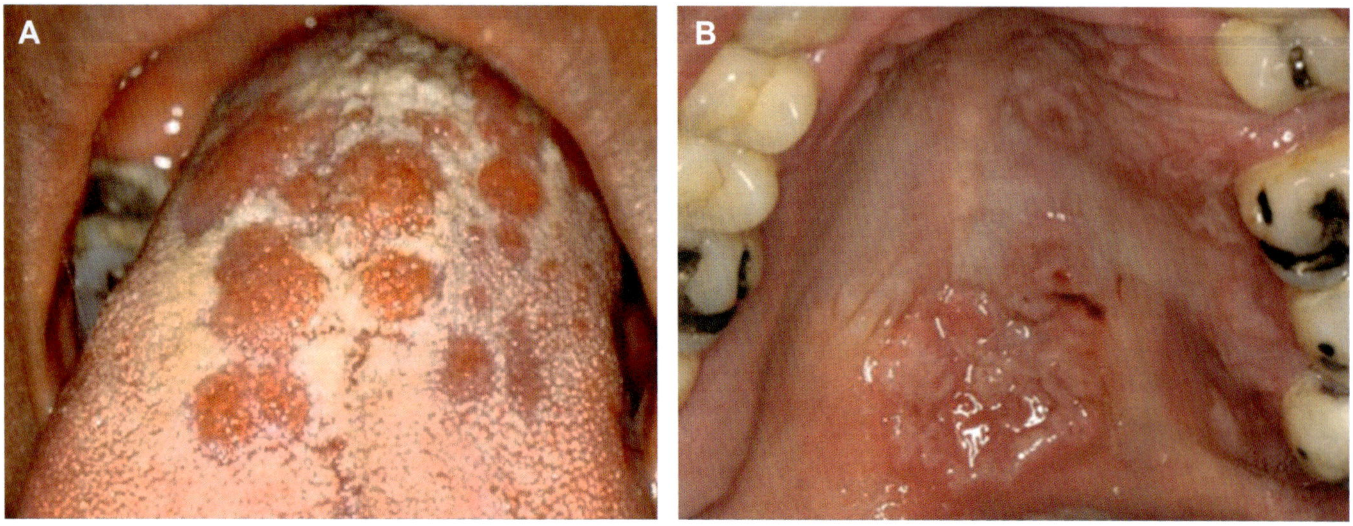

Fig. 5 Secondary syphilis. (*A*) Papular syphilitic lesions on the dorsal surface of the tongue. (*B*) Elevated plaques surrounded with erythematous zone (mucous patch) on palate. (*Reproduced from* Ramirez-Amador V, Anaya-Saavedra G, Crabtree-Ramirez B, et al. Clinical spectrum of oral secondary syphilis in HIV-infected patients. J Sex Transm Dis 2013;2013:892427.)

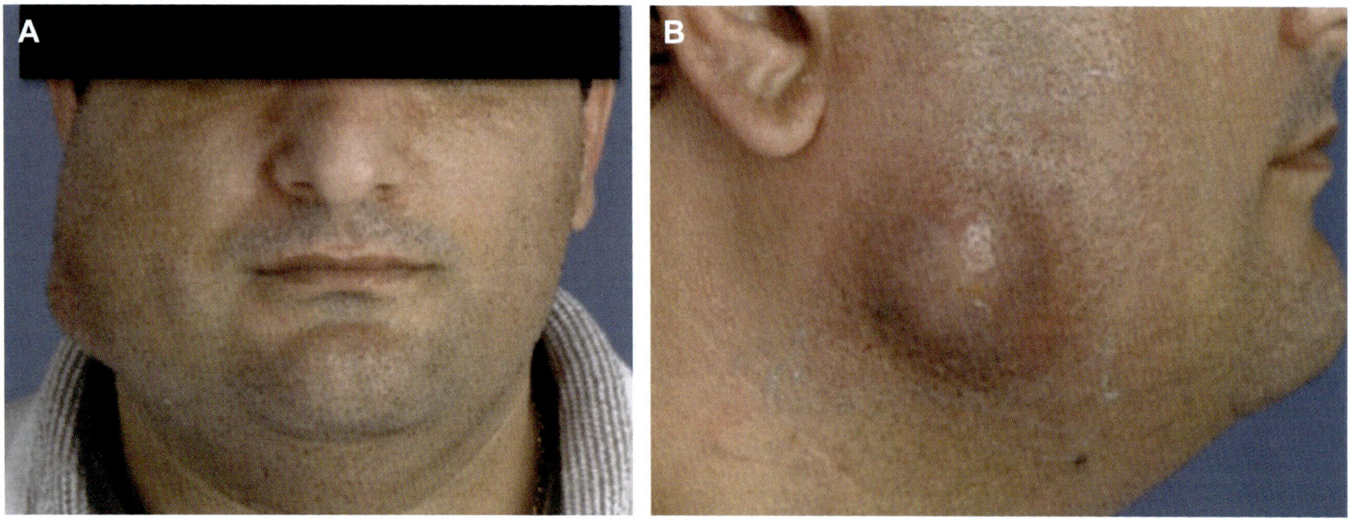

Fig. 6 Cervicofacial actinomycosis. (*A, B*) Indurated swelling on the right cheek. (*Reproduced from* Moghimi M, Salentijn E, Debets-Ossenkop Y, et al. Treatment of cervicofacial actinomycosis: a report of 19 cases and review of literature. Med Oral Patol Oral Cir Bucal 2013;18(4):e627–32.)

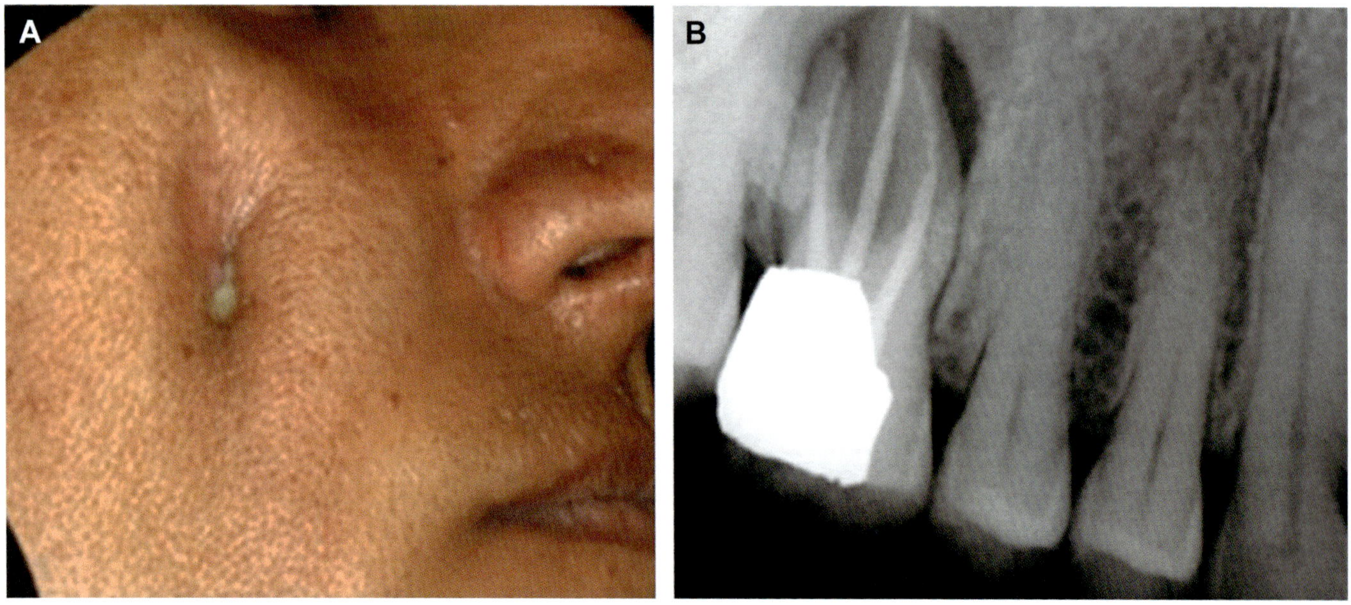

Fig. 7 Periapical actinomycosis. (*A*) Draining fistula of the right cheek. (*B*) Periapical radiograph showing a radiolucent lesion associated with tooth #16. (*Reproduced from* Jamshidi D, Moazami F, Sobhnamayan F, et al. Clinical and histopathologic investigation of periapical actinomycosis with cutaneous lesion: a case report. J Dent (Shiraz) 2015;16(3 Suppl):286–90.)

Manifestations of the head and neck region

Submandibular lymph nodes are the most commonly affected followed by preauricular and submental lymph nodes (Fig. 8). Cervical lymph nodes and parotid tail lymphadenopathy has been reported. Overlying skin shows erythematous discoloration in most cases with tenderness on palpation. Scratch on the eyes by infected cat may be associated with unilateral conjunctivitis with either preauricular or submandibular lymphadenopathy known as Parinaud oculoglandular syndrome.[23–25]

Diagnosis

Diagnostic modalities may include serologic test (IgG and IgM antibodies to *B henselae* antigen), molecular methods (enzyme-linked immunosorbent assay and PCR), and special microorganisms stain of infected lymph node (Warthin-Starry stain).[3,24]

Histopathology

There is hyperplasia of the affected lymph node with central necrotic area surrounded by neutrophils and histiocytes.[3]

Differential diagnosis

In head and neck region, other infections, such as TB, sialadenitis, salivary gland tumors, lymph node malignancy (lymphoma) should be considered.

Treatment

In most cases, swelling of affected lymph node resolves within 9 weeks. However, a few cases may take up to 12 months. Aspiration or drainage may help relieve suppurative lymph nodes. Antibiotics, such as azithromycin, erythromycin, doxycycline, or ciprofloxacin, may be required in some cases especially with medically compromised population.[3]

Uncommon bacterial infections associated with oral manifestations

Erysipelas, impetigo, and scarlet fever are rarely seen bacterial infections that are associated with some oral manifestation. Table 3 summarizes details about these infections.

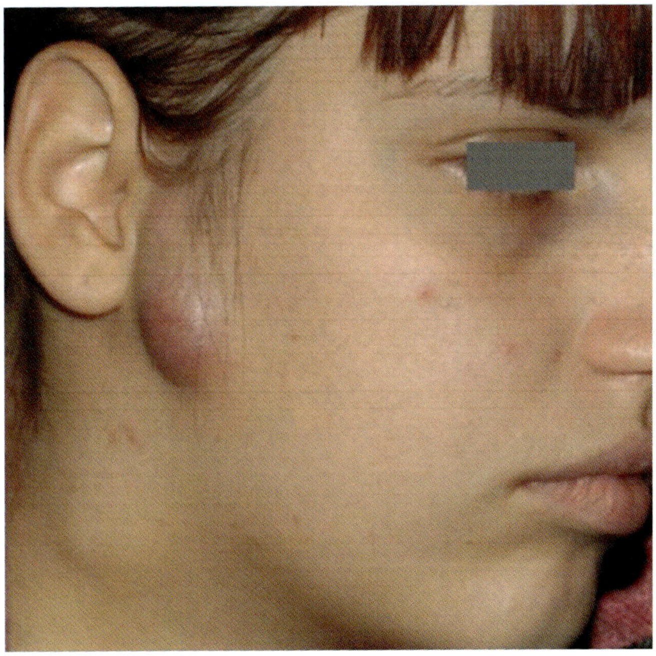

Fig. 8 Cat-scratch disease: preauricular lymphoadenopathy after a scratch on the eyelid from a kitten. (*Reproduced from* Stanimirov P, Dimitrov M. Cat scratch disease: follow up of a clinical case. Int J Sci Res 2014;11(3):2319–7064.)

Fungal infections

Oral candidiasis

Up to 60% of healthy individuals harbor candida organisms as part of their normal oral flora.[28] Oral candidiasis is the most common opportunistic infection of the oral mucosa (primary candidiasis). Several predisposing factors ;may increase the risk of oral candidal infection including use of systemicantibiotics, poor denture hygiene, hyposalivation, and immunocompromised status of the

Table 3 Oral manifestations of uncommon bacterial infections

	Erysipelas	Impetigo	Scarlet Fever
Causative pathogen	• *Streptococcus pyogenes* (β-hemolytic streptococci group A)[26]	• Nonbullous impetigo is caused by mixture of β-hemolytic streptococci (*S pyogenes*) and *Staphylococcus aureus* • Bullous impetigo is caused mainly by *S aureus*	• Group A β-hemolytic streptococci[3]
Mode of transmission	• Infection spreads via skin trauma/ abrasion, surgical incision, skin disease, or local skin infection[26]	• Bacterial colonization on the skin of poor hygiene children • Most common in tropical or subtropical climates • More common in low socioeconomic communities • Damaged skin, such as trauma or insects bite, may help in intradermal inoculation of the pathogen[26]	• Associated with streptococcal pharyngitis • Pathogen elaborates toxin that attack blood vessel causing skin rash[3,26]

(*continued on next page*)

Table 3 (*continued*)

	Erysipelas	Impetigo	Scarlet Fever
Clinical presentation	• Superficial skin infection • Common in infants, young children, and older adults • Lower extremities are the most commonly affected sites followed by the face • Skin lesions are well-demarcated, erythematous, swollen and raised with red margins • Facial erysipelas affects mostly the butterfly area (cheeks and nose bridge) and advanced lesions can cause eyes swelling • Fever, chills, and toxicity are reported[26]	• Superficial skin infection • Common in children <15 y[27] • Face and lower extremities are commonly affected • Start as skin papules that enlarges gradually forming vesicles • 4–6 d later, vesicles break forming thick crust • Regional lymphadenitis may occur[26]	• Diffuse skin red bluish popular rash appears second day of clinical illness • Sandpaper skin texture caused by blocked sweat glands • Petechiae (fragile capillary) • Skin desquamation may occur later Oral manifestations: • Exudative pharyngitis and tonsillitis • Petechiae on the palate • Initially, tongue covered with white coating with red papillae (white strawberry tongue) • Later, tongue becomes red (red strawberry tongue)[26]
Treatment	• Penicillin is the treatment of choice • Alternative antibiotics may be considered in penicillin-allergic patients[3,26]	• Remove the crust and clean the area • Topical antibiotic with localized lesion • Systemic antibiotic that effective against *S pyogenes* and penicillin-resistant *S aureus* including cephalexin, flucloxacillin, and augmentin[3]	• Early treatment is required to prevent late complications • Oral penicillin V or amoxicillin is the first-line treatment • Alternative antibiotics can be used with penicillin-allergic patients • Antipyretic may be used to reduce the fever[3]

Table 4 Clinical presentation of oral candidiasis

	Clinical presentation
Pseudomembranous candidiasis	• Affected population ○ Patients taking antibiotics or immunosuppressant drugs ○ Patients with compromised immune system, such as those with HIV and hematologic malignancies ○ Young children and infants with immature immune system • Creamy-white plaque (cottage cheese appearance), which consist of debris, desquamative epithelium, and fungal organisms (Fig. 9) • Can be wiped off leaving an inflamed area • Can be acute (with antibiotics and immunosuppressive therapy) or chronic (with impaired immunity)[3,29]
Erythematous candidiasis	• Diffuse erythematous macule (no wipeable white plaque) • Several clinical patterns: Acute atrophic candidiasis (antibiotic sore mouth) • Mostly associated with antibiotic therapy • Erythematous plaque, which might be accompanied by burning sensation • Tongue is commonly affected[3] Median rhomboid glossitis • Asymptomatic well-demarcated erythematous lesion in the center or posterior dorsal tongue (Fig. 10) • Erythematous appearance is caused by atrophy of the filiform papillae • Increased risk with smoking, inhalation of steroid • Contact between the affected tongue and the palate may result in palatal erythema (kissing lesions) (see Fig. 10)[3,29] Angular cheilitis • Erythematous fissured lesion affects the mouth corners (Fig. 11) • Mostly caused by mixture of *Candida albicans* (80%) and *Staphylococcus aureus* (20%) • Predisposing factors include loss of vertical dimension, vitamin B_{12} deficiency, and iron deficiency[3,29] Denture Stomatitis • Erythematous lesion is localized to the denture-bearing area of the maxillary removable partial denture • May present as localized erythema, diffuse erythema, or granular lesion[3,29]
Chronic hyperplastic candidiasis (candidal leukoplakia)	• Uncommon form of candida infection • Characterized by white patch that cannot be wiped off • Anterior buccal mucosa is the most common site[3]
Mucocutaneous candidiasis	• Immunologic disorder associated with candidal infections of nails, skin, and mucosal surfaces affects young children • Oral lesions present as nonremovable white patches (hyperplastic candidiasis) • Associated with IL-17 gene mutation[3]

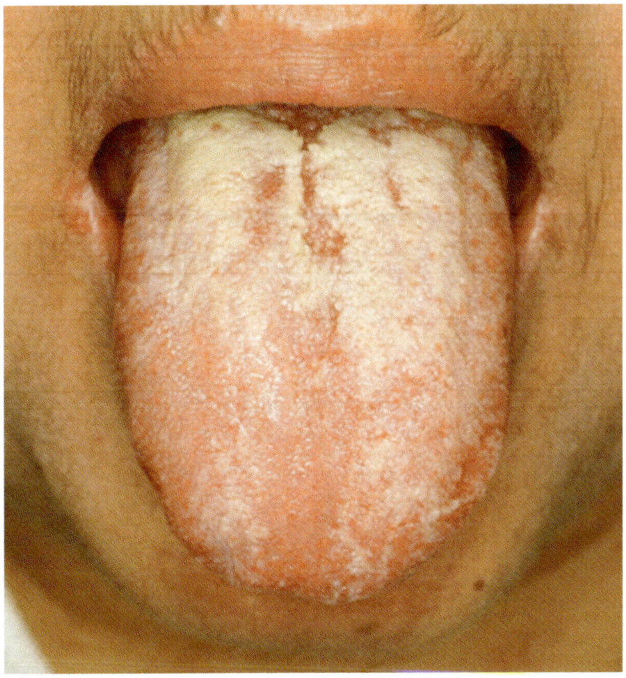

Fig. 9 Pseudomembranous candidiasis (thrush) of HIV patient. Creamy-white plaque resembles cottage cheese on the dorsal surface of the tongue. (*From* Millsop JW, Fazel N. Oral candidiasis. Clin Dermatol 2016;34(4);487–94; with permission.)

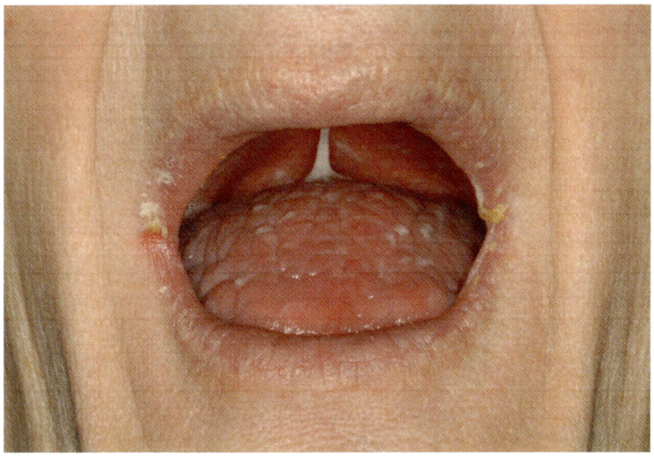

Fig. 11 Erythematous candidiasis. Angular cheilitis, erythematous fissured lesion affects the mouth corners. (*Courtesy of* Dr Mark Lerman, Division of Oral Pathology, Department of Diagnostic Sciences, Tufts University School of Dental Medicine, Boston, MA.)

patients. On rare occasions, infection may spread and cause systemic mucocutaneous manifestations (secondary candidiasis).[29]

Causative pathogen

Candida albicans, *Candida tropicalis*, and *Candida glabrata* are associated with 80% of candidal infection. *C albicans* is strongly linked to oral candidiasis because of its ability to form filamentous shape and invades the mucosal surface.[29]

Clinical presentation

Table 4 summarizes the different clinical patterns of oral candidiasis.

Diagnosis

Diagnosis can be made by biopsy and special microorganisms stain (periodic acid–Schiff or Gomori methenamine silver) and cytology smear (scrape the lesion and smear it on glass slide).[3,29]

Histopathology

Candidal infection may show hyperparakeratosis of the surface epithelium in conjugation with elongation of rete ridges. Small collections of neutrophilis in the parakeratin layer are accompanied with chronic inflammation in the underlying connective tissue.[3,29]

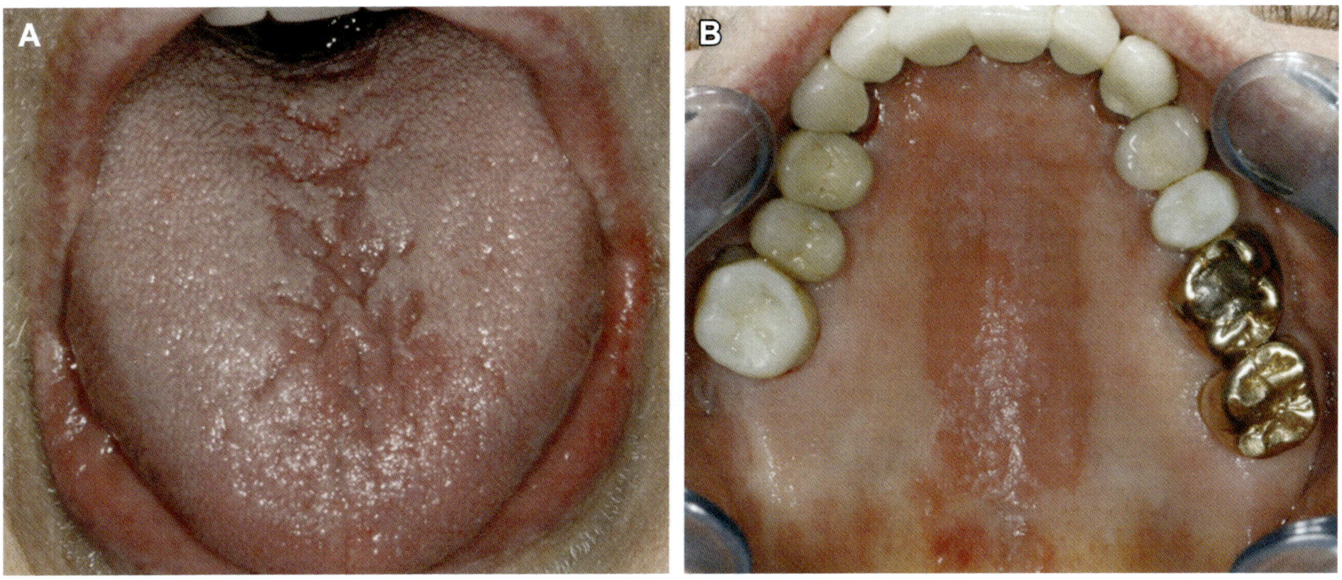

Fig. 10 Erythematous candidiasis. (*A*) Median rhomboid glossitis, well-demarcated erythematous lesion in the center of posterior dorsal tongue. (*B*) Palatal erythema results from contact with the infected tongue (kissing lesion). (*Courtesy of* Pooyan Refahi, DMD, MS, TUSDM Department of Periodontology, Boston, MA.)

Table 5 Antifungal therapies

Antifungal	Dosage
Clotrimazole (Mycelex oral troches)	1 troche (10 mg) 5 times daily for 10–14 d
Nystatin (Mycostatin oral suspension)	Switch and expectorate 4 times daily for 2 wk
Nystatin combined with triamcinolone acetonide cream	For angular cheilitis; apply topically 3–4 times daily
Fluconazole (Dipluran tablets)	Two tablets (200 mg) on the first day followed by one 100-mg tablet daily for 1–2 wk[3,29]

Differential diagnosis

For chronic hyperplastic candidiasis, frictional keratosis, chemical burn, and dysplasia should be included. For erythematous candidiasis, thermal burn, erythroplakia, and vitamin B_{12} or iron deficiency should be considered.[3]

Treatment

The most common antifungal medications used for the treatment of oral candidiasis are listed in Table 5.

Deep fungal infections

Oral manifestations of systemic fungal infections are not commonly encountered. Tables 6 and 7 summarize the details

Table 6 Summary of deep fungal infections

	Histoplasmosis	Mucormycosis
Causative organism	• *Histoplasma capsulatum*[3]	• *Rhizopus arrbizus*[29]
Transmission mode	• Inhalation of airborne spores[30]	• Spores inhalation or enter through traumatic wound[29]
Clinical presentation	• Most common systemic fungal infection in the United States[31] • In most patients (90%), the infection is subclinical and self-limited • Immunocompromised patients or inhalation of large quantity of spores may develop: • Acute pulmonary histoplasmosis: Characterized by dyspnea, cough, chest pain, joint pain for 1–2 wk[32] • Chronic pulmonary histoplasmosis: Mostly occur in older and smoker males.[33] Patients develop persistent productive cough, dyspnea, chest pain and weight loss. Cavitation of the lung and calcification of the surrounding lymph node may be detected in chest radiograph.[34] • Disseminated histoplasmosis: In immunosuppressed or older patients, pathogen may spread via blood outside the lung to other body organs (occurs during the acute infection stage)[3,35]	• Opportunistic infection found in nose, throat, and mouth of healthy individual • Immunocompromised patients can be affected (especially uncontrolled type 1 diabetes) • Organisms can invade the arteries and form emboli, which result in necrosis of the involved tissue • Sinus, pulmonary, and rhinocerebral structures can be affected[29]
Oral Manifestation	• Most commonly detected in HIV-infected patients • Begins as erythematous macule then forms a painful ulcerative lesion indistinguishable from malignancy • Common in gingiva, palate, and tongue	• Rhinocerbral mucromycosis may be associated with nasal obstruction, epistaxis, facial pain, and visual disturbance • Maxillary sinus involvement can present as intraoral swelling of maxillary ridge or palate. If left untreated, palatal destruction and necrosis may occur.[3,29]
Diagnosis	• Culture of the sputum • Histopathology and microorganism stain (GMS or PAS) • PCR[32]	• Histopathology and microorganism stain (GMS or PAS)[3]
Histopathology	• Granulomatous inflammation consists of macrophages, plasma cells, multinucleated giant cells, and lymphocytes • Sometimes, organisms can be identified in hematoxylin-eosin stain[3]	• Necrotic tissue with predominant neutrophils. Numerous branching nonseptate hyphae can be identified.[3]
Treatment	• Only chronic and disseminated histoplasmoses require treatment • Antifungal therapy, such as amphotericin B and itraconazole[3]	• Surgical debridement of the infected tissue followed by amphotericin B[3]

Abbreviations: GMS, Gomori methenamine silver; PAS, periodic acid–Schiff.

Table 7 Summary of deep fungal infections

	Aspergillosis
Causative organism	• *Aspergillus fumigatus* is the most common pathogen (sinus infection) • *Aspergillus flavus* is associated with invasive infection[36]
Transmission mode	• Inhalation spore[36]
Clinical presentation	• Most prevalent opportunistic infection after candida • Infection may present as superficial infection without invasion, allergic reaction, or invasive infection • Infection can be acquired from the hospital (nosocomial infection)[3,36]
Oral manifestation	• Can be manifested as allergic fungal sinusitis or aspergilloma (mass of fungal hyphae in the maxillary sinus) • In immunosuppressed patients, pathogen may spread and invade the oral mucosa forming yellow-black necrotic area; most common sites are in palate and tongue[36]
Diagnosis	• Histopathology and microorganisms staining • Culture of sputum or blood[36]
Histopathology	• Infiltration of inflammatory cells, necrotic tissue, and large number of branching septate hyphae[3]
Treatment	• Debridement of noninvasive aspergilloma • Systemic antifungal therapy (voriconazole, triazole, and amphotericin B) with invasive infection[3]

of the most common deep fungal infections and their clinical presentations.

References

1. Falsetta ML, Klein MI, Colonne PM, et al. Symbiotic relationship between *Streptococcus mutans* and *Candida albicans* synergizes virulence of plaque biofilms in vivo. Infect Immun 2014;82(5):1968–81.
2. World Health Organization. Global tuberculosis report 2013, in Nonserial Publications. Geneva (Switzerland): World Health Organization; 2013. 1 online resource (p. 303).
3. Neville BW, Damm DD, Allen CM, et al. Oral and maxillofacial pathology. St. Louis (MO): Elsevier; 2016.
4. Lee SH. Tuberculosis infection and latent tuberculosis. Tuberc Respir Dis (Seoul) 2016;79(4):201–6.
5. Kakisi OK, Kechagia AS, Kakisis IK, et al. Tuberculosis of the oral cavity: a systematic review. Eur J Oral Sci 2010;118(2):103–9.
6. Brook I. The bacteriology of salivary gland infections. Oral Maxillofac Surg Clin North Am 2009;21(3):269–74.
7. Bhatty MA, Piggot TA, Soames JV, et al. Chronic non-specific parotid sialadenitis. Br J Plast Surg 1998;51(7):517–21.
8. Cascarini L, McGurk M. Epidemiology of salivary gland infections. Oral Maxillofac Surg Clin North Am 2009;21(3):353–7.
9. Schlossberg D. Clinical infectious disease, in Cambridge medicine. Cambridge, United Kingdom: University Printing House; 2015. p. 1470.
10. WHO Guidelines for the Treatment of *Treponema pallidum* (Syphilis). Geneva (Switzerland): 2016. Available at: http://apps.who.int/iris/bitstream/10665/249572/1/9789241549806-eng.pdf. Accessed December 15, 2016.
11. Leao JC, Gueiros LA, Porter SR. Oral manifestations of syphilis. Clinics (Sao Paulo) 2006;61(2):161–6.
12. Laskaris G. Oral manifestations of infectious diseases. Dent Clin North Am 1996;40(2):395–423.
13. Meyer I, Shklar G. The oral manifestations of acquired syphilis. A study of eighty-one cases. Oral Surg Oral Med Oral Pathol 1967;23(1):45–57.
14. Brown DL, Frank JE. Diagnosis and management of syphilis. Am Fam Physician 2003;68(2):283–90.
15. Belmont MJ, Behar PM, Wax MK. Atypical presentations of actinomycosis. Head Neck 1999;21(3):264–8.
16. Valour F, Sénéchal A, Dupieux C, et al. Actinomycosis: etiology, clinical features, diagnosis, treatment, and management. Infect Drug Resist 2014;7:183–97.
17. Jeansonne BG. Periapical actinomycosis: a review. Quintessence Int 2005;36(2):149–53.
18. Chen TC, Lin WR, Lu PL, et al. Cat scratch disease from a domestic dog. J Formos Med Assoc 2007;106(2 Suppl):S65–8.
19. Nelson CA, Saha S, Mead PS. Cat-scratch disease in the United States, 2005-2013. Emerg Infect Dis 2016;22(10):1741–6.
20. Kordick DL, Hilyard EJ, Hadfield TL, et al. *Bartonella clarridgeiae*, a newly recognized zoonotic pathogen causing inoculation papules, fever, and lymphadenopathy (cat scratch disease). J Clin Microbiol 1997;35(7):1813–8.
21. Kradin RL. Diagnostic pathology of infectious disease. , Philadelphia: Saunders Elsevier; 2010. p. xiii. 644 p.
22. Carithers HA. Cat-scratch disease. An overview based on a study of 1,200 patients. Am J Dis Child 1985;139(11):1124–33.
23. Lindeboom JA. Pediatric cervicofacial lymphadenitis caused by *Bartonella henselae*. Oral Surg Oral Med Oral Pathol Oral Radiol 2015;120(4):469–73.
24. Munson PD, Boyce TG, Salomao DR, et al. Cat-scratch disease of the head and neck in a pediatric population: surgical indications and outcomes. Otolaryngol Head Neck Surg 2008;139(3):358–63.
25. Loftus MJ, Sweeney G, Goldberg MH. Parinaud oculoglandular syndrome and cat-scratch fever. J Oral Surg 1980;38(3):218–20.
26. Stevens DL, Bryant AE. Impetigo, erysipelas and cellulitis, In: Ferretti JJ, Stevens DL, Fischetti VA, editors. *Streptococcus pyogenes*: basic biology to clinical manifestations. Oklahoma City (OK): 2016. p. 723–40.
27. Carapetis JR, Steer AC, Mulholland EK, et al. The global burden of group A streptococcal diseases. Lancet Infect Dis 2005;5(11):685–94.
28. Fotos PG, Vincent SD, Hellstein JW. Oral candidosis. Clinical, historical, and therapeutic features of 100 cases. Oral Surg Oral Med Oral Pathol 1992;74(1):41–9.
29. Glick M. Burket's oral medicine. Shelton (Connecticut): People's Medical Publishing House USA; 2014.
30. Horwath MC, Fecher RA, Deepe GS Jr. *Histoplasma capsulatum*, lung infection and immunity. Future Microbiol 2015;10(6):967–75.
31. Chu JH, Feudtner C, Heydon K, et al. Hospitalizations for endemic mycoses: a population-based national study. Clin Infect Dis 2006;42(6):822–5.
32. Wheat LJ, Azar MM, Bahr NC, et al. Histoplasmosis. Infect Dis Clin North Am 2016;30(1):207–27.

33. Wheat LJ, Wass J, Norton J, et al. Cavitary histoplasmosis occurring during two large urban outbreaks. Analysis of clinical, epidemiologic, roentgenographic, and laboratory features. Medicine 1984;63(4):201–9.
34. Kennedy CC, Limper AH. Redefining the clinical spectrum of chronic pulmonary histoplasmosis: a retrospective case series of 46 patients. Medicine 2007;86(4):252–8.
35. Kauffman CA. Histoplasmosis: a clinical and laboratory update. Clin Microbiol Rev 2007;20(1):115–32.
36. Warnakulasuriya S, Tilakaratne WM. Oral medicine and pathology: a guide to diagnosis and management. First edition. New Delhi: Jaypee Brothers Medical Publishers (P) Ltd; 2014. p. xix. 563 pages.

Oral Complications of Dermatologic Disorders

Paolo G. Arduino, DDS, MSc, PhDs

KEYWORDS

- Autoimmune dermatologic oral conditions • Oral lichen planus • Mucous membrane pemphigoid • Pemphigus vulgaris

KEY POINTS

- The oral lesions in dermatologic diseases may be the early aspects of the disease itself, the most significant clinical appearance, or the only sign or symptom; sometimes lesions can occur simultaneously in the skin and in the oral cavity.
- Although in most instances cutaneous lesions of lichen planus are self-limiting, causing merely itching, oral lesions are persistent, potentially premalignant, hardly ever undergo spontaneous remission, and are habitually a source of morbidity.
- From a diagnostic and therapeutic point view, it might be of significant advantage to discriminate a clinical subset of mucous membrane pemphigoid, termed oral pemphigoid, in which the disease is mainly limited to the oral cavity and patients have a better prognosis compared with other variants.
- Gingival lesions caused by autoimmune dermatologic disorders are described with diffuse erythematous lesions, blisters, erosions, or ulcerations, mainly located on the attached gingiva and on the palate; the occurrence of epithelial desquamation, erythema, and erosive lesions on the gingival tissue is described in literature as "desquamative gingivitis."
- Oral manifestations and dental involvement of epidermolysis bullosa vary in frequency and severity according to the form. Intraoral manifestations include multiple carious lesions affecting almost the entire dentition, with severe gingival inflammation, microstomia, ankyloglossia, and obliteration of oral vestibule.

Introduction

Skin and oral mucosa are analogous and comparable structural tissues, composed of specialized stratified epithelium functioning as a first-line barrier against dissimilar types of chemical or physical injuries. Stratified squamous epithelia are complex compound structure, mainly comprising of keratinocytes (KCs) adherent to each other, and to the underlying epithelial basement membrane and connective tissue. Cohesion among KCs is needed for preserving the tissues' structure and epithelial functions. Three functional types of junctional structures interconnect KCs: (1) anchoring junctions (including desmosomes and adherens junctions), (2) occludens junctions (tight junctions), and (3) nexus junctions (gap junctions). Much of the oral mucosa is resulting embryologically from an invagination of the ectoderm and, not surprisingly, it may become involved in disorders that are mostly associated with the skin.

The oral lesions in dermatologic diseases may be the early aspects of the disorder itself, or the most significant clinical appearance; other times, they are the only sign or symptom, or sometimes lesions can occur simultaneously in the skin and in the oral cavity. A wide range of dermatologic disorders can affect the mouth, although the more common are oral lichen planus (OLP), mucous membrane pemphigoid (MMP), pemphigus vulgaris (PV), epidermolysis bullosa (EB), and psoriasis.

The proper diagnosis of this oral condition should be made through clinical findings, assessment of subepithelial or intraepithelial blister by histopathology, detection of autoantibodies in the mucosal samples by direct immunofluorescence, and binding to the roof and/or floor of the blister of salt-split skin by indirect immunofluorescence. Commercially available enzyme-linked immunosorbent assays, based on proteins involved in dermoepidermal or chorioepithelial adhesion, are also usually used for serologic diagnosis.

Oral lichen planus

OLP is a chronic inflammatory disease, affecting roughly 1.5% to 2% of the total population, women almost more than twice as men. Patients of all ages could be interested, frequently in the fifth to sixth decades of life, usually at an earlier age in men. Patients with OLP usually show no increased prevalence of cigarette smoking or alcohol consumption.

To date, the defined cause remains unknown. Immune dysregulation plays a critical role in the development and progression of this disease; however, it is unlikely to be caused by a single antigen, given that studies of T-cell receptor variable region genes from lesional OLP T cells have not revealed the use of a restricted number of different variable region genes. Probably, OLP is the outcome of the influence of a limited range of extrinsic antigens or altered self-antigens. In a

Disclosure Statement: The author confirms no relationship with any commercial company that has a direct financial interest in subject matter or materials discussed in the article.

Department of Surgical Sciences, CIR-Dental School, University of Turin, Via Nizza 230, Turin 10100, Italy
E-mail address: paologiacomo.arduino@unito.it

Atlas Oral Maxillofacial Surg Clin N Am 25 (2017) 221-228

http://dx.doi.org/10.1016/j.cxom.2017.04.013

minority of patients, precipitating factors have been identified, including dental materials, medications (eg, nonsteroidal anti-inflammatory drugs and angiotensin-converting enzyme inhibitors), stress, trauma, and various infectious agents. Different authors have demonstrated an association of OLP and hepatitis C in southern Europe and in Asia, reporting that viral sequences could be also discovered in the serum of patients with OLP; moreover, the virus was also shown to occasionally replicate in OLP tissues. The possible association of hepatitis C virus infection with OLP may necessitate the importance of virus screening in such patients, especially in some regions.

The oral manifestations of OLP are satisfactory recognized. To date, six clinical forms of have been described (white [reticular, plaque-like, popular], or red [atrophic, erosive, and bullous]). Although white forms are generally asymptomatic (counting usually for 60% of total cases) (Fig. 1), atrophic and erosive (Fig. 2) lesions could result in profound discomfort. The gingiva is one of the most prevalent oral sites (Figs. 3 and 4), after the buccal mucosa and the tongue (Fig. 5). Skin lesions characteristically present as flat-topped, polygonal, violaceous papules regularly covered by a network of fine lines affecting usually wrists, ankles, and genitalia. Although in most instances cutaneous lesions of lichen planus are self-limiting, causing merely itching, oral lesions are persistent, potentially premalignant, hardly ever undergo spontaneous remission, and are habitually a source of morbidity. One of the most important complications of OLP is the potential development of an oral squamous cell carcinoma (Fig. 6), although this is a reasonably controversial matter. The rate of transformation in individual studies ranged from 0% to 3.5%. However, it should be judicious for clinicians to pursue continued regular observation and follow-up in patients with OLP with these conditions, even if they do not fit a traditional high-risk category for oral cancer (eg, female and nonsmokers). In patients followed up for a long period, it has been published that less than 3% of them had a complete and definitive healing of oral lesion, whereas most showed a stable clinical appearance (more than 75%) and a minority of patients got worse (less than 10%).

Numerous drugs have been used to treat this condition, with variable results; however, even if the best treatment remains high-potency topical corticosteroids, management is commonly empirical, with no adequate control groups or corrected study designs. Treatment is usually undertaken with the goal of achieving control of symptoms with minimal side effects. Clobetasol propionate 0.05% seemed to be one of the most effective topical steroids, because in an adhesive base it led to complete remission in almost 75% of patients with symptomatic forms, but strong evidence on its efficacy is lacking. However, independently from the active principle used and the way of administration, more than half of the responsive patients showed yet again active painful disease, and can need a new therapeutic approach, confirming the OLP chronic course and the symptomatic character of therapeutic treatments. Moreover, some patients are refractory to steroid medication and could need a different approach. The nonsteroidal topical calcineurin inhibitors are important treatment option and are indicated in cases where the use of topical steroids is unsuitable, or have failed to adequately control OLP, especially in the acute phase, similarly to other dermatologic conditions. Pimecrolimus and tacrolimus ointments seemed to be a treatment of choice, safe and easy, for patients with atrophic-erosive OLP, previously treated with topical steroids but unresponsive. Low-level laser therapy (LLLT) is an approach increasingly used in medicine, which also has potential biostimulating effects if applied to oral tissues by improving wound healing. LLLT has also been showed to be a feasible treatment choice for patients with unresponsive symptomatic OLP, but small data from limited studies are available.

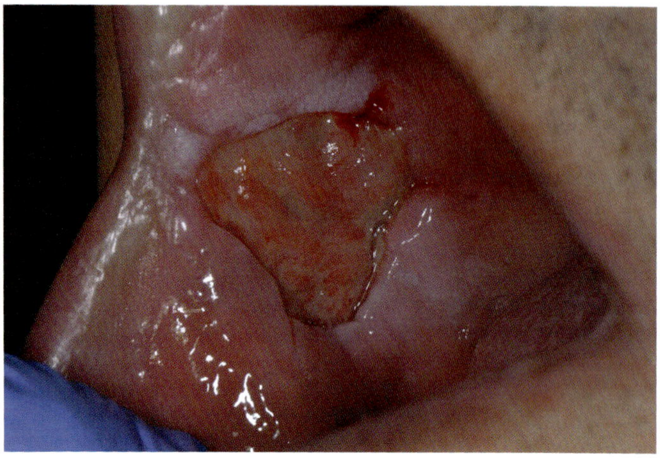

Fig. 2 Oral lichen planus. Red erosive lesion on the right buccal mucosa.

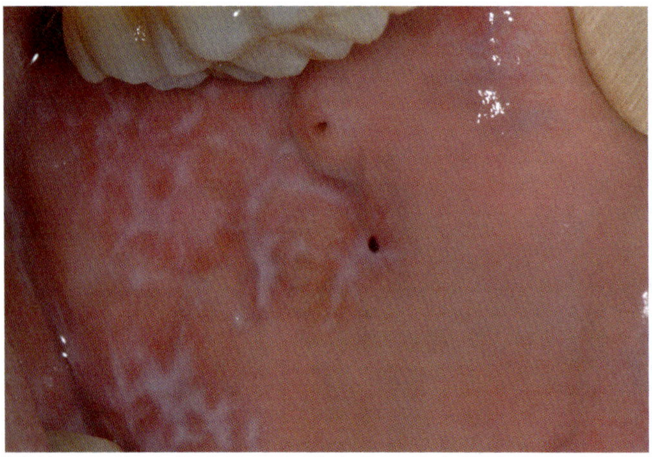

Fig. 1 Oral lichen planus. White reticular lesions on the left buccal mucosa.

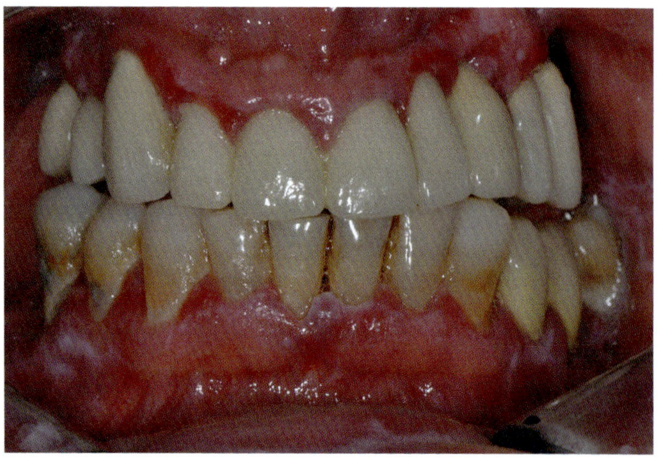

Fig. 3 Diffuse gingival involvement (desquamative gingivitis) in a patient with diagnosed oral lichen planus (mainly erythematous).

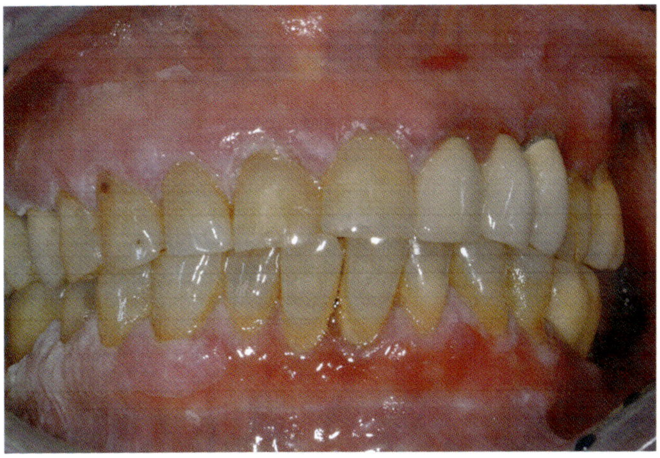

Fig. 4 Diffuse gingival involvement (desquamative gingivitis) in a patient with diagnosed oral lichen planus (mainly hyperkeratotic).

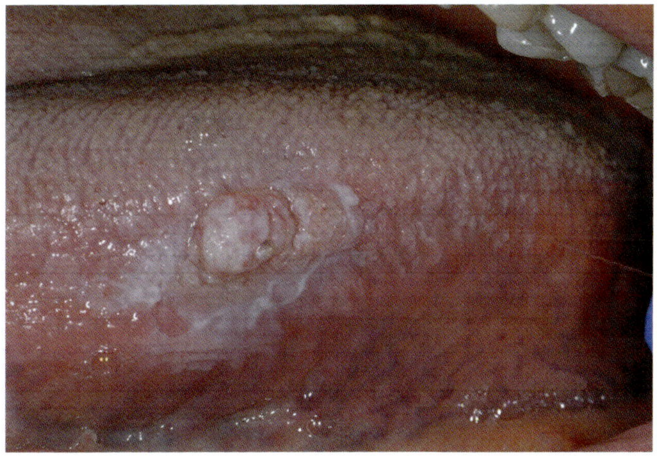

Fig. 6 A case of oral squamous cell carcinoma of the lateral border of the tongue developed in a patient with previously diagnosed oral lichen planus.

Mucous membrane pemphigoid

MMP describes an assorted group of chronic and inflammatory diseases clinically presenting with countless oral, ocular, skin, genital, naospharyngeal, and laryngeal lesions. MMP is essentially a subepithelial blistering disease, histologically characterized by linear deposition of immunoglobulins (essentially IgG or C3) along the epithelial basement membrane zone. Moreover, at least in some patients, circulating IgG and/or IgA autoantibodies could be present, targeting several basement membrane zone components, including the bullous pemphigoid antigens of 180 kDa (BP180) and 230 kDa (BP230), $\alpha_6\beta_4$ integrin, laminin 332, and type VII collagen. BP180 and BP230 are components of the junctional adhesion complex called "hemidesmosome"; BP230 is a cytoplasmic protein implicated in the organization of the keratin filament network and BP180 is a transmembrane protein that, by interaction with $\alpha_6\beta_4$, contributes to the assembly and stabilization of hemidesmosomes. Moreover, $\alpha_6\beta_4$ integrin mediates cell adhesion to extracellular matrix, and laminin 332 and type VII collagen play an important role in the maintenance of epithelial cell anchorage to the underlying connective tissue. In ex vivo and in vivo models it has been demonstrated that autoantibodies against laminin 332 and β_4 integrin could have a role in the pathogenesis of MMP.

There is a marked degree of variability in the clinical and immunologic characters of MMP, suggesting the existence of different phenotypic variants. From a diagnostic and therapeutic point view, it might be of significant advantage to discriminate a clinical subset of MMP, termed oral pemphigoid, in which the disease is mainly limited to the oral cavity (Fig. 7) and patients have a better prognosis compared with other variants. Moreover, the oral cavity has been described as the only site of involvement or as the first manifestation of the disease in different reports, being the gingival tissues often involved, but usually this has been detailed in limited case series. Gingival lesions caused by MMP (Figs. 8 and 9) are described with diffuse erythematous lesions, blisters, erosions, or ulcerations, mainly located on the attached gingiva and on the palate; the occurrence of epithelial desquamation, erythema, and erosive lesions on the gingival tissue is described in literature as "desquamative gingivitis," a typical clinical picture of autoimmune bullous diseases (mostly MMP and PV).

MMP does not have a predictable natural history. In some reported cases, the disease is localized and has a slowly progressive course without complications; in others, it is

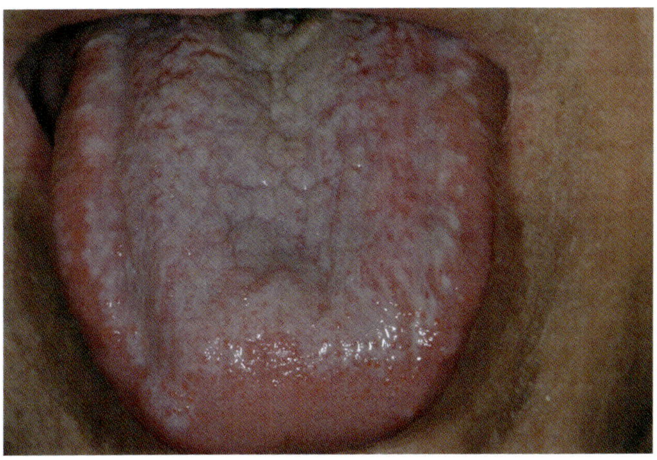

Fig. 5 Typical aspect of the dorsum of the tongue in a patient with diagnosed oral lichen planus.

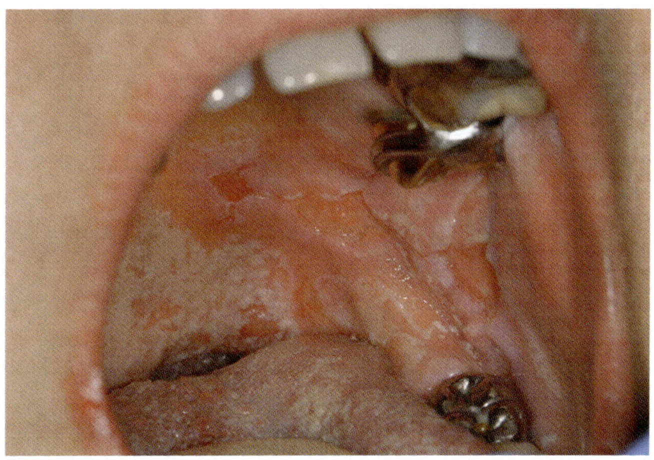

Fig. 7 Diffuse palatal erosive lesions in a patient with diagnosed mucous membrane pemphigoid.

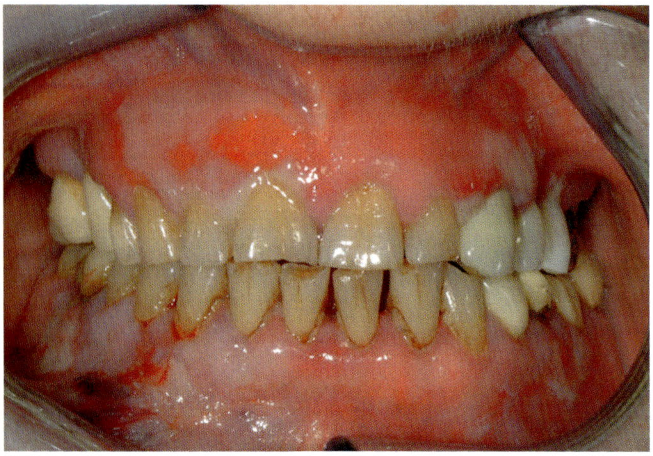

Fig. 8 A typical case of mucous membrane pemphigoid gingival lesion in a male patient.

devastating, with strict morbidity. There have been no large-scale, well-controlled studies regarding therapy for MMP and most of the therapeutic experience is from studies on cutaneous bullous pemphigoid. The choice of agents for its treatment is mainly based on the sites of involvement, clinical severity, and disease progression.

To date, the treatment of intraoral lesion of MMP still represents a confusing therapeutic challenge but high-potency corticosteroids remain the most reliable and effective modality. Patients who demonstrate only intraoral lesions usually respond effectively to topical corticosteroids alone.

Some recent reports also suggested that LLLT seemed to be a possible treatment of some patients with oral erosive lesions caused by MMP, also giving a notable analgesic effect.

Pemphigus vulgaris

Pemphigus is a group of potentially life-threatening and organ-specific autoimmune diseases, characterized by cutaneous and/or mucosal blistering, with an established immunologic basis. Pemphigus is classified into four types: (1) PV, (2) pemphigus vegetans, (3) pemphigus erythematosus, and (4) pemphigus foliaceus. In addition, new entities of pemphigus have been more recently described: paraneoplastic pemphigus and IgA pemphigus.

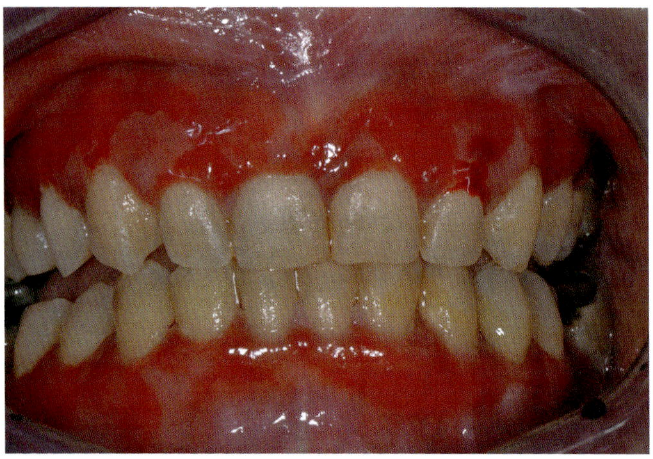

Fig. 9 A typical case of mucous membrane pemphigoid gingival lesion in a female patient.

PV, the most common variant, is characterized by circulating IgG antibodies directed against desmoglein 3 (Dsg3), with about half the patients also having Dsg1 autoantibodies. There is a fairly strong genetic background, and it affects 0.1 to 0.5 patients per 100,000 population per year.

There are two controversial concepts about the pathogenesis of pemphigus. The monopathogenic theory explains intraepidermal blistering through the "Dsg compensation" hypothesis, according to which an antibody-dependent disabling of Dsg1- and/or Dsg3-mediated cell-cell attachments of KCs is sufficient to disrupt epidermal integrity and cause blistering. The multipathogenic theory explains intraepidermal blistering through the "multiple hit" hypothesis stating that a simultaneous and synchronized inactivation of the physiologic mechanisms regulating and/or mediating intercellular adhesion of KCs is necessary to disrupt epidermal integrity. The major premise for a multipathogenic theory is that a single type of autoantibody induces only reversible changes, so that affected KCs can recover because of self-repair. The damage, however, becomes irreversible when the salvage pathway and/or other cell functions are altered by a partnering autoantibody and/or other pathogenic factors. Future studies are needed to (1) corroborate these findings, (2) characterize in detail patient populations with non-Dsg-specific autoantibodies, and (3) determine the extent of the contribution of non-Dsg antibodies in disease pathophysiology.

The lesions of PV characteristically occur first in the oropharyngeal mucosa and later in the skin; other mucosa (eg, genitalia and conjunctiva) also may be involved.

Oral lesions of pemphigus are seen in up to 18% of patients at dermatology clinics, but despite the frequency of oral involvement (in more than 70% of cases the oral lesion have been described as the first manifestation of the disease), and novel therapeutic approaches, there are unexpectedly not many recent studies of either the oral manifestations of pemphigus or their long-term management, and delays in diagnosis are still frequent. Many patients are at first misdiagnosed, frequently as having aphthous or gingivostomatitis or candidosis, and erroneously treated for a long period.

The oral lesions at first comprise small asymptomatic blisters (Fig. 10), although these are thin-walled and easily rupture, giving rise to painful and hemorrhagic erosions (Figs. 11 and 12). Although the lesions are located anywhere within the oral cavity, they are most often found in areas subjected to friction trauma, such as the cheek mucosa, tongue, palate, and lower lip. Gingival lesions (Fig. 13) are less frequent than those of MMP, but usually are more difficult to treat and tend to be long-standing.

In PV cases, the Nikolsky sign is usually present, resulting as a bulla development after a delicate tangential distress (ie, air in the oral cavity) is performed (Fig. 14). The invariably fatal outcome of PV has changed dramatically with the advent of corticosteroids. However, there is a lack of consensus in the literature about the treatment of this disorder, this issue further complicated by the fact that therapy has to be individualized.

Epidermolysis bullosa

EB is a rare group of genetically heterogeneous diseases, characterized by deficiencies in the synthesis of proteins

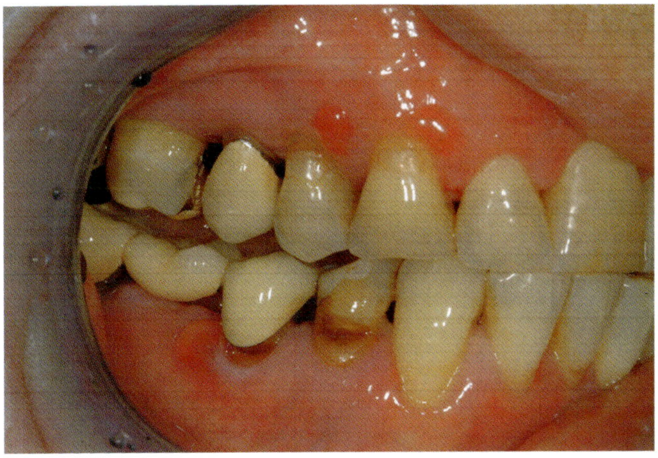

Fig. 10 Three small asymptomatic bullae on the gingiva of a patient with diagnosed pemphigus vulgaris.

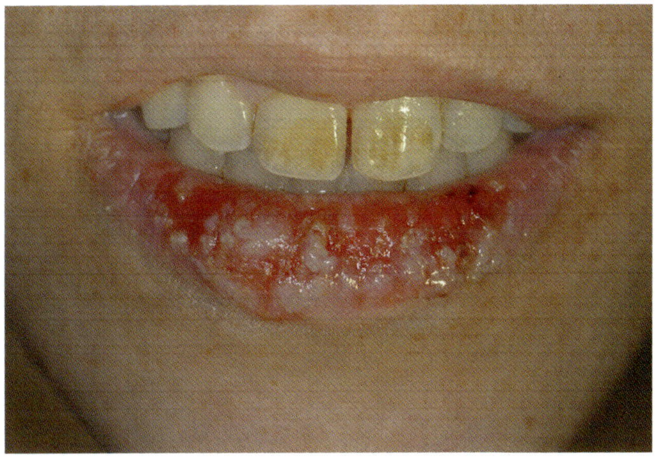

Fig. 12 Diffuse labial erosive lesions in a patient with diagnosed pemphigus vulgaris.

involved in the adhesion of the connective tissue to the epithelium. The common clinical manifestations are mechanical fragility of the skin and mucosae, with blister formation and abnormal wound healing, the severity of the lesions depending on the distinct type.

There are four major forms: (1) simplex, (2) junctional, (3) dystrophic, and (4) Kindler syndrome, with more than 20 distinctive clinical subtypes. The dystrophic EB has two subtypes: recessive and dominant.

It seems that the cause of EB is related to abnormal enzyme activity and collagen degradation. Specific genetic mutations are well characterized for most of the different EB subtypes and variants.

Oral manifestations and dental involvement of EB vary in frequency and severity according to the form. Intraoral manifestations include multiple carious lesions affecting almost the entire dentition, with severe gingival inflammation, microstomia, ankyloglossia, and obliteration of oral vestibule (Fig. 15).

In the simplex form the teeth usually are not affected; however, the dystrophic types often display malformed teeth caused by enamel hypoplasia, early caries development, and gingival inflammation caused by plaque accumulation because of impaired oral hygiene. The most common oral mucosal manifestations of EB are painful blisters affecting all the oral surfaces.

The approach to dental treatment of patients with EB, in particular for those with the more severe types, has changed dramatically during the last 30 years. At the beginning, it was stated that extractions should be the treatment of choice. This view completely changed in 1999, when authors started to declare that it was possible to manage dental abnormalities successfully with a combination of anesthetic and restorative techniques, and caries could be successfully prevented by continuous follow-up aimed at dietary advice, oral hygiene habits, frequent professional cleaning, and fluoride therapy. Thus, a preventive protocol is today's dental management approach of choice. Dental treatment is an important part of the multidisciplinary care of patients with EB, especially the severe types. Maintaining a functional dentition reduces the potential for oral and esophageal soft tissue damage through more efficient mastication and favors nutrition.

The only level of evidence available to support most recommendations is case reports and a few case series. The oral cavity is frequently involved but, although oral bullae, ulcers, and erosions are common, there is only one published study of

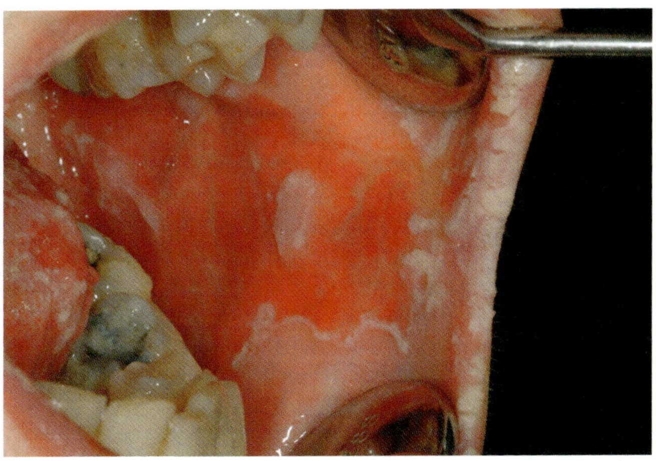

Fig. 11 Diffuse mucosal erosive lesions in a patient with diagnosed pemphigus vulgaris.

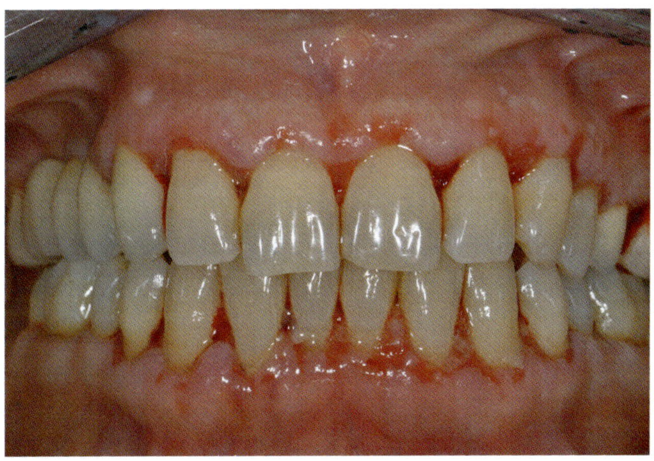

Fig. 13 A mild typical case of pemphigus vulgaris gingival lesion in a female patient.

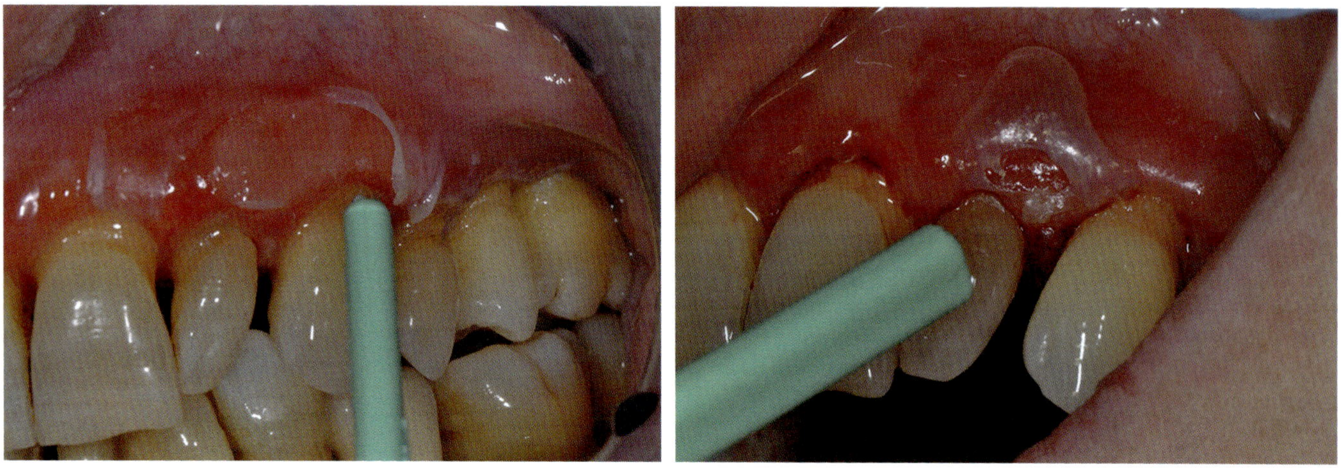

Fig. 14 Positive Nikolsky sign on an upper gingival site.

therapy, reporting that sucralfate suspension can reduce the development and duration of blisters and ulcers, reduce the associated pain, and improve indices of gingival inflammation.

The oral mucosa in patients with EB is affected with different lesions and degrees of severity, even if their patterns are still unclear. Using long-term therapies, such as a topical medication (eg, topical corticosteroid as used for other oral bullous diseases), within the mouth in EB is challenging especially for patients with compromised hand movements. Recently, the effectiveness of cord blood platelet gel and LLLT has been showed in reducing intraoral discomfort from ulcerations in patients with dystrophic EB, being effective also in the long-term.

Psoriasis

Psoriasis is a common chronic inflammatory cutaneous disease with characteristic and sharply demarcated red squamous plaques, generally restricted to distinct sites or disseminated over the skin surface. With a variable frequency of 2% to 5% in the white population, it is one of the most common chronic inflammatory skin diseases. Whereas 80% of patients present with circumscribed or disseminated typical plaques referred to as plaque psoriasis, 20% show sterile pustules on erythematous ground with scaling to a varying extent.

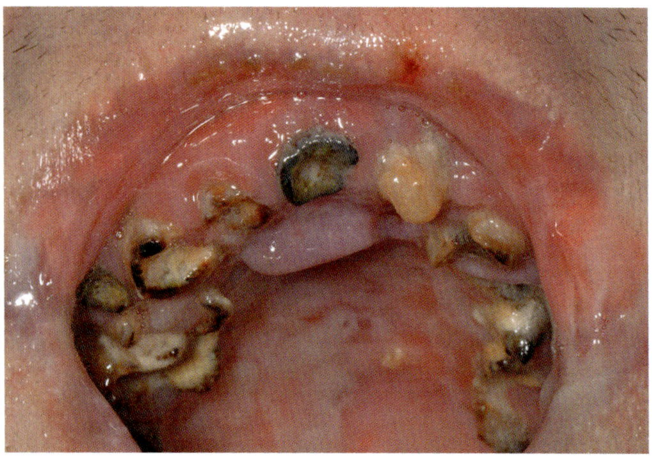

Fig. 15 Diffuse oral and dental involvement in a pediatric case with diagnosed epidermolysis bullosa.

Although clinically well described, the exact etiologic and pathogenic mechanisms are still not known. Present understanding indicates distinctive and unique overlap to other inflammatory and autoimmune conditions. Conversely, the one or more relevant autoantigens could not be characterized so far; however, several autoimmune diseases were shown to be frequently associated. In addition, serologic autoimmune phenomena, namely diverse circulating detailed autoantibodies, could be demonstrated in the past. A matter of current debate is if psoriasis is a primary autoimmune disease or secondarily evolving into autoimmunity as seen in other chronic inflammatory diseases.

The issue of whether psoriasis can manifest itself in the oral mucosa has been debated for many years, but to date no definitely data are stated, and the prevalence of oral manifestations in patients with cutaneous psoriasis is absolutely unreliable. There are currently no definite accepted clinical or histopathologic criteria by which an oral lesion can be unequivocally associated with psoriasis.

Psoriatic involvement of the vermilion border and perioral region is rare, but it may present with diffuse erythema, fissuring, silvery scales, and desquamation, which start from the commissures and spread to involve both lips. Occasional bleeding, serous exudate, and itching and discomfort aggravated by movements may also be present.

There is no consensus regarding the authentic oral manifestations of psoriasis. Different patterns have been described, including diffuse, intense mucosal erythema associated with acute "psoriatic" flares; well-defined, annular, white or yellowish lesions; and mixed, ulcerative, vesicular, pustular, and indurated objects. Manifestations of psoriasis may involve the oral cavity in a variety of locations with the buccal mucosa most commonly affected. The palate and gingiva are unusual sites. Oral findings are frequently transient, migratory, and fluctuate daily in prominence parallel to exacerbation or remission of cutaneous lesions. A higher prevalence of benign migratory glossitis (Fig. 16) and fissured tongue (Fig. 17), compared with the general population, has also been reported.

In patients with known cutaneous psoriasis, routine examination should also include the oral mucosa, with the meaning to identify subtle changes. Management of oral psoriasis is not well described primarily because, unlike cutaneous psoriasis,

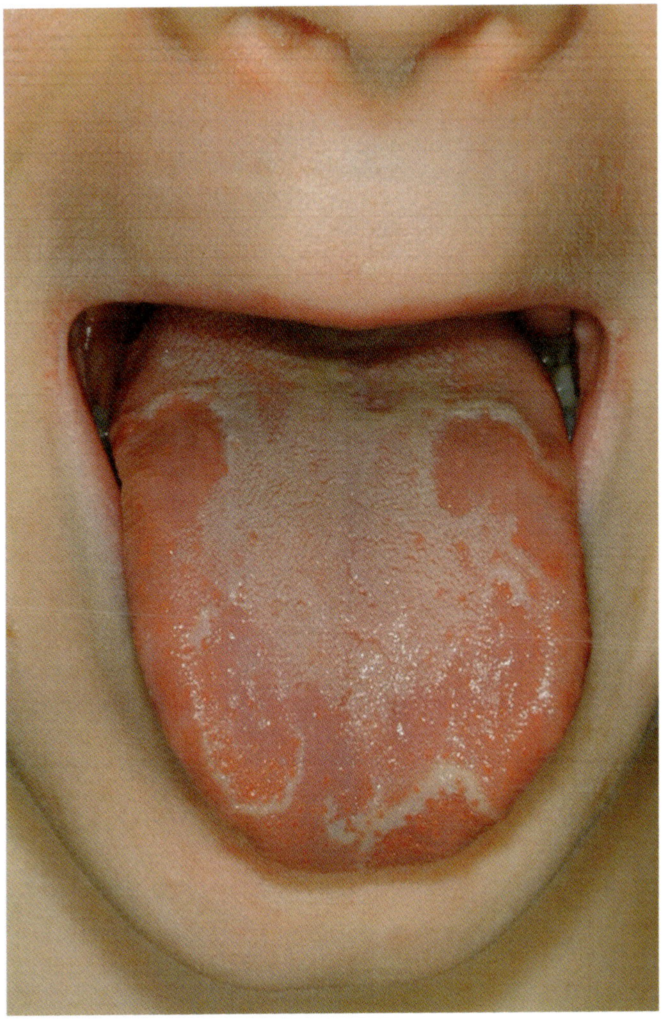

Fig. 16 Typical case of geographic tongue.

most cases are asymptomatic, transient, and not requiring precise interventions. Also, control of cutaneous disease often helps resolve symptomatic oral psoriasis, which may occur during a flare. Typical symptoms, when present, may include oral pain, burning, or changes in taste perception. Patients may also express concern about the malignant potential of lesions or the unsightly appearance of the affected visible mucosa.

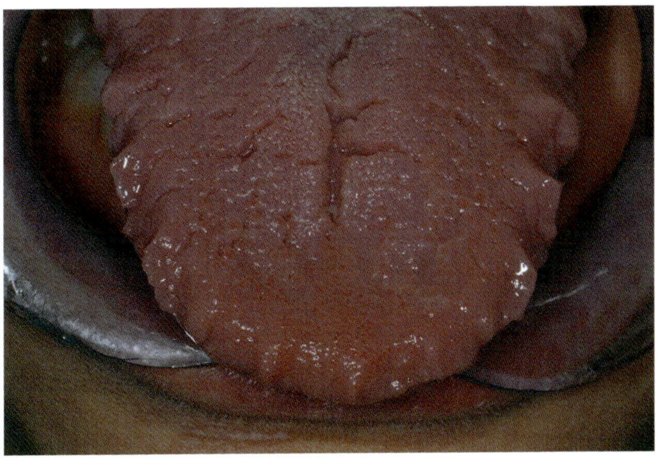

Fig. 17 Typical case of fissured tongue.

Although many of the therapeutic modalities for cutaneous psoriasis are not appropriate for use in the oral cavity, a variety of approaches have been documented. Administration of topical or intralesional steroids guided by the severity of symptoms and localization of lesions is generally efficacious. Despite efficacy, several medications used to treat systemic treatments for severe cases may lead to adverse effects within the oral cavity; examples include xerostomia associated with retinoids, gingival enlargement with cyclosporine, and ulcerations associated with methotrexate.

Patients with arthritis or severe cutaneous involvement may also have difficulty holding a toothbrush or performing acceptable oral hygiene procedures. Therefore, regular oral evaluations are necessary for these patients.

Further readings

Ahmed AR, Carrozzo M, Caux F, et al. Monopathogenic vs. multipathogenic explanations of pemphigus pathophysiology. Exp Dermatol 2016;25:839–46.

Alwan W, Nestle FO. Pathogenesis and treatment of psoriasis: exploiting pathophysiological pathways for precision medicine. Clin Exp Rheumatol 2015;33:S2–6.

Arduino PG, Broccoletti R, Sciannameo V, et al. A practical clinical recording system for cases with desquamative gingivitis. Br J Dermatol 2016. http://dx.doi.org/10.1111/bjd.15075.

Arduino PG, Carbone M, Della Ferrera F, et al. Pimecrolimus vs. tacrolimus for the topical treatment of unresponsive oral erosive lichen planus: a 8 week randomized double-blind controlled study. J Eur Acad Dermatol Venereol 2014;28:475–82.

Arduino PG, Farci V, D'Aiuto F, et al. Periodontal status in oral mucous membrane pemphigoid: initial results of a case-control study. Oral Dis 2011;17:90–4.

Baccaglini L, Thongprasom K, Carrozzo M, et al. Urban legends series: lichen planus. Oral Dis 2013;19:128–43.

Black M, Mignogna MD, Scully C. Number II. Pemphigus vulgaris. Oral Dis 2005;11:119–30.

Cafaro A, Arduino PG, Massolini G, et al. Clinical evaluation of the efficiency of low-level laser therapy for oral lichen planus: a prospective case series. Lasers Med Sci 2014;29:185–90.

Cafaro A, Broccoletti R, Arduino PG. Low-level laser therapy for oral mucous membrane pemphigoid. Lasers Med Sci 2012;27:1247–50.

Calabresi V, Carrozzo M, Cozzani E, et al. Oral pemphigoid autoantibodies preferentially target BP180 ectodomain. Clin Immunol 2007; 122:207–13.

Carbone M, Arduino PG, Carrozzo M, et al. Course of oral lichen planus: a retrospective study of 808 northern Italian patients. Oral Dis 2009; 15:235–43.

Carbone M, Arduino PG, Carrozzo M, et al. Topical clobetasol in the treatment of atrophic-erosive oral lichen planus: a randomized controlled trial to compare two preparations with different concentrations. J Oral Pathol Med 2009;38:227–33.

Carbone M, Broccoletti R, Gambino A, et al. Clinical and histological features of gingival lesions: a 17-year retrospective analysis in a northern Italian population. Med Oral Patol Oral Cir Bucal 2012;17: e555–61.

Carrozzo M, Dametto E, Fasano ME, et al. Cytokine gene polymorphisms in hepatitis C virus-related oral lichen planus. Exp Dermatol 2007; 16:730–6.

Carrozzo M, Uboldi de Capei M, Dametto E, et al. Tumor necrosis factor-alpha and interferon-gamma polymorphisms contribute to susceptibility to oral lichen planus. J Invest Dermatol 2004;122:87–94.

Chan LS, Ahmed AR, Anhalt GJ, et al. The first international consensus on mucous membrane pemphigoid: definition, diagnostic criteria, pathogenic factors, medical treatment, and prognostic indicators. Arch Dermatol 2002;138:370–9.

Cozzani E, Di Zenzo G, Calabresi V, et al. Autoantibody profile of a cohort of 78 Italian patients with mucous membrane pemphigoid:

correlation between reactivity profile and clinical involvement. Acta Derm Venereol 2016;96:768–73.

David JO. Fine inherited epidermolysis bullosa. Orphanet J Rare Dis 2010;5:12.

Di Zenzo G, Carrozzo M, Chan LS. Urban legend series: mucous membrane pemphigoid. Oral Dis 2014;20:35–54.

Fatahzadeh M, Schwartz RA. Oral psoriasis: an overlooked enigma. Dermatology 2016;232:319–25.

Fitzpatrick SG, Hirsch SA, Gordon SC. The malignant transformation of oral lichen planus and oral lichenoid lesions: a systematic review. J Am Dent Assoc 2014;145:45–56.

Krämer SM. Oral care and dental management for patients with epidermolysis bullosa. Dermatol Clin 2010;28:303–9.

Krämer SM, Serrano MC, Zillmann G, et al. Oral health care for patients with epidermolysis bullosa: best clinical practice guidelines. Int J Paediatr Dent 2012;22(Suppl 1):1–35.

Leao JC, Ingafou M, Khan A, et al. Desquamative gingivitis: retrospective analysis of disease associations of a large cohort. Oral Dis 2008;14:556–60.

Ljibojevic S, Lipozencic J, Brenner S, et al. Pemphigus vulgaris: a review of treatment over a 19-year period. J Eur Acad Dermatol Venereol 2002;16:599–603.

Mattsson U, Warfvinge G, Jontell M. Oral psoriasis-a diagnostic dilemma: a report of two cases and a review of the literature. Oral Surg Oral Med Oral Pathol Oral Radiol 2015;120:e183–9.

Migliari DA, Penha SS, Marques MM, et al. Considerations on the diagnosis of oral psoriasis: a case report. Med Oral 2004;9:300–3.

Mustafa MB, Porter SR, Smoller BR, et al. Oral mucosa manifestations of autoimmune skin diseases. Autoimmun Rev 2015;14:930–51.

Raychaudhuri SK, Maverakis E, Raychaudhuri SP. Diagnosis and classification of psoriasis. Autoimmun Rev 2014;13:490–5.

Scully C, Bagan JV, Black M, et al. Mucosal disease series. Epithelial biology. Oral Dis 2005;11:58–71.

Scully C, Lo Muzio L. Oral mucosal diseases: mucous membrane pemphigoid. Br J Oral Maxillofac Surg 2008;46:358–66.

Sindici E, Astesano S, Fazio L, et al. Treatment of oral lesions in dystrophic epidermolysis bullosa: a case series of cord blood platelet gel and low-level laser therapy. Acta Derm Venereol 2017;97(3):383–4.

Sheridan
Hanover, PA USA
July 31, 2019